D0780831

DECISION MAKING IN NURSING

EDITORS

Rebecca A. Patronis Jones, D.N.Sc., R.N., C.N.A.A.

Director and Associate Professor of Nursing
Department of Nursing and Health Sciences
Texas A & M University - Corpus Christi
6300 Ocean Drive
Corpus Christi, TX 78412

Sharon E. Beck, D.N.Sc., R.N.

Assistant Professor
La Salle University
School of Nursing
1900 West Olney
Philadelphia, PA 19141

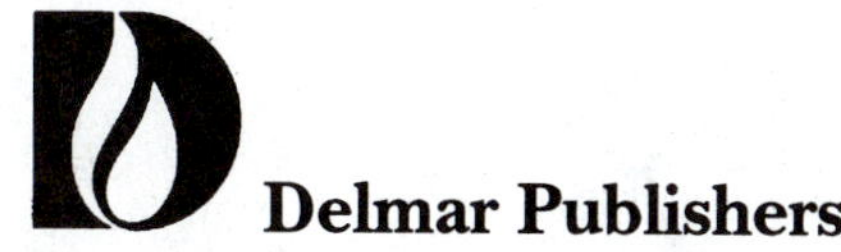

Delmar Publishers

I(T)P® An International Thomson Publishing Company

Albany • Bonn • Boston • Cincinnati • Detroit • London • Madrid • Melbourne
Mexico City • New York • Pacific Grove • Paris • San Francisco • Singapore • Tokyo
Toronto • Washington

Cover Design: Associated Graphics

Delmar Staff

Publisher: Diane L. McOscar
Senior Acquisitions Editor: Bill Burgower
Senior Marketing Manager: Hank Bertsch
Assistant Editor: Debra M. Flis
Project Editor: Judith Boyd Nelson
Production Coordinator: James Zayicek
Art and Design Coordinator: Timothy J. Conners
Editorial Assistant: Chrisoula Baikos

For more information, contact:

Delmar Publishers
3 Columbia Circle, Box 15015
Albany, NY 12212-5015

International Thomson Publishing Europe
Berkshire House 168-173
High Holborn
London WC1V7AA
England

Thomas Nelson Australia
102 Dodds Street
South Melbourne, 3205
Victoria, Australia

Nelson Canada
1120 Birchmount Road
Scarborough, Ontario
Canada M1K 5G4

International Thomson Editores
Campos Eliseos 385, Piso 7
Col Polanco
11560 Mexico D F Mexico

International Thomson Publishing GmbH
Königswinterer Strasse 418
53227 Bonn
Germany

International Thomson Publishing Asia
221 Henderson Road
#05-10 Henderson Building
Singapore 0315

International Thomson Publishing—Japan
Hirakawacho Building, 3F
2-2-1 Hirakawacho
Chiyoda-ku, Tokyo 102
Japan

1 2 3 4 5 6 7 8 9 10 XXX 01 00 99 98 97 96 95

Library of Congress Cataloging-in-Publication Data

Decision making in nursing / editors, Rebecca A. Patronis Jones and Sharon E. Beck.
p. cm.
Includes bibliographical references and index.
ISBN 0-8273-5684-6
1. Nursing—Decision making. 2. Nursing services—Administration—Decision making. I. Jones, Rebecca A. Patronis. II. Beck, Sharon E.
[DNLM: 1. Nursing Care—methods. 2. Decision Making—nurses' instruction. 3. Nurse Administrators. WY 100 D294 1995]
RT42.D43 1996
610.73—dc20
DNLM/DLC
for Library of Congress

94-42417
CIP

DEDICATION

Rebecca dedicates this book to her husband, Robert, and daughter, Aislan, who have spent numerous hours of family time without her; to her loving and supporting parents, Jim and Ada Lee, for all of their words of encouragement; and to the nurses from three generations in her family, Alice, Zelma, Jean, Patty, and Ginger who have provided countless stories about their decision making in nursing.

Sharon dedicates this book to her husband, Morton, her children Paul and Lisa, and her parents Ruth and Al Bralow. Their loving support, patience, and help has made this book possible.

Rebecca and Sharon would also like to acknowledge all of the chapter authors who worked very hard through many edits to perfect their work. They have made this a book to be proud of.

CONTENTS

Preface ix
Contributors xi

PART I FOUNDATIONS

Chapter 1 Processes and Models 3
Rebecca A. Patronis Jones

Introduction 3
Significance 4
Routine Process 4
Creative Process 7
Emergency Process 8
Multiattribute Utility Model 9
Intuitive Process 10
Diagnostic Decision Making 12
Collaborative Model 16
Assisting Patients with Decision Making 18
Scope of Practice Model 21

Chapter 2 Organizational Models 25
Rebecca A. Patronis Jones

Introduction 25
Rational Model 26
Political Model 28
Collegial Model 31
Bureaucratic Model 33
Garbage Can Model 36
Cybernetic Model 38

Chapter 3 Strategies 43
Sharon E. Beck

Introduction 43
Quantitative Strategies 44
Psychological Strategies 51

Chapter 4 Individual Decision Making 59
Alice Donahue and Suzanne G. Martin

Introduction 59
What Is Decision Making? 60
The Role of the Nurse 60
Decision Stages 61
The Individual Decisionmaker 62
Myers-Briggs Type Indicator 63
Rational Decision Making 65

Modified Rational Approach 66
Risk and Decision Making 67
Conflict and Decisions 68
The Role of Stress 68
Other Issues 72
Wrong Decisions 73
Monitoring Decisions 73

Chapter 5 Group Decision Making 77
Sandra M. Gomberg and Teresa A. Long

Introduction 77
The Individual as a Group Member 77
Group Process 79
Oermann's Model 80
Tuchman and Jensen's Model 82
The Committee as a Group 85

Chapter 6 The Effects of Cultural Factors 87
Ellie Mack

Introduction 87
Gender as a Culture 88
The Influence of Culturalism on Communication Style 89
The Culture of Nursing 92
Culturalism and Nursing Administration 92
Hospital Culture 93

Chapter 7 Ethical Decision Making: The Morally Reflective Practitioner 97
Patricia Hentz Becker

Introduction 97
Sphere of Ethics: Ethical Theory 99
Ethical Principles as Guides in Decision Making 102
Moral Development Theory 103
Nursing Theory: Human Connection 104
The Social/Interactional Sphere and Nursing 106
The Patient's Role 107
The Contextual/Situational Sphere 108
Guide for Ethical Decision Making 108

Chapter 8 Computer-Assisted Decision Support 113
Terry B. McGoldrick and Elisabeth T. Hallman

Introduction: The Past and Present 113
Computer Magic? 114
Computer Applications for Nursing Care 115
Coordination of Care 116
Bedside Decision Making: Artificial Intelligence or Expert System? 117
How Computers Make Decisions 118

The Problems with Expertise 120
Making the Decision to Automate 121
The Way We Need to Be 125

PART II MANAGING NURSING RESOURCES

Chapter 9 The Strategic Planning Process 131
Christina M. Fitz-Patrick and DeEtta F. Hayes

Introduction 131
Operational versus Strategic Planning 131
The Strategic Planning Process 133
Decision-Making Models 139
Nursing's Role in the Strategic Planning Process 141

Chapter 10 Financial Decision Making in Nursing 143
Elisabeth T. Hallman and Robin B. Allen

Introduction: The Past in Perspective 143
Definitions of Various Budgets 144
The Present: The Process of Budget Development 146
The Future 162

Chapter 11 Human Resource Management 163
Robin B. Allen and Linda A. Sinesi

Introduction 163
The Selection Process: Hiring 163
Performance Appraisals/Evaluation 168
Counseling and Discipline 171
Recruitment and Retention 175

Chapter 12 Leadership 179
Robin W. Wells

Introduction 179
Leadership Theory 180
The Boss's Leadership Style 186
Strengths of Subordinates 186
Group Behavior 187
Other Situational Considerations 187
Decision-Making Obstacles 188

Chapter 13 Empowerment 193
Yvonne Troiani Sweeney and Sharon M. McLane

Empowerment and Autonomy 193
Team Building 195
Creating a Mission and a Vision of Leadership 198
Traditional Leadership 199
Participative Management 199

Professional Practice Models 201
Shared Governance 201

Chapter 14 Computer-Supported Decision Making for the Nurse Manager 207
Patricia M. Haynor

Introduction 207
Need Definition 208
Decision Data 209
Data Manipulation 212
Additional Software Applications 216
Information Sharing Systems 216
Using Technology to Support Decisions 217

PART III APPLICATIONS IN CLINICAL PRACTICE

Chapter 15 Critical Care 225
Teresa A. Long and Sandra M. Gomberg

Introduction 225
Regulatory Bodies Governing Decision Making 225
Factors Affecting Clinical Decision Making 228
Legal Issues 232
Ethical Issues 234
Leadership Factors 236
Staffing Issues 238
Communication Skills and Decision Making 239

Chapter 16 Acute Care 243
Luann K. Lavin and Susan M. Low

Introduction 243
Patient Advocacy 244
Competent versus Incompetent 245
Allocation of Beds 248
Room Changing 249
Nursing Care Hours versus Bed Allocation 250
Decreasing Length of Stay 252
Delegation 253
Formulating Opportunities 255
Intuitive Decision Making 256

Chapter 17 Maternal and Child Care 259
Susan L. McCulley and Sandra M. Gomberg

Introduction 259
Oversight by Regulatory Bodies 260
Clinical Decision Making 262
Legal Issues 268

Ethical Issues 270
Leadership 272

Chapter 18 Oncological Nursing 277
Jeanne L. Held and Anne Robin Waldman

Introduction 277
Crucial Factors 278
Decision Making during the Treatment Process 280

Chapter 19 The Psychiatric Setting 283
Gary E. Bilski

Introduction 283
Decision Influencers in the Psychiatric Setting 284
Clinical Decision Making 287
Pitfalls 293

Chapter 20 The Rehabilitation Setting 295
Julie Hensler-Cullen, Elaine Flynn, and Julie Hyland

Introduction 295
Theories in Clinical Decision Making 296
Team Function and Decision Making 300
The Use of Preceptors/Mentors 300

Chapter 21 The Primary Care Setting 305
Renee P. McLeod

Introduction 305
Definitions 306
Collaboration with the Patient: The Hunt for All the Facts 307
Using Clinical Skills to Gather Supporting Data 310
Therapeutic Decision Making: Involving the Patient in the Treatment Plan 313
Deciding When to Close the Patient Encounter 315
Improving Clinical Decision-Making Skills 316

Appendix A 318

Appendix B 319

Index 321

Preface

The professional practice of nursing today requires the practitioner to be adept at many complex skills, both technical and cognitive. Because technology continues to advance at increasingly rapid rates, the nurse is constantly challenged to learn and master new skills that will aid in patient care. Computer technology provides the nurse with sources of information that can be utilized and evaluated to solve patient care problems. New research and theory development provide the nurse with other sources of information on which to evaluate clinical assessments and determine appropriate interventions for care. Thus the ability to be competent in problem solving and decision making becomes an essential part of nursing practice.

The nurse manager is also required to be a competent decisionmaker in many different arenas. He or she is expected to be an expert clinician as well as an expert in budgeting, human resource development, leadership strategies, and team building. It is our belief that decision making is developed through theory and strategy acquisition and then continual practice of the new skills. Therefore, understanding basic decision-making models and strategies for the practicing nurse and manager are the foundations upon which to develop new skills. Nursing practice also requires that the nurse be able to make decisions both individually and in group or team situations. These strategies may at times be the same or different. The ability to decide when one needs help in making a decision is also very important. Once the basic skills have been mastered, they need to be adapted to the unique practice situations in which the nurse or manager finds him or herself. Specific strategies that have been useful in a particular practice setting can help the nurse or manager who is new to a setting, or a nurse who is new to nursing, or perhaps who is challenged by wanting to give up old practices and try something new.

This book is written for the student at the undergraduate and graduate levels, the practicing nurse, and the nurse administrator in a variety of clinical settings. It is an attempt to provide both theory and strategies based on theory that can be learned and implemented in practice. Scenarios provide contemporary situations in which the nurse finds him- or herself needing to know how to make an appropriate decision. Tables and figures are used throughout the chapters to illustrate applications of decision making. Reviews of the newest nursing research and theory in clinical decision making are contained in reference lists. Practical applications are included in each chapter to help nurses and managers feel more competent in this important nursing skill. Individual chapters are written by clinicians, educators, and administrators in the field to provide unique and expert reviews.

Several terms are used interchangeably throughout the chapters. Patient(s) and client(s), and nurse(s), professional nurse(s), and registered nurse(s) may be found in various chapters to address the same individuals or groups.

In Part 1, Foundations, the first three chapters review decision-making theory and strategies, with practical examples and scenarios from daily nursing practice. The traditional routine decision-making process is reviewed and applied to emergency situations and situations requiring creative decision making. The quantitative multiattribute decision-making model is reviewed; then clinical diagnostic reasoning processes are addressed to include models and theories that nurses use to help patients make decisions. Chapter 2 approaches decision making from the organizational perspective with a review of models for decision making in rational, political, collegial, and bureaucratic organizations. A more realistic model, garbage can decision making, is suggested as the way that organizations really function. Last, an evaluation model is presented. Once the theoretical foundation has been laid for decision making, both qualitative and quantitative decision-making strategies are discussed, including the latest techniques from both philosophical approaches. Advantages and disadvantages for each strategy are provided. These decision-making theories, processes, and strategies are applied throughout the subsequent chapters.

The individual decision-making process is reviewed from the Myers-Briggs Type Indicator theory, and the role that stress and conflict play in decision making, as espoused by Janis and Mann. Chapter 5 provides readers with a view of the stages that groups or teams move through during the decision-making process. Chapter 6 includes cultural settings that affect decision making, to include gender, nursing, nursing administration, and hospitals. The ethics of decision making are discussed in Chapter 7 from the perspectives of both ethical and nursing theory. Chapter 8 provides an in-depth view of how computers work, to include their role in artificial intelligence and expert systems for clinical nursing practice. A process for selecting and implementing computers is reviewed.

The new few chapters in Part 2, Managing Nursing Resources, focus on topical areas of interest to nurse administrators and include models, strategies, and scenarios that pertain to strategic planning, financial and human resource management, and the use of computers in nursing administration. Chapter 12 reviews decision making from the perspective of leader and follower, including the various leadership styles that individuals may possess. Next, in Chapter 13, leadership is explored in conjunction with the concept of empowerment and how the move to professional practice and shared governance models has impacted decision making in nursing organizations. Chapter 14 reviews the use and application of computers in making decisions for all aspects of nursing management.

In Part 3, Applications in Clinical Practice, the last six chapters pertain to decision making in the clinical nursing specialities of critical care for adults and neonates, acute care, maternal and child health, oncology, psychiatry, rehabilitation, and the primary care setting. The latest theoretical and research pieces pertaining to each specialty are reviewed and included in reference lists. Regulatory, legal, ethical, and clinical influences are discussed. Real-life scenarios from practical experiences of clinical experts are provided. We hope that the reader will find this book both enlightening and enjoyable to read.

Contributors

Robin B. Allen, M.S.N., M.B.A., R.N., C.N.A.A.
Vice President of Nursing
Methodist Hospital
Philadelphia, Pennsylvania

Sharon E. Beck, D.N.Sc., R.N.
Assistant Professor, Nursing Administration, Psychiatry
La Salle University
School of Nursing
Philadelphia, Pennsylvania

Patricia Hentz Becker, Ed.D., R.N.
Associate Professor, Psychiatry, Education
La Salle University
School of Nursing
Philadelphia, Pennsylvania

Gary E. Bilski, M.B.A., R.N., C.N.A.
Assistant Administrator
The Horsham Clinic
Horsham, Pennsylvania

Julie Hensler-Cullen, M.S.N., R.N.
Assistant Director of Nursing Education and Research
Moss Rehabilitation Hospital
Philadelphia, Pennsylvania

Elaine Flynn, M.S.N., C.R.R.N.
Nursing Quality Improvement Coordnator
Clinical Instructor
Moss Rehabilitation Hospital
Philadelphia, Pennsylvania

Alice Donahue, M.S.N., R.N.
Associate Administrator Clinical Services
Atlantic City Medical Center
City Division
Atlantic City, New Jersey

Christina M. Fitz-Patrick, M.S.N., R.N.
Director of Nursing
Nazareth Hospital
Philadelphia, Pennsylvania

Sandra M. Gomberg, M.S.N., R.N.C.
Pediatric Program Manager
Kimberly Quality Care
West Conshohocken, Pennsylvania

Elisabeth T. Hallman, M.B.A., R.N., C.N.A.
Administrator, Perinatal Services
Albert Einstein Medical Center
Philadelphia, Pennsylvania

DeEtta F. Hayes, M.S.N., R.N.
Consultant
Management Services
Moorestown, New Jersey

Patricia M. Haynor, Ph.D., R.N.
Associate Professor, Nursing Adminitration
School of Nursing
Department of Nursing Administration
Villanova University
Bryn Mawr, Pennsylvania

Jeanne L. Held, M.S.N., R.N.C.S.
Clinical Nurse Specialist, Medical Oncology
Albert Einstein Medical Center
Philadelphia, Pennsylvania

Julie Hyland, M.S.N., R.N., C.N.A.
Associate Administrator of Hospital Services
Moss Rehabilitation Hospital
Philadelphia, Pennsylvania

Rebecca A. Patronis Jones, D.N.Sc., R.N., C.N.A.A.
Formerly:
Associate Professor, Nursing Administration
La Salle University
School of Nursing
Philadelphia, Pennsylvania
and
Associate Director of Nursing Services
Albert Einstein Medical Center
Department of Nursing
Philadelphia, Pennsylvania

Luann K. Lavin, M.S.N., R.N.
Clinical Faculty
School of Nursing
Mercer Medical Center
Trenton, New Jersey

Teresa A. Long, M.S.N., R.N., C.C.R.N., C.R.R.N, C.N.A.
Clinical/Case Manager Intensive Care Continuum
Montgomery Hospital
Norristown, Pennsylvannia

Susan M. Low, B.S.N., R.N.C., C.N.A.
Clinical Staff Nurse
Albert Einstein Medical Center
Department of Nursing
Philadelphia, Pennsylvania

Ellie Mack, M.S., M.Ed., R.N.C.
Director of Cancer Outreach
Albert Einstein Medical Center
Breast Cancer Program
Philadelphia, Pennsylvania

Suzanne G. Martin, M.S.
Director of Administrative Services, Nursing
Albert Einstein Medical Center
Department of Nursing
Philadelphia, Pennsylvania

Susan L. McCulley, M.S.N., R.N., C.N.A.
Assistant Director of Nursing
Operations
Moss Rehabilitation Hospital
Philadelphia, Pennsylvania

Terry B. McGoldrick, M.S.N., R.N.
Director of Nursing for Professional Development
Albert Einstein Medical Center
Department of Nursing
Philadelphia, Pennsylvania

Sharon M. McLane, M.B.A., R.N.,
C.N.A.A.
Director of Nursing Services
Albert Einstein Medical Center
Department of Nursing
Philadelphia, Pennsylvania

Renee P. McLeod, M.S.N., R.N., R.N.C.
Nurse Practitioner Primary Care
and
Doctoral Candidate
Widener University
Chester, Pennsylvania

Linda A. Sinesi, M.S., R.N., C.N.A.A.
Director of Nursing
HCA Neurological Hospital
Beaumont, Texas

Yvonne Troiani Sweeney, M.S.N., R.N.
President and Consultant
YTS Professional Resource Development
Langhorne, Pennsylvania

Anne Robin Waldman, M.S.N., R.N.C.,
O.N.C.
Clinical Nurse Specialist, Oncology
Albert Einstein Medical Center
Philadelphia, Pennsylvania

Robin W. Wells, M.S.N., R.N., C.N.A.
Nurse Consultant
Bates and Associates
Bala Cynwood, Pennsylvania

PART I

FOUNDATIONS

Rebecca A. Patronis Jones

CHAPTER 1

Processes and Models

Choices are the spice of life.
—*Anonymous*

INTRODUCTION

Discussion in clinical, academic, and administrative nursing circles today revolves around the topics of problem solving, decision making, critical thinking, and critical analysis. Some authors use problem solving and decision making to describe the same process. For the purposes of this book, decision making is a process that involves steps or actions that one might take in solving problems relevant to the discipline of nursing. Tappen (1989) clarifies the relationship of critical thinking and critical analysis in relation to the decision-making process: Critical thinking is a skill developed in looking for alternative solutions to problems and adopting a questioning approach. Critical analysis is a tool used in critical thinking and may involve asking the following questions:

- What is the central issue?
- What are the underlying assumptions?
- Is there valid evidence?
- Are the conclusions acceptable?

These questions help analyze the steps in the decision-making process.

Decision making applies to many disciplines. Discussions of decision-making models can be found in economics, operations theory, philosophy, political science, psychology, sociology, business administration, healthcare administration, healthcare policy, and nursing. This chapter discusses models that are applicable to problems within the discipline of nursing. Models specific to ethical decision making or topics specific to clinical specialties will be discussed in the respective chapters.

SIGNIFICANCE

Decision making is important to the discipline of nursing for dealing with problems arising in the management of nursing resources and clinical practice. Nurse administrators must determine the best courses of action for managing staff members, budgets, supplies, and in governance decisions concerning the nursing department within the larger organization. Decisions must be made concerning the nursing actions that may be required by a group of patients with similar medical and nursing diagnoses and demographic and psychosocial characteristics. Nurses also assist patients in making decisions concerning health care. Nurses in both of these roles can make a significant impact on the delivery of health care by learning to make the best decisions.

ROUTINE PROCESS

Table 1-1 illustrates five steps that are applicable to individual or group decision making (Marriner-Tomey, 1992; Sullivan and Decker, 1992).

Step 1

Step 1 involves the **identification** of the problem that needs a solution by answering several questions:

- What is the story or issue?
- How long has the problem existed?
- What is the history of the problem?
- What is wrong?
- What improvement is needed?

The identification phase should include an analysis of the situation in which the problem occurs by gathering all of the pertinent facts. Facts may be determined by answering several questions:

- What is the desirable situation?
- What are the presenting symptoms of the problem?
- What are the discrepancies?
- What are the related issues?
- Who is involved?
- When?
- Where?
- How?

Table 1-1 • **Decision-Making Process**

Routine Process	Creative Process
1. Problem Identification • situation analysis • pertinent facts and related issues • decision goals and criteria	1. Felt Need
2. Seek Alternatives • apply criteria	2. Preparation
	3. Incubation
3. Select Alternative	4. Illumination
	5. Verification
4. Implement Decision	6. Implement Decision
5. Evaluation	7. Evaluation

Adapted from A. Marriner-Tomey, Guide to Nursing Management *(Philadelphia: Mosley Year Book, 1992) and E.J. Sullivan and P.J. Decker,* Effective Management in Nursing *(New York: Addison-Wesley Publishing Company, 1992).*

The identification phase involves establishing goals for the decision by asking:

- Why is a decision necessary?
- What specific aspects of the decision need to be determined?
- What is the purpose of the decision?

The goal of the decision may be further defined by setting and weighting criteria. Criteria are comprised of certain standards that should be met when the decision is made. Typical criteria for alternative solutions to nursing problems might include cost, practicality, feasibility, quality of patient care, and satisfaction for both the nurse and patient (Graham, 1987). Each criterion may be weighted by assigning orders of importance to the specific goals set for the decision.

Step 2

The second step involves **seeking alternatives** from which to select appropriate decisions or solutions for the issue at hand. Alternatives involve various courses of action that may fulfill the criteria for the goal of the decision. Once alternatives are generated, they are tested using the preestablished, weighted criteria. The most desirable alternatives are determined.

Step 3

Selection of an alternative is the third step. Based on the work completed in Step 2, rank-ordered alternatives should make the selection process an easy task.

Step 4

The fourth step involves **implementing the decision**, when a timeline should be established and tasks assigned to accountable parties.

Step 5

The last step is **evaluation** of the solution implemented; decisionmakers must determine if the decision made was effective in solving the issue or problem. Determinations are also made as to how efficient the solution was for the initial problem.

Scenario 1-1

A problem concerning a nurse shortage in a 200-bed community hospital is presented. Creek Memorial Hospital (CMH) is a community hospital located 30 miles from a major city in the deep South. Nurse administrators at CMH consist of three clinical nurse managers, an assistant director, and a director. Nurse managers have been spending two full weeks preparing a six-week nursing time schedule for all units within the Department of Nursing. This time commitment to schedule preparation has existed for the last six months. Some directors have noted that although they have permanent and part-time staff members, they still do not have enough members to cover all shifts for a six-week period.

The nursing administration staff would like to reduce the time needed to prepare a six-week time schedule to one week. They have also decided that staffing levels are appropriate for the census and acuity of patients on each unit and would like to keep their personnel budgets on target with annual projections. The nursing administrative staff identifies a nurse shortage as the problem *(Step 1)* at a meeting one morning. The director of nursing spends the next week searching for possible solutions to the nurse shortage. She calls three different nurse staffing agencies for skill levels and salaries of agency nurses and requests information on a computerized nurse staffing and scheduling system *(Step 2)*. Bearing in mind the nursing personnel budgets, staffing levels, and time commitment set for schedule preparation, she chooses Agency A. Agency A has the cheapest rates and nurses experienced in the specialties that CMH has the greatest need for (*Step 3*). This option will also speed time schedule preparation as nurse managers need only give a list of needs to Agency A, who will guarantee staff for the next six weeks. A computerized staffing and scheduling system would take six months to implement and train staff to use. The director is pleased with being able to solve her department's shortage and still meet the proposed annual personnel budget.

The nursing administration staff are informed of the solution at the next morning meeting and instructed how to complete the next six-week time schedules *(Step 4)*. The nurse managers complete the schedules within one week's time, budget projections are met, and only the critical care area is left with vacancies, which the nurse manager plans to cover herself *(Step 5)*. Everyone is pleased with the solution.

CREATIVE PROCESS

Marriner-Tomey (1992) has proposed a creative decision-making process, outlined in Table 1-1, that is similar to the routine process, except the focus is on creating unique solutions as opposed to generating choices of solutions.

Step 1

The first step in the creative process is a **felt need** for generating unique solutions. This step is similar to Step 1, problem identification, in the routine process, as the individual or group recognizes that a problem exists.

Step 2

The second step in the creative process is **preparation**, similar to the second step in the routine process, seeking alternatives. However, emphasis is placed on innovation in exploring numerous potential solutions and considering the relationship of each of these solutions. Marriner-Tomey (1992) suggests that the individual involved in the creative process would use the library extensively to generate creative solutions during the preparation phase. The emphasis is on generating numerous creative alternatives rather than focusing on alternatives that would adequately meet the goals for the decision.

Step 3

The third step in the creative process is **incubation**: taking time to review the problem and data collected once a point has been reached where no new alternatives are being generated. This step occurs before Step 3 in the routine process, and represents an additional step.

Step 4

The fourth step is **illumination** and involves the discovery of a solution. This step is comparable to the Step 3 in the routine process. Illumination differs from selecting an alternative, as the individual or groups take time off to incubate and illumination may occur apart from work time.

Step 5

The fifth step in the creative process is **verification**. During this step the solution is refined, and criteria are used to assess the advantages and disadvantages of the chosen alternative. This step is comparable to Step 2 in the routine model, where criteria are applied to determine the best solution. The last steps are identical to the routine model. The chosen solution is implemented and evaluated.

Similarities of Routine and Creative Processes

The creative process includes some of the same steps as the routine process. The major differences are that the focus initially is on creating numerous innovative solutions before criteria are used to verify the appropriateness of the chosen solution. In the creative model, individuals and groups allow incubation, or time off from working on the problem, so that illumination may occur before selecting a solution.

Scenario 1-2

To illustrate the creative process, the same nursing shortage scenario may be used. The nursing administrative staff identifies the same problem, a nurse shortage, after reviewing the situation *(Step 1)*. The director calls a special administrative meeting for the nursing administration staff to brainstorm alternatives. The assistant director conducts a review of the literature on the shortage. This time the group comes up with the same list of alternatives and one additional alternative concerning the initiation of a hospital flexi-pool *(Step 2)*. The meeting convenes and all staff are asked to consider the alternatives and generate a list of advantages and disadvantages for each alternative for the next monthly meeting *(Step 3, incubation)*. All group members come to the same conclusion on off-duty time *(Step 4, illumination)*. At the next meeting, the group verifies the flexi-pool alternative as the cheapest, least time consuming, and the best match for nursing specialty needs *(Step 5, verification)*. The nursing administration staff creates a time-line and assigns responsibilities for establishing the flexi-pool before the next time schedule preparation is due *(Step 6, implementation)*. During the evaluation two time periods later, the staff assesses that only one week was spent on time schedule preparation, budget projections were met, all staffing levels were met, and the critical care nurse manager does not need to cover shifts.

EMERGENCY PROCESS

The decision-making process adapted from Marriner-Tomey (1992) and Sullivan and Decker (1992) can be applied to decisions made by nurses in both routine and emergency situations involving patients. In emergency situations, the same steps occur, but at a much more rapid pace. Problem identification *(Step 1)* involves a rapid assessment of the situation. In the case of an adult nonpregnant female choking victim, this assessment might include blueness around the mouth, clutching at the throat, and inability to speak as signs and symptoms. Decision goals are based on the potential for loss of life or limb. Seeking alternatives *(Step 2)* is based on a quick assessment of interventions with similarities to other situations in the nurse's knowledge base for application to the patient problem. For our choking victim, this might include the Heimlich maneuver or chest thrusts, depending on the age of the victim. Selecting the alternative *(Step 3)* occurs almost simultaneously with implementation of the decision *(Step 4)*. Our victim is an adult nonpregnant female, thus the Heimlich maneuver is applied. Solution evaluation *(Step 5)* occurs immediately after implementation of the solution. After the Heimlich maneuver has been applied several times, the choking victim is asked if she can speak, and the mouth is checked for blueness. The choking victim coughs up a piece of steak and states, "I can breathe OK now." Thus, the decision-making process in the emergency situation was a success.

MULTIATTRIBUTE UTILITY MODEL

Huber (1980) has proposed a multiattribute utility (MAU) model for decision making involving multiple goals or criteria. Before explaining this model, we will first define the concepts of **attribute** and **utility**. Huber defines an attribute as a characteristic of an alternative or potential solution for a problem. The utility for an alternative or problem solution involves assigning criteria that demonstrate usefulness. Utilities may include worth, payoff, psychological value, or level of satisfaction. The overall utility might be defined as the extent to which an alternative or problem solution satisfies a criterion or goal defined for the decision-making session, using one or more utility criteria assigned a number value (Huber, 1980). Utilities derived from the individual criteria of a decision situation may be weighted and aggregated to determine a problem solution or alternative with the highest overall multiattribute score. This model is most clearly understood by applying four steps to Scenario 1-3.

Attribute

Suppose you want to select a nurse manager from three potential candidates. First, identify the attributes for the nurse manager. Suppose the three most important attributes for this decision situation are

- education
- previous experience
- leadership style

Utility

Next, a utility (u) score for each attribute is determined. The following scores are assigned for education:

- Master's degree = 1
- Bachelor's degree = 2
- Diploma = 3
- Associate's Degree = 4

The following scores are assigned for experience:

- 10 years or more of experience = 1
- 5 to 9 years of experience = 2
- 2 to 4 years experience = 3
- 1 year or less of experience = 4

The following scores are assigned for leadership style:

- participatory = 1
- consultative = 2
- laissez faire = 3
- autocratic = 4

Weight

Now the importance or weight (w) of each attribute is weighted on a scale of 0 to 100. Leadership style is weighted 50 percent, and education and years experience each receive a 25 percent weighting.

Formula

The above steps are combined into a formula: utility score times weighted importance for attribute 1 plus utility score times weighted importance for attribute 2 plus utility score times weighted importance for attribute 3 equals the overall multiattribute score or ([u1 × w1] + [u2 × w2] + [u3 × w3] = MAU).

Scenario 1-3

If candidate 1 received an education score of 1, a years experience score of 1, and a leadership style score of 1, then the MAU score would be (1 × .50) + (1 × .25) + (1 × .25) = 1. If candidate 2 received an education score of 1, a years experience score of 2, and a leadership style score of 4, then the MAU score would be (1 × .50) + (2 × .25) + (4 × .25) = 2. If candidate 3 received an education score of 3, a years experience score of 3, and a leadership style score of 2, then the MAU score would be (3 × .50) + (3 × .25) + (2 × .25) = 2.75. In the current system, 1 is considered to be the best score, so candidate 1 would be rated overall as the best candidate for the nurse manager position.

INTUITIVE PROCESS

All of the above authors view the decision-making process as comprised of a series of steps or questions. Benner and Tanner (1987) have taken a different approach. They view the nurse's decision-making process based on Benner's (1984) study of nursing competencies. In this study, nurse competencies are described for the novice, advanced beginner, competent nurse, proficient nurse, and expert nurse (Benner, 1984). Nurses move along this same continuum of competence in their decision-making skills (Table 1-2).

The novice and advanced beginner rely heavily on rules, procedures, maxims, and principles. The decision-making process at this level may be characterized from a rationalist perspective: A rational, step-by-step analytic approach to clinical judg-

Table 1-2 • Intuitive Process

Intuitive Judgment	Nurse Competency				
	Novice	*Advanced Beginner*	*Competent Nurse*	*Proficient Nurse*	*Expert Nurse*
Pattern Recognition	>	>>	>>>	>>>>	>>>>>
Similarity Recognition	>	>>	>>>	>>>>	>>>>>
Common Sense Understanding	>	>>	>>>	>>>>	>>>>>
Skilled Knowhow	>	>>	>>>	>>>>	>>>>>
Sense of Salience	>	>>	>>>	>>>>	>>>>>
Deliberate Rationality	>	>>	>>>	>>>>	>>>>>

KEY > = gradual increase

Adapted from P. Benner and C.A. Tanner. Clinical Judgment: How Expert Nurses Use Intuition, *American Journal of Nursing, 87(7), (1987), 23–31, and H. Dreyfus and S. Dreyfus,* Mind over Machine: The Power of Human Intuition and Expertise in the Era of the Computer *(New York: Free Press, 1985).*

ment is evident here. One such model described by Elstein, Shulman, and Sprafka (1978) included four steps:

1. Identifying the problem through initial, available clues
2. Formulating diagnostic hypotheses to explain the initial clues
3. Gathering more data to provide support or nonsupport and refinement of the diagnostic hypotheses
4. Evaluating the hypotheses

However, nurses at the proficient and expert level perceive the patient's situation as a whole in which only selected bits of information are relevant, yet the nurse is fully involved in the situation. At this level, the nurse demonstrates intuition versus an analytical step-by-step approach. Benner and Tanner (1987) define intuition as an understanding or synthesis of events without rationale or analysis, based on clinical observations that may not be expressed as a diagnosis.

Aspects of Intuitive Judgment

Various levels of intuition are evident in nurses' decision-making processes. The Dreyfus and Dreyfus (1985) model of skill acquisition proposes six key aspects of intuitive judgment:

- Pattern recognition
- Similarity recognition

- Common sense understanding
- Skilled know how
- Sense of salience
- Deliberate rationality

Benner and Tanner (1987) suggest that these six key aspects of intuitive judgment are evident in the decision-making processes of all nurses, depending on their level of competence. They propose the following definitions: **Pattern recognition** is defined as a perceptual ability to recognize configurations and relationships among variables in a situation without having explicitly stated these variables and their relationships before the situation occurs. **Similarity recognition** is the ability to recognize similarities and differences in the objective aspects of past and current situations. **Common sense understanding** is a deep grasp of the culture and language of an illness experience from direct observations of patients' carrying out routine activities of daily living. **Skilled knowhow** involves juggling many considerations during the decision-making process. A **sense of salience** means recognition of events as more or less important in combination with other extraneous events in describing a patient's condition. **Deliberate rationality** is defined as selective attention that involves viewing certain aspects of the current situation in light of past situations (Benner & Tanner, 1987). Thus, clinical nurse decision making may be described based on evidence of the six key aspects of intuitive judgment in varying degrees, depending on the nurse's competence level. While a rational step-by-step process may be evident in a novice's decision-making process, these steps become more difficult to distinguish in the decision-making processes of expert nurses. Thus, key aspects may be more helpful in distinguishing competency levels among nurse decisionmakers. Readers are referred to Benner's classic (1984) work for descriptions of novice to expert decision making by nurses.

DIAGNOSTIC DECISION MAKING

Building on the work of Elstein and associates (1978), Carnevali and Thomas (1984, 1993) have further advanced a rational model of decision making for nursing. Carnevali and Thomas (1984, 1993) define the diagnostic reasoning process for nursing as a complex, sometimes unconscious integration of critical thinking and data collecting processes used by clinicians to identify and classify phenomena in presenting clinical situations. These phenomena provide the foundation for subsequent treatment decisions. Carnevali and Thomas's (1984, 1993) decision-making model may be classified as a process model. Carnevali and Thomas (1993) describe the process as nonlinear due to the retrieval and consideration of diagnostic possibilities, making diagnostic judgments, and adjusting interventions sooner than they might appear in an actual situation. As a result of this nonlinear process, the model is best described by elements and their potential pattern in Figure 1-1. The model may also be classified as an intuitive decision-making model, as Carnevali recognizes the differences between novice and expert nurses' use of the model.

Carnevali (1984), in her extension of Elstein and associates' (1978) model of decision making, includes the idea that nurses must diagnose in two domains. Diagnosis in the nursing domain includes accountability for making judgments

Collection of Pre-Encounter Data about Patient Situation*

*** Entry into the Patient Situation**

Make a quick overview
Do an urgency scaling for data collection or action
Determine strategies for gathering patient data
Structure role and nursing perspective for patient

*** Collection of Data Using Screening or Problem-Oriented Approach**

*** Coalescing of Data into Related Chunks in Working Memory**

*** Selection of Cue or Cue Cluster of Highest Priority for Initial Diagnosing**

*** Retrieval of Possible Diagnostic Explanations or Patient Instances from Long-Term Memory**

Move from generic to specific
Consider competing or alternative diagnostic explanations

*** Utilization of Recognition Features Associated with the Retrieved Diagnostic Concepts as Guides for Observation of Patient and Situation**

*** Comparison of Data in Patient Situation to Recognition Features in Diagnostic Concept, Problem Script, or Patient Instances**

*** Assignment of a Diagnosis** if the data fit the recognition features of one of the retrieved diagnoses, problem scripts, or patient instances.

Or If None Fit

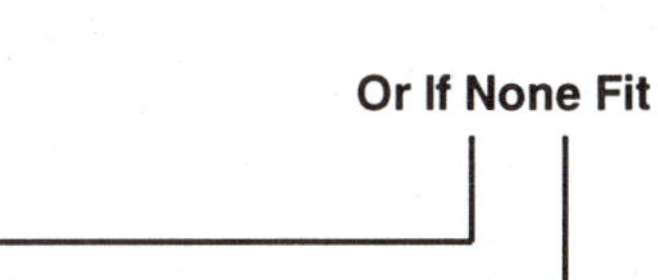

* Pre-encounter data may or may not involve clinical judgment. If information is deliberately sought out by the nurse, judgment is involved. If the nurse is exposed to data without taking initiative no clinical judgment is involved.

Figure 1-1 Clinical Diagnostic Reasoning Model. *Source: D.L. Carnevali and M.D. Thomas,* Diagnostic Reasoning and Treatment Decision Making in Nursing *(Philadelphia: J.B. Lippincott Co., 1993). Reprinted with permission.*

regarding the status of the patient's and family's daily living as it affects or is affected by the health status (Carnevali, 1984). Diagnosis in the biomedical domain consists of delegated responsibilities by the physician to make accurate, appropriate clinical judgments on the patient's pathophysiologic health status (Carnevali, 1984). These judgments concern decisions about whether the patient can provide self-care, is in need of nursing management, or requires a physician referral for medical diagnosis and treatment or altered medical regimes.

Pre-Encounter Data

The following application to the clinical diagnostic reasoning model has been taken from readings in both Carnevali (1984) and Carnevali and Thomas (1993). Carnevali and Thomas (1993) describe the nurse's clinical diagnostic reasoning process using nine basic elements combined in the following pattern. The first element consists of **pre-encounter data** (Figure 1-1). These are early limits set on the data space by using available patient data before actually meeting the patient in a clinical encounter. These data may consist of age, sex, or other demographic variables available from a previous patient history. By setting early limits, the nurse helps to reduce cognitive strain and the infinity of the presenting situation. In the example that follows, the medical record indicates that Tim is a 2-year-old male with normal growth and development who has presented to the pediatric clinic with numerous bouts of otitis media. Jane is a pediatric clinical nurse specialist employed by Dr. Johns to work in the clinic.

Entry into the Assessment Situation

The second element in the process is **entry into the data field.** Nurses usually begin with a known starting point and complete a quick overview or visual scanning of the patient from head to toe, verbal questioning about the chief complaint or other key information, and observation of specific body parts with palpation. Next, standard patterns for the specific clinical specialty are usually followed, the nurse begins to focus on high risk areas, or other strategies for data collection are selected. The patient's and family's role in data collection is also determined. In Tim's case, the mother explains that Tim has been crying and irritable, with a runny nose, dry cough, fever, and loss of appetite for the past twenty-four hours. She has been giving him Tylenol® every four hours, which reduced his fever from 101°F to 98°F, but it was up again to 102°F this morning so she brought him to the clinic. Jane includes the mother's report in her assessment and proceeds with a physical examination. Jane finds reddened, bulging ear drums, and rales in both upper lobes of the lungs.

Collection of the Data Base

The third element in the process is **collection of the database**. During the previous element, Jane used the focused or problem-oriented approach to begin her data entry into assessment. Now, Jane focuses her attention on the collection of a more comprehensive database using a nursing database form designed specifically for the clinic and arranged by body systems and developmental phases of children and adolescents.

Cue Clusters

Cues collected from the first three elements are placed into **cue clusters** or chunks in the fourth and fifth elements. Cues may consist of risk indicators associated with specific health problems, strength indicators concerning the patient or family's effectiveness in performing activities of daily living and available resources to meet these needs, objective signs collected from the physical examination, and subjective symptoms provided by the patient during the patient interview or history-taking sessions (Carnevali, 1984). During this element the nurse must be aware of irrelevant clues. These may be determined by the clinical specialty in which the nurse is functioning. Nurses must also learn to collect pivotal cue clusters, as patients may present with more than one health problem or diagnosis. Jane concludes that all clues from the physical exam and mother's history fit into a respiratory syndrome. In this case, the patient, Tim, has only a primary problem up to this point in time.

Diagnostic Explanations or Concepts

Once pertinent cues are assimilated into clusters or chunks, the sixth through eighth elements concerning **diagnostic explanation** or concepts are activated. Carnevali and Thomas's (1993) description of the cue cluster elements most reflects the intuitive process. The novice's use of clues is slow and tentative. Novices tend to generate multiple clusters which contain fewer clues, while experts generate fewer clusters containing more clues in each cluster. During these elements, the nurse attaches tentative problem labels that are subject to change to the clusters of cues. In addition to the patient data field cues, each nurse maintains a cerebral library or long-term memory of knowledge packets containing problem labels or diagnostic classifications, lists of characteristics or features to include risk factors, signs and symptoms, and sets of associated actions. Carnevali and Thomas (1984, 1993) describe processing these elements as a mental shuffle between the cerebral library, patient data field, and recognition features to activate potential hypotheses. These searches or mental shuffles assist the nurse in developing relationships among hypotheses. These relationships may be hierarchical, consisting of signs and symptoms associated with risk factors from general to specific diagnoses, or competing hypotheses that may be alternate explanations at both the general and specific levels.

Jane assesses Tim's problem as a repeat otitis media, viral upper respiratory infection, or bacterial pneumonia. Jane has been given protocols by Dr. Johns to treat Tim's recurrent otitis media or viral upper respiratory infections; however, bacterial infections must be referred for further diagnostic workup. In Jane's search of the mother's history, physical exam, and associated signs and symptoms for her three diagnostic hypotheses, she is unable to make a definitive diagnosis. Jane decides to refer Tim to Dr. Johns for further diagnostic workup.

Diagnosis

The ninth element consists of **assigning a diagnosis**. During this element, the nurse matches the diagnosis with antecedent or patterned events, associated risk factors, signs and symptoms, complications and possible treatment alternatives, and prognoses. This usually leads to the final element where a definitive diagnosis is made and treatment decided upon. Dr. Johns orders a chest X-ray, which indicates bilateral pneumonia. A throat and nasal cultures are ordered, and Tim is placed on antibiotics and instructed to call the clinic in 72 hours for lab results.

No Fit

If a definitive diagnosis cannot be made, a **no fit situation** exists. The nurse may begin data collection or retrieval of diagnostic explanations again. Thus the process is repeated from the third or sixth element on. Possible diagnostic explanations are retrieved. Another alternative is to reshape the direction of the data gathering and start the entire process again from the third element, data collection. In the case example, the culture results confirm the diagnosis of bacterial pneumonia with appropriate antibiotic therapy. Thus, activating additional diagnostic hypotheses or initiating data collection again are not necessary.

Both Elstein et al. (1978) and Carnevali and Thomas (1984, 1993) have provided excellent models to potentially explain the diagnostic reasoning process of nurses. Elstein et al. (1978), in extensive testing of their model, have not been able to differentiate between expert and nonexpert physicians during the medical reasoning process. Westfall, Tanner, Putzier, and Padrick (1986) also found statistically insignificant differences when testing these models on nurses and nursing students. Elstein et al. (1978) have attributed these results to differences in an individual's repertoire of experiences organized in long-term memory as opposed to differences in problem-solving rules. Much work remains to be done in the research testing of these models.

COLLABORATIVE MODEL

Building on the work of Elstein and associates (1978) and Carnevali (1984), a collaborative model is proposed for today's healthcare environment. This model is most applicable to the clinical staff nurse in the inpatient setting and includes five major steps (Table 1-3) that may be repeated by nurse, physician, or other healthcare provider.

The Problem

A patient presents with a manifestation, chief complaint, or symptoms to the physician. The physician takes a history from the patient, performs a physical exam, and orders diagnostic tests. Mr. Tap is a 50-year-old Hispanic male who presents himself to Dr. Kutz with a complaint of radiating chest pain that increases on exertion. Mr.

Table 1-3 • **Collaborative Model**

Steps	Process
1	Assessment of the Problem
2	Differential Diagnosis
3	Diagnostic Workup
4	Care Plan Formulation and Implementation
5	Final Diagnosis and Treatment

Tap gives a history of the following symptoms for the past twenty-four hours: shortness of breath, nausea, and sweating. Dr. Kutz finds tachycardia on physical examination and orders an electrocardiogram, which indicates premature ventricular beats. Further diagnostic workup indicates abnormal cardiac enzymes.

Differential Diagnosis

Dr. Kutz generates a list of potential causes for Mr. Tap's chest pain and concludes that Mr. Tap is experiencing a myocardial infarction, angina, costochondritis, or hiatal hernia. Dr. Kutz proceeds to the next step in collaborative decision making.

Diagnostic Workup

Dr. Kutz admits Mr. Tap to the medical unit with the following orders: bed rest up ad lib to the bathroom, cardiac diet, cardiac enzymes every 8 hours times 3, repeat electrocardiogram to be interpreted by the cardiologist, and echocardiogram.

Care Plan Formulation

The admitting nurse, Mr. Tip, receives Mr. Tap on the unit and orients him to his room. While Mr. Tap is changing into hospital pajamas, nurse Tip reviews the physician's history, physical exam, and orders in the medical record. Nurse Tip returns to Mr. Tap's room to assess *the problem* from the nursing perspective. A nursing history, physical exam, and chief complaint analysis are conducted to investigate Mr. Tap's ability to meet activities of daily living and the level of psychosocial and emotional support available. Findings are similar to Dr. Kutz's. The history reveals the following additional information: Mr. Tap is a car salesman with a sixth-grade education who works six days a week for commissions with a supportive wife; he consumes a diet high in cholesterol and salt, leads a sedentary lifestyle with bowling once a month as the only exercise, and has a smoking history of one pack of cigarettes per day for the past thirty-five years. Mr. Tap expresses no understanding of cholesterol and salt content in the list of foods that he has generated, and believes that walking to the end of his driveway two to three times per week for the daily newspaper is a vigorous exercise routine. Nurse Tip formulates the following nursing diagnoses:

- Alteration in nutrition manifested as more than body requirements related to lack of basic nutritional knowledge
- Knowledge deficit about cardiac risk factors and healthy lifestyle related to lack of education and new medical condition
- Ineffective individual coping related to career pressures manifested as stress

Care Plan Implementation

Nurse Tip *implements the plan of care* designed thus far. High levels of collaboration occur from this point on between Dr. Kutz, Nurse Tip, and other healthcare providers. Nursing-dependent functions that involve carrying out Dr. Kutz's orders are implemented. Nursing-independent interventions are also implemented. Nurse Tip begins teaching Mr. Tap about the diagnostic tests ordered and cardiac risk factors. A referral is completed to the dietitian to begin teaching a cardiac diet. A physical therapy referral is completed for the therapist to teach the cardiac exercise program. The occupational therapist is contacted to begin a stress reduction program for Mr. Tap. Nurse Tip monitors the patient for additional symptoms, abnormal diagnostic tests, or physical findings and reports these to Dr. Kutz daily during his morning rounds and to the healthcare team at the weekly discharge planning meeting.

Final Diagnosis

Dr. Kutz diagnoses Mr. Tap as having a myocardial infection with the assistance of the diagnostic workup findings and Nurse Tip's reports.

Treatment

Dr. Kutz discharges Mr. Tap with a progressive exercise program, continuation of stress clinic, cardiac diet, and appropriate vasodialator and antiarhythmic medications with orders to return to clinic in one week. Nurse Tip explains the discharge treatment plan and gives Mr. Tap the clinic nurse's phone number for further questions.

ASSISTING PATIENTS WITH DECISION MAKING

Corcoran (1988) has adapted the decision-making process as described in Table 1-1 for nurses serving in a patient advocacy role, assisting patients with the decision-making process. Corcoran's model is summarized in Table 1-4, and is based on the use of decision theory with Gadow's (1980) model of ethical decision making.

Corcoran (1988) defines the nurse's advocacy role in decision making as helping another to decide while providing relevant information. This process, as described by Gadow (1980), involves five steps.

Table 1-4 • **Nurse as Patient Advocate in the Decision-Making Process**

Steps	Process
1	Assure Relevant Information
2	Enable Patient Selection of Information
3	Disclose Personal View
4	Assist Patient with Value Determination
5	Assist Patient in Attaching Meaning to Decision

Adapted from S. Corcoran, Toward Operationalizing an Advocacy Role, *Journal of Professional Nursing, 4(4), (1988), 242–248.*

Scenario 1-4

Step 1 involves ensuring relevant information (Gadow, 1980). Corcoran (1988) proposes the use of decision analysis to provide relevant information. By taking alternatives, chance events associated with each alternative, the probabilities for chance events occurring, outcomes, and values for each alternative, a decision tree of relevant information may be constructed for the patient's current situation. (See Corcoran (1986) for further information on how to construct a decision tree.) Probabilities would come from the health literature while values would be supplied by the involved patient.

Nurse Jane has a 65-year-old black female patient present to the neighborhood nursing center for her annual flu shot. The patient, Mrs. M, tells Jane that she has smoked for the past twenty years since she quit working. Mrs. M inquires about the influence of smoking on lung infections. Jane constructs a decision tree (Figure 1-2) to help Mrs. M consider health options, chance events, outcomes, and values. Mrs. M's options are to continue or quit smoking. The chance events for each option are to contract lung cancer or remain cancer free with a 9 to 1 or 1 to 9 ratio depending on the option chosen. Outcomes associated with the options are death or early cancer detection, in which the patient responds to treatment with minor associated symptoms. Values are left for Ms. M to establish as she and Jane continue with the decision-making process.

Step 2 involves enabling the patient to select information (Gadow, 1980). Corcoran (1988) advises that this may be done by carefully talking with the patient to determine how much information he or she needs and wants to make the decision, as well as coordinating information that will be provided by other members of the healthcare team. In this scenario, Jane shares the decision analysis tree for a patient who smokes with Mrs. M. Jane also provides Mrs. M with pamphlets on lung cancer and smoking cessation clinics.

Step 3 involves disclosing the nurse's view (Gadow, 1980). During this step the nurse should share his or her personal views and opinions of the information in the decision tree to assist the patient with values clarification. However, Corcoran (1988) cautions that nurses should be careful in communicating values so that the patient is not persuaded to adopt the nurse's point of view.

In Step 3, Jane shares with Mrs. M that she has never smoked; however, she watched her husband smoke for twenty years and understands how difficult it is to quit. Jane tells Mrs. M that based on the probabilities in the decision analysis tree, she would choose the smoking cessation option.

Step 4 involves helping the patient determine her own values (Gadow, 1980). Values for alternatives may have already been determined in construction of the decision tree in Step 1. Now the nurse and patient might also wish to consider risks and benefits for the consequences of each option.

Jane and Mrs. M continue to discuss the decision analysis tree, and while considering the outcomes, Mrs. M decides to place a high value on smoking cessation and a low value on smoking continuation. Mrs. M. decides to quit smoking cigarettes and to attend the smoking cessation clinic for assistance.

The last step, *Step 5*, involves assisting the patient to determine meaning (Gadow, 1980). In this step the nurse assists the patient in attaching his or her own individuality to the decision that has been made, so that closure for the decision-making process is obtained. In this scenario, Mrs. M tells Jane that she feels she has made a wise decision for her health and advises her that she should cease to have her morning cough.

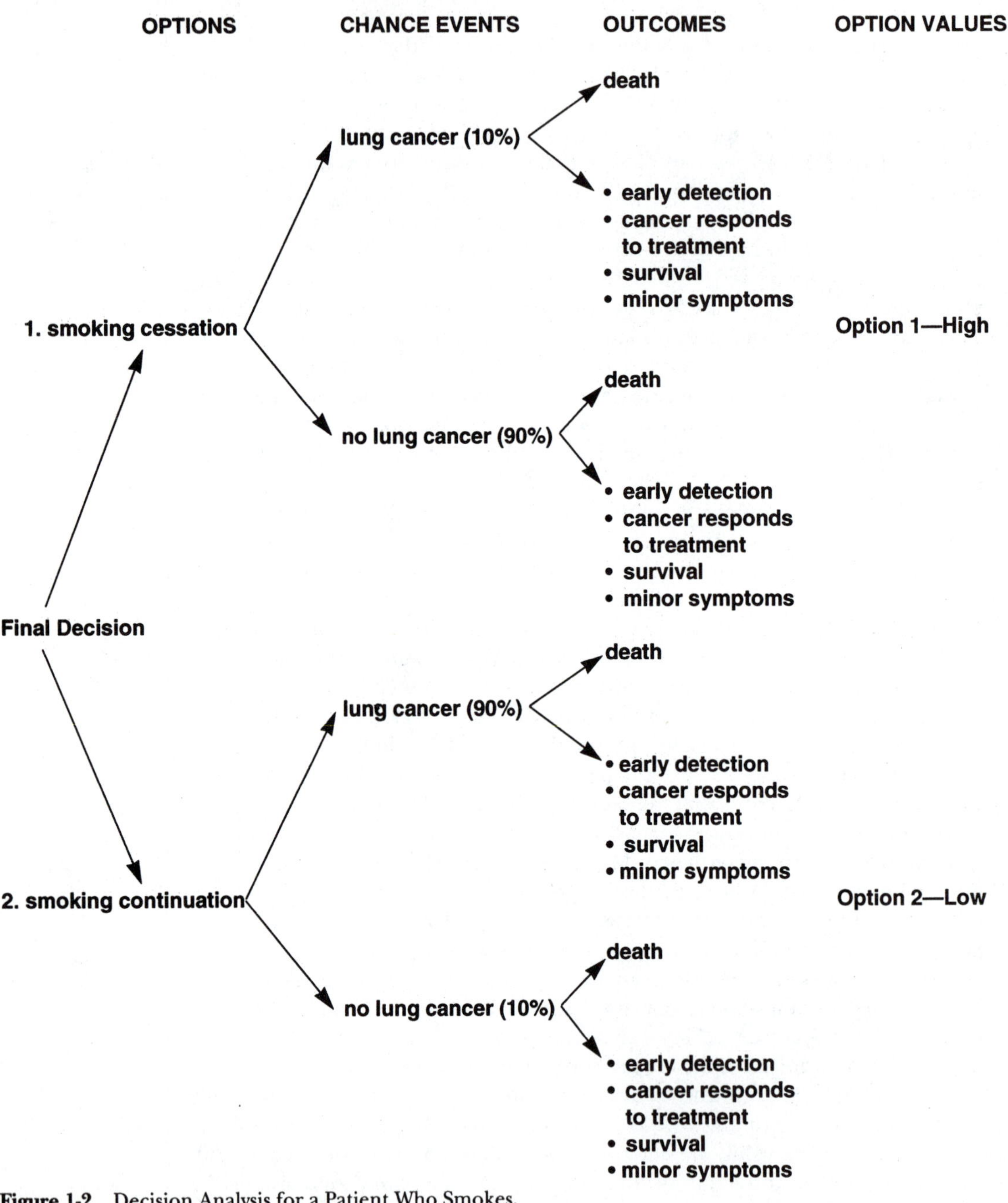

Figure 1-2 Decision Analysis for a Patient Who Smokes.

Thus, by focusing on information including alternatives that the patient needs and values to make a decision, the nurse may assist the patient in the decision-making process.

SCOPE OF PRACTICE MODEL

The Pennsylvania Nurse (1992) has proposed a model for determining the registered nurses' and licensed practical nurses' scopes of practice (Figure 1-3). The model consists of a series of steps involving questions requiring yes or no answers.

Scenario 1-5

Step 1 is to identify the act that is to be performed and see if it is addressed in your state nurse practice act. A new registered nurse graduate, David, has recently passed the national council licensing examination and wants to test the model. He asks if he is licensed to conduct a physical examination on a patient.

In *Step 2*, if the answer to whether this act is addressed by one's state nurse practice act is no, then the decision process is ended and the act is not within the nurse's scope of practice. If the answer is yes, then the individual needs to answer yes to the following questions outlined in *Steps 5* through *8*, proposed by *The Pennsylvania Nurse* (1992), before considering the act within his or her scope of practice:

Step 5 Do you possess the depth and breadth of knowledge to perform the act through your initial licensing program or continuing education?

Step 6. Do you possess clinical competence to perform the act safely?

Step 7. Is performance of the act within the accepted standard of care for similar situations by nurses with similar training and experience?

Step 8. Are you prepared to accept accountability for your actions in performing the act?

If the answer is no to any of the above questions, then the nurse should consider the act outside the limits of his or her scope of practice and end the decision-making process at that step.

Upon review of his copy of the nurse practice act, David finds that he is licensed to collect complete and ongoing data to determine nursing care needs (*Rules and Regulations,* 1983). He possesses both depth and breadth of knowledge to perform a physical assessment as he completed a physical assessment, course in his baccalaureate program and applied these skills throughout all of his clinical rotations. Thus, David feels that he possesses clinical competence to perform the act safely. Performance of this act is an accepted standard of care for all registered nurses on the medical-surgical unit where David currently works. David is willing to accept accountability for his actions in performing the act, which is reinforced in his hospital philosophy statement.

In *Step 3*, if one is unsure whether an act is explicitly covered by the nurse practice act, then that individual should determine if specialized education is needed as *Step 3*. If the answer is no to this question, then the act may be within the scope of practice of a registered nurse or licensed practical nurse. If the answer is yes, then the act may be within the scope of practice of the registered nurse or certified registered nurse practitioner.

To verify his thought processes thus far, as physical exam is not explicitly mentioned in the nurse practice act, David considers Step 3. Specialized education is not needed, thus performance of a physical exam is within the scope of practice of a registered nurse.

Step 4 involves determining if the act is consistent with scopes of practice as determined by standards of practice of a national nursing organization, conclusive data in nursing research literature, or policies and procedures established by the employing institution. If the answer is no to Step 4, then the decision-making process is ended. If the answer is yes, then questions 5 through 8 should be answered before making the final determination of whether the act is included within one's scope of practice.

To continue with reinforcement for the correct decision, David also reviews the questions in Step 4. He finds that performance of a physical exam as a part of the database in determining nursing care needs is addressed in the standards of practice and policies and procedures available on David's unit. These formal institutional documents reference the American Nurses' Association standards of practice.

SUMMARY

In this chapter, the process of decision making has been reviewed from several different perspectives. Steps in the traditional, creative, emergency, and multiattribute utility processes of decision making were discussed and scenarios or examples were included. The next group of decision-making processes discussed were more applicable to clinical situations, and involved the intuitive, diagnostic, and collaborative processes. Processes were reviewed for assisting patients with decision making and making decisions about one's scope of practice. By applying these models and processes to both administrative and clinical situations, readers should be able to gain a wider perspective of how decisions may be made during daily nursing activities. Through understanding the process, hopefully, readers will be able to improve decision-making skills.

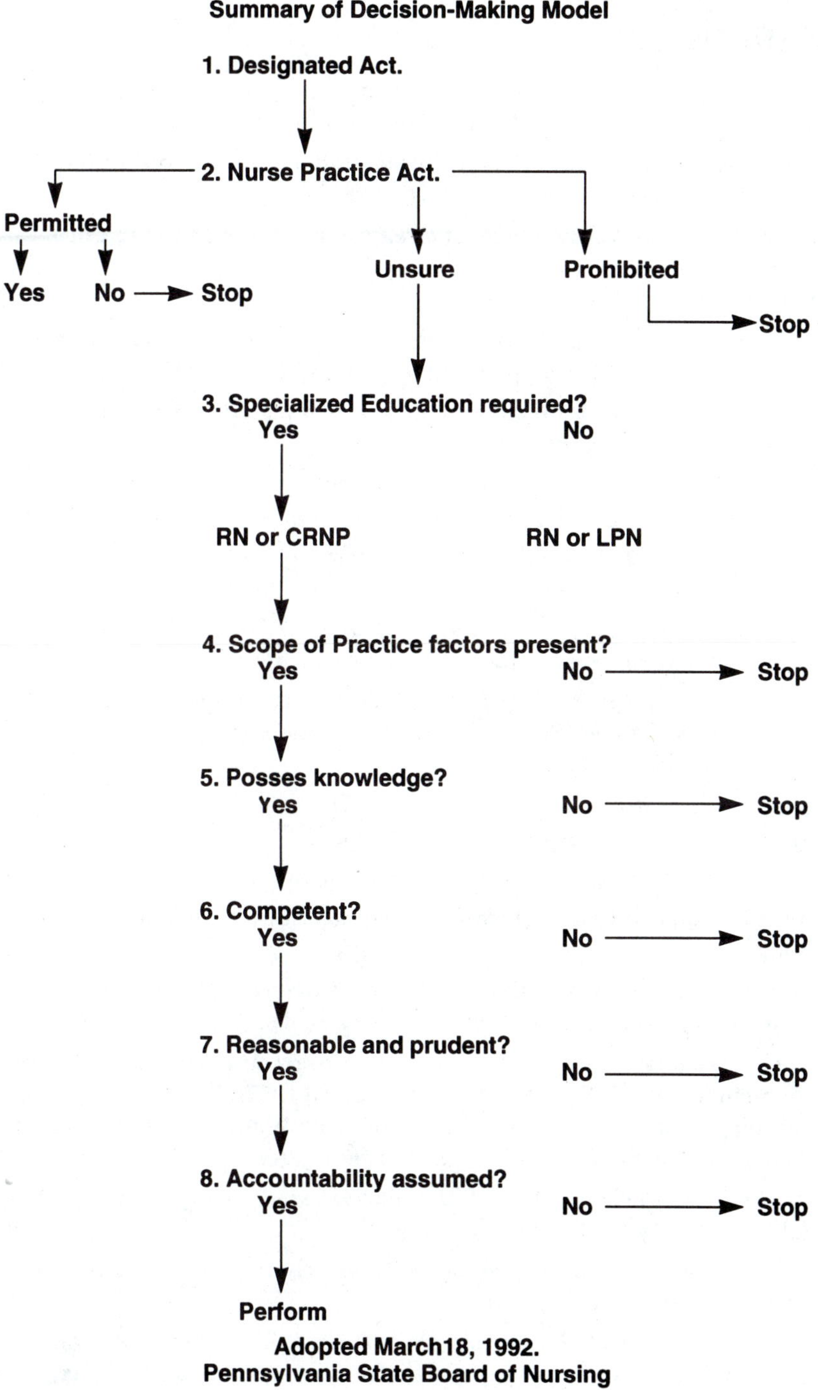

Figure 1-3 Decision-Making Model for Scope of Practice. *Source: Pennsylvania Nurses' Association, 1992,* Perspectives on Practice: State Board Adopts a Decision Tree, *The Pennsylvania Nurse, June (1992), 8. Reprinted with permission. Acknowledgments: Original model developed by the Kentucky State Board of Nursing. Other Contributors: Florida State Board of Nursing; North Carolina State Board of Nursing; South Dakota State Board of Nursing; The National Council of State Boards of Nursing, Inc.*

REFERENCES

Benner, P. (1984). *From novice to expert: Excellence and power in clinical nursing practice.* Menlo Park, CA: Addison-Wesley Publishing Co.

Benner, P., & Tanner, C.A. (1987). Clinical judgment: How expert nurses use intuition. *American Journal of Nursing, 87*(7), 23–31.

Carnevali, D.L. (1984). The diagnostic reasoning process. In D.L. Carnevali, P.H. Mitchell, N.F. Woods, & C.A. Tanner (Eds.), *Diagnostic Reasoning in Nursing.* Philadelphia: J.B. Lippincott Co.

Carnevali, D.L., & Thomas, M.D. (1993). *Diagnostic reasoning and treatment decision making in nursing.* Philadelphia: J.B. Lippincott Co.

Corcoran, S. (1986). Decision analysis: A step-by-step guide for making clinical decisions. *Nursing and Health Care, 7,* 149–154.

Corcoran, S. (1988). Toward operationalizing an advocacy role. *Journal of Professional Nursing, 4*(4), 242–248.

Dreyfus, H., & Dreyfus, S. (1985). *Mind over machine: The power of human intuition and expertise in the era of the computer.* New York: Free Press.

Elstein, A.S., Shulman, L.S., & Sprafka, S. (1978). *Medical problem solving: An analysis of clinical reasoning.* Cambridge, MA: Harvard University.

Gadow, S. (1980). Existential advocacy: Philosophical foundation of nursing. In S. Spikes and S. Gadow (Eds.), *Nursing: Images and ideals* (pp. 79–101). New York: Springer-Verlag.

Graham, S.M. (1987). Decision making: The multi-attribute model. *Nursing Management, 18*(3), 18–19.

Huber, G.P. (1980). *Managerial decision making.* Glenview, IL: Scott, Foresman and Co.

Marriner-Tomey, A. (1992). *Guide to nursing management.* Philadelphia: Mosby Year Book.

Pennsylvania Nurses' Association. (1992). Perspectives on practice: State Board adopts a decision tree. *The Pennsylvania Nurse, June,* 8.

Rules and regulations of the State Board of Nurse Examiners for Registered Nurses. (September 16, 1983). Pa. B. Doc. No. 83-1257. Commonwealth of Pennsylvania, Department of State, Bureau of Professional and Occupational Affairs, State Board of Nurse Examiners, Harrisburg, PA.

Sullivan, E.J., & Decker, P.J. (1992). *Effective management in nursing.* New York: Addison-Wesley Publishing Company.

Tappen, R. (1989). *Nursing leadership and management: Concepts and practice,* 2nd edition. Philadelphia: S.A. Davis Co.

Westfall, U.E., Tanner, C.A., Putzier, D., & Padrick, K.P. (1986). Activating clinical inferences: A component in diagnostic reasoning in nursing. *Nursing in Research & Health, 9,* 269–277.

Rebecca A. Patronis Jones

CHAPTER 2

Organizational Models

> There comes a moment when you have to stop revving up the car and shove it into gear.
>
> —*David Mahoney (cited in Safire and Safir, 1990).*

INTRODUCTION

A system may be defined as a group of regularly interacting, interdependent individuals who function under an organized set of doctrines, ideas, or principles usually intended to explain the arrangement of the whole organization (Webster's, 1977). Healthcare organizations may be viewed as systems with individuals and groups within them comprising subsystems. It is important to understand the interactions of individuals or groups both internal and external to the systems and subsystems.

Nursing as a science is ever evolving. Although some work has been done in the field, describing models for use in management and patient care decisions, much work is still needed. The organizational-level models presented here came from the field of academic administration. Because nursing organizations are moving toward shared governance models, it seems reasonable to assume that these models may have more relevance to nursing than those from other disciplines.

Chaffee (1983) describes the organizational-level decision-making process using three major components:

- The decision
- Underlying features
- Change features

The decision choice consists of the control an individual or group has over the decision that must be made, even though the need to make a decision may arise from forces beyond individual or group control. The actual decision choice has several underlying features:

- Values of the organization and individuals internal and external to the organization
- Alternative courses of action for consideration
- Premises or givens that guide the consideration of alternatives

The decision that is made results in change features, consisting of:

- Implementation of a procedure for carrying out the decision
- Results of changes both internal and external to the organization
- Feedback that acts as both output and input by providing information concerning the outcomes of the choice and guiding future choices

The entire process, based on the underlying features, decision, and consequences, is active and deliberate and involves interactions among people over time. Other key components of organizational-level decision making include:

- Consideration of key players
- Supporting organizational structure
- Goals
- Type of information available
- Timing allowed for the decision

Descriptions of the rational, political, collegial, bureaucratic, and garbage can organizational-level models are taken from Chaffee (1983) and Baldridge, Curtis, Ecker, and Riley (1977). Descriptions will be accompanied by an application of each model to nursing units that must make a decision on how to promote nurse-physician collaboration.

RATIONAL MODEL

The **rational model** consists of making deliberate decisions through a sequential analytical process (Table 2-1).

Underlying Features and Process

In the rational model, values are known beforehand and ranked into a single preference list consistent with some superordinate organizational goal for the decision. For the Medical Intensive Care Unit (MICU), the superordinate organizational goal is to deliver quality cost-effective care. Since nurse-physician collaboration is necessary to achieve this goal, all members of the unit highly value collaboration. The alternative courses of action constitute methods to achieve the goals implied by the values. For the MICU, these include implementation of a joint practice committee, primary nursing, or an integrated patient record. The premises for the rational model are common goals, congruent ideas and attitudes, understood

Table 2-1 **• Rational Model**

Underlying Features	*Values:* Individual consistent with organizational *Alternatives:* Methods to achieve goals *Premises:* Common goals Technical competence Sequential process
Process	*Decision:* Active, conscious, deliberate action of selecting the best alternative to achieve the goal
Change Features	*Implementation:* Carrying out details of the decision with unified support *Results:* Cause-effect *Feedback:* Understanding of causal relations Input for future decisions
Other Components	*Key Players:* Individuals or groups with similar analytic styles using any leadership style *Organizational Structure:* Hierarchical *Goals:* Common and unified *Information:* Known cause-effect relationship *Timing:* Adequate, lengthy

Adapted from E.E. Chaffee, Rational Decisionmaking in Higher Education *(Boulder, CO: National Center for Higher Education Management Systems, 1983), p. 12. Reprinted with permission.*

cause-effect relationships, technical competence, and a view of the decision-making process as sequential. For MICU nurses on this unit, everyone supports the organizational mission, values collaboration, and has used the sequential steps in the decision-making process to effectively solve numerous problems in the past. In rational decision making, the decision is an active, conscious, deliberate action and involves selecting the alternative that will maximize achievement of goals. Nurse members of the MICU staff review the alternatives at their next staff meeting. Members decide that primary nursing is too costly for the unit to implement. Process improvement teams have already been established, due to changes mandated by the Joint Commission on Quality Assurance standards. These teams focus primarily on joint practice issues. However, an integrated patient record does not exist for the unit. During the weekly nursing staff meeting, members review the pros and cons for each alternative and decide to implement integrated patient records.

Change Features

Implementation in the rational model is straightforward and involves carrying out the details of the decision with unified support of all organizational members. A timeline for implementation of the integrated patient record is developed for the

MICU staff, and it includes steps and responsible parties. The results are intended consequences in which causal relations are understood. Specific goals for each step are also included on the integrated patient record timeline. Feedback provides information useful for understanding the causal relations and nature of the problem; it is also applied analytically for use in future input in the rational model. Feedback on the MICU unit consists of reviewing the program timeline to assure that the goals are being achieved.

Other Components

The key players may be individuals or groups with similar analytical skills. For our MICU staff, several individuals live in the same neighborhoods and work the same shifts, thus, pairs of nurses sign up for various aspects of the project. Leadership roles may include players with any style in rational models. Maria is the informal organizational leader in the MICU unit and assumes overall responsibility for the project as project director. The organizational structure for rational organizations may tend to be hierarchical with distinct lines of authority. Appointment of project directors has been delegated by the nurse manager to the members of the MICU staff. The goals for the process are common and unified. Everyone in the MICU agrees that the integrated patient record is appropriate to the progress notes only in the MICU, so there is little debate over the steps required for implementation of the project. The information available implies that all cause and effect relationships concerning the problem are known in the rational model. The MICU staff reviewed the literature and chose their alternatives from recommendations made by several authors on implementing nurse-physician collaboration. Thus, the potential solutions were thought to represent all aspects of causes and effects in the search for a solution. In the rational model, the sequential process would occur in steps with adequate time to process each step. For our MICU staff, solutions are presented at one staff meeting, and reviewed and implemented over the course of several weeks. Due to the nature of the decision that must be made there is no specific time limit for the process in the MICU unit.

Pros and Cons

The disadvantages include unrealistic expectations concerning how the decision-making process works, excess amounts of time if all sequential steps are followed, and narrow interactions and thought processes that may become counterproductive. An advantage of the model involves unification of actors with the goals of the organization.

POLITICAL MODEL

The **political model** is often referred to as a conflict resolution model (Chaffee, 1983). This is due to participants' having multiple conflicting values and objectives determined by their self-interests. The political model may be a more appropriate model for interdepartmental decisions that occur within an organization (Table 2-2).

***Table 2-2* • Political Model**

Underlying Features	*Values:* Multiple, conflicting *Alternatives:* Generated based on individual self-interest *Premises:* Win-win situation Diversity of interests and power evenly dispersed Available forums
Process	*Decision:* Lobby majority
Change Features	*Implementation:* Verify and monitor details of decision *Results:* Organizational changes based on negotiated consequences of decision Lack of causal link to objectives *Feedback:* Change in constituent power bases
Other Components	*Key Players:* Statesmen with political skills *Organizational Structure:* Shared governance, fragmented loosely connected departments of professionals *Goals:* Organizational may not be supported by individual *Information:* Supplied by leading statesman *Timing:* Less than for models using group consensus

Adapted from E.E. Chaffee, Rational Decisionmaking in Higher Education *(Boulder, CO: National Center for Higher Education Management Systems, 1983), p. 19. Reprinted with permission.*

Underlying Features and Process

Values of members in a political model are multiple and based on individual self-interests. These values may or may not support superordinate goals of the organization. In the pediatric unit, some members value independent nursing practice, while others believe that nursing practice should be primarily physician dependent, that is, carrying out the physicians' orders. Alternatives are generated based on the participant's self-interest and may be determined largely by items that the stakeholder may gain or lose from the decision. Participants who generate alternatives usually are interested in the topic or are more likely to act as a statesman for the group (Baldridge et al., 1977). In the pediatric unit, John favors independent nursing practice and Sue favors nursing practice dependent solely on physician orders. Thus, John suggests individual clinical decision making by nursing while Sue proposes a joint practice committee to promote physician input concerning how nurses should carry out doctors' orders. Premises of the political model include the provision of a win-win situation, diversity and power dispersed enough among the participants to support coalitions, and available forums for negotiation and ratification of decisions.

The premises of the political model are evident in the pediatric unit situation. Whichever alternative is chosen, both John and Sue will be able to lobby staff members to support his or her chosen alternative and continue to practice nursing according to his or her views. The pediatric unit has weekly meetings, with adequate time for discussion of alternatives. The decision is made by lobbying a majority of the members to support one's individual position through negotiation and bargaining in the political model. John and Sue would each attempt to negotiate his or her chosen alternative with the other during the weekly staff meeting. Sue's alternative for a joint practice committee wins as John sees how he will be able to further promote individual clinical decision making by nurses through this committee.

Change Features

Implementation of the choice is characterized by verifying and monitoring details in the political model. Both John and Sue discuss the details of implementing a joint practice committee and set up the date, time, place, and invitation list for the first committee meeting. Results are characterized by changes in the organization based on the negotiated consequences of the choice. There may be little or no causal linkage between objectives and results. Although there were no formal objectives set by the pediatric unit in making this decision, the alternative of the joint practice committee does support organizational goals for delivery of quality, cost-effective care. Both John and Sue continue to practice nursing according to their perceptions. Feedback in the political model is characterized by changes in participants' strengths within the organization. In the pediatric unit, John gradually begins to sway members toward more independent nursing practices when they see that physicians on the joint practice committee are willing to delegate these activities to nurses.

Other Components

Key players in the political model would be statesmen who rally others to support a cause. Both John and Sue in this situation acted as statesmen by rallying others to their causes. This type of leader would have skills in political strategies, interpersonal dynamics, and coalition management (Baldridge et al., 1977).

The organizational structure fostering this model of decision making may consist of fragmented, professional groups with numerous individual values in a shared governance structure. It just so happens that the pediatric unit in this situation is a professional practice unit with two informal leaders, John and Sue, who set the pace for practices on the unit. The goals established for the decision by key players may or may not support organizational goals in the political model. In the pediatric unit situation, fortunately both alternatives would have supported organizational goals. Information available for making the decision would be supplied by the leading statesmen in the political model. Both John and Sue rallied for their alternatives by focusing on the advantages in the group meeting. Time required for the process in this model may be less than time required for models relying on group consensus. This was true of the pediatric unit, due to the two informal leaders with camps of pre-established supporters versus a group of individuals rallying for several different solutions.

Pros and Cons

The political model does not always foster support of organizational goals. Results are unpredictable and may not be linked to objectives or ultimately serve the interests of any parties. Solutions generated may be limited and narrowed to the lobbyer's view point (Baldridge et al., 1977). Advantages of the model consist of drawing attention to critical interests within an organization that might not otherwise be recognized. The model may be more efficient than others requiring group consensus, because less time is spent on reaching a decision and decisions can be implemented in spite of differences among the participants in the organization. This model may also foster creative solutions with majority support.

COLLEGIAL MODEL

The **collegial model** of decision making involves the full participation of a community of peers and has been named after the academic community (Table 2-3).

Table 2-3 • **Collegial Model**

Underlying Features	*Values:* Shared responsibility for organizational goals *Alternatives:* Generated based on professional back ground and interests of participants *Premises:* Group consensus Mutual respect Ample time
Process	*Decision:* Support general welfare
Change Features	*Implementation:* By effected individuals with widespread commitment *Results:* Smooth organizational change *Feedback:* Through participant observation and priorities
Other Components	*Key Players:* Professionals *Organizational Structure:* Shared governance *Goals:* Organizational, supported through shared responsibility *Information:* Diverse, specialized *Timing:* Lengthy, numerous group meetings

Adapted from E.E. Chaffee, Rational Decisionmaking in Higher Education *(Boulder, CO: National Center for Higher Education Management Systems, 1983), p. 17. Reprinted with permission.*

Underlying Features and Process

In the collegial model, shared responsibility, based on shared organizational goals and processes, is valued. In the rehabilitation unit, all nursing staff highly value shared decision making. Many forums exist where staff are allowed to participate in decisions to support goals for the delivery of nursing care that assists the patient to achieve his optimum level of wellness. Alternatives are determined by the backgrounds and interest of the participants and through interaction and iteration. Thus, a wide range of alternatives is likely to be produced. In the rehabilitation unit, a joint practice committee, computer support, role clarification and team building sessions, clinical care maps, and luncheon are suggested as alternatives. The collegial nature of this unit has definitely produced more alternatives than our previous two models. The guiding premise for choices in collegial models is group consensus with mutual respect for individuals. Ample time and opportunity must also be available for the process. Participants are willing to take the time to defend, explain, receive new information, and be open to change their minds throughout time-consuming meetings and discussion. In the rehabilitation unit, each staff member who proposed an alternative is given time to describe his or her alternative and state the advantages and disadvantages. Three staff meetings are planned to hear debates on all alternatives before a vote is made to choose an alternative. The decision is made based on alternatives generated that satisfy most, if not all, participants. Compromises are made for the general welfare. When all members of the rehabilitation unit voted, the alternatives received the following ranking:

1. Computer support
2. Clinical care maps
3. Joint practice committee
4. Luncheon
5. Role clarification and team building sessions

The majority of members voted for computer support and clinical care maps.

Change Features

The decision is implemented by the delegated or affected individuals with widespread commitment in a collegial model. Members decided that computer support might facilitate the implementation of clinical care maps as the next project for the unit. The member who proposed computer support is nominated as the project director and several rehabilitation unit staff members volunteer to serve on the steering committee. Results are characterized by organizational change with smooth transitions. The project coordinator and steering committee review and select computer hardware and software and set up an inservice program for all staff members, with total implementation of the project lasting for six months. Feedback is informal and depends on the participants' observations and priorities in collegial models. Issues and problems with the computer support are placed on the agenda at subsequent staff meetings. Overall, the majority of staff members are pleased with the work of the steering committee.

Other Components

Key players are individuals and groups within the organization who possess professional authority in collegial models. The member who proposed the computer support alternative and was nominated as the project coordinator was completing a doctoral degree in nursing informatics. Leadership is assumed by the individual who is considered a first among equals with the ability to persuade and negotiate with experts in the collegial model. This type of leader facilitates and allows for consensus decisions. This leadership type is evident in the staff member who proposed the winning alternative. Collegial decision making is unlikely to occur in a bureaucratic or autocratic organizational structure, but may be fostered by a shared governance organizational structure. The rehabilitation unit in this situation has implemented a shared governance organizational structure with all decision making vested in committees. Organizational goals are usually supported through shared responsibility in the collegial model. This occurred when several members volunteered for the task force in the rehabilitation unit.

Information available for the decision process is likely to be diverse and specialized in the collegial model. The information available for the rehabilitation unit came from staff nurses with various interests, as evidenced by the nature of the alternatives suggested. In a collegial model, the process requires large amounts of participant time for meeting and discussion; however, members tend to maintain higher levels of job satisfaction than in other types of organizational decision-making models.

Pros and Cons

Although the rehabilitation unit took longer to review alternatives than the members of previous models discussed, the final implementation of the chosen alternative proceeded in a smooth and rapid manner.

BUREAUCRATIC MODEL

The **bureaucratic model** is probably the model most commonly applied to healthcare organizations. The model consists of deciding by structured interaction patterns and standard operating procedures (Table 2-4) that are dictated by the organization's hierarchical structure (Chaffee, 1983). Operational efficiency is valued in this model of decision making.

Underlying Features and Process

On the surgical unit, operational efficiency is highly valued, as patients must be admitted, receive preoperative workups and surgical procedures, and recover sufficiently for a timely discharge to produce revenue from the Diagnostic Related Grouping–based prospective payment system. The alternatives are generated from the history of the institution and are based on traditions in a bureaucratic model. The number of alternatives generated are usually small. There is little search for creative alternatives outside the routine. In the surgical unit, alternatives generated consist of a joint practice committee and joint patient care record review, since

Table 2-4 • Bureaucratic Model

Underlying Features	*Values:* Operational efficiency
	Alternatives: Based on history, tradition
	Premises: Historical norms Operating routines
Process	*Decision:* Based on organizational outputs or goals
Change Features	*Implementation:* Through routines determined by policy and procedure Widespread commitment
	Results: Predictable from organizational structure
	Feedback: Routine Slight adaptation to operations
Other Components	*Key Players:* Dictated by organizational structure
	Organizational Structure: Hierarchical bureaucracy
	Goals: Organizational supported by history
	Information: Historical, tradition, norms
	Timing: Depends on efficiency of operation

Adapted from E.E. Chaffee, Rational Decisionmaking in Higher Education *(Boulder, CO: National Center for Higher Education Management Systems, 1983), p. 22. Reprinted with permission.*

other units have implemented these strategies effectively to promote nurse-physician collaboration. The underlying premise for making a decision is the historical norm that it worked before and the results are predictable. Premises also include the existence of standard operating routines, the ability to adapt routines slightly to the current situation, and a system for initiating routines as the need arises. The choice of alternatives is made based on an identification of the outputs of the procedure. The focus is more on the procedure itself as opposed to the decision. The surgical unit reviews the two alternatives at the next monthly staff meeting. A joint patient care record review is already being conducted at the surgical department Quality Assessment and Improvement (QA&I) committee by nurses and physicians to identify potential process problems. Thus, the joint patient care record review alternative is suggested by the nurse manager and chosen by the staff based on her recommendation. The QA&I procedure can be slightly adapted to review clinical problems of interest to both nurses and physicians. Surgical staff nurses feel confident that since other units have implemented this strategy, they will have even higher levels of success because the forum and procedure already exist on their unit.

Change Features

In the bureaucratic model, the decision is implemented through a series of routines determined by organizational policies and procedures. On the surgical unit, the record review procedure of the QA&I committee is adapted by the staff nurse member to accommodate joint clinical problems. Results are predictable from the organization's structure and rules of interaction as organizations are slow to change in bureaucratic models. For the surgical unit, the joint record review process proceeds smoothly. However, little collaboration occurs. The physician takes care of medical problems and the nurse attends to nursing problems, with little collaboration on patient problems that might require the expertise of both participants. Feedback is informal and consists of repetition of routines and processes with slight adaptations to the current situation in bureaucratic models. When the nurse manager reviews the minutes of the surgical department's QA&I committee, she reports at the next nursing staff meeting that the decision-making process has been a success and nurse-physician collaboration has been promoted. Joint record review is occurring according to procedures outlined. She is unaware of the lack of collaboration on joint problems.

Other Components

Key players in the model would consist of persons with direct responsibility, authority, and accountability for whatever system or subsystem of the organization was responsible for the routine or process selected in the decision. The leader would be the top individual in the organizational hierarchy, even though leaders under him or her may be delegated responsibility for implementing the decision. The leader is viewed as a hero with expert rational decision-making skills by subordinates. In our surgical unit example, the nurse manager is viewed as the formal and informal leader with expert skills, although she has delegated responsibility for attending the QA&I committee to a staff nurse. The nurse manager still maintains ultimate responsibility for assuring that the procedures are occurring according to plan.

The organizational structure would be a hierarchical bureaucracy that may be centralized or decentralized in a bureaucratic model. Our surgical unit example is organized as a centralized bureaucracy. Organizational goals would be supported through the selection of decisions based on history that would foster those goals in this model. The surgical unit chose strategies that had proven effective over time, thus goal accomplishment was easily attained. The information available for making the decision would consist of formal historical documents as well as traditions and norms in a bureaucratic model. The surgical unit definitely based its decision on history and norms within the institution. Timing for the decision-making process in this model would be largely determined by how efficiently the organization operated. For the surgical unit, since decisions are largely made by the nurse manager with little staff nurse input, the unit tends to function very efficiently.

Pros and Cons

There are probably more disadvantages than advantages for this model. The model does not recognize informal channels of communication or power. Alternatives generated are very limited and depend on the historical success of the organization. Some organizations do not have formal channels of communication, policies, procedures, or routines that have fostered adequate decision making in the past. Thus, the organization may tend to flounder in its inefficient state. The model also ignores any political struggles or informal struggles for control and power. The case example presented does not exemplify any of these disadvantages. Advantages would include arousal of little conflict throughout the process due to understood norms and routines. If the organization had a history of efficient operation, then chances are current decisions would also be made and implemented efficiently.

GARBAGE CAN MODEL

This model draws its name from a classic article written by Cohen and March (1974) in which organizations were described as "collections of choices looking for problems, issues and feelings looking for decision situations in which they might be aired, solutions looking for issues to which they might be the answer, and decision makers looking for work" (Cohen and March, 1974, p. 85). The **garbage can model** (Table 2-5) is based on deciding by accident.

Underlying Features and Process

The values of the actors are diffuse and multiple, and come into play as they present opportunities for making a choice among alternatives. On the psychiatric unit, some members value collaborative practice, some quality care, and some perceive the cost of care as more important. Alternatives for the decision are generated from lists of floating problems and solutions with no common goal or criteria that may be plucked from a garbage can. The psychiatric unit staff have read in the latest nursing journals that product lines and case managed care are the wave of the future. In

Table 2-5 • Garbage Can Model

Underlying Features	*Values:* Diffuse, multiple opportunities
	Alternatives: Floating problems and solutions
	Premises: Pure accident
Process	*Decision:* Unplanned, coincidental
Change Features	*Implementation:* Incidental with no preplanning
	Results: Occur by chance May repeat errors
	Feedback: New problems, solutions, and actors
Other Components	*Key Players:* Actors perceiving opportunity Weak leaders who negotiate
	Organizational Structure: Organized anarchy, adhocracy, matrix
	Goals: Organizational supported by chance
	Information: Dependent on key player creativity
	Timing: Continuous, accidental

Adapted from M.D. Cohen and J.G. March, Leadership and Ambiguity: The American College President *(New York: McGraw-Hill Book Company, 1974).*

garbage can models, the guiding premise for the choice is pure accident, governed by chaotic actions of the participants with no consideration of causal relations. The choice of alternatives is made by coincidence with no major purpose in mind. Although the alternatives generated by the psychiatric unit have not been specifically cited as strategies for improving nurse-physician collaboration, staff members feel that it is logical to assume that these new care delivery strategies will naturally promote collaboration as well.

In garbage can models, decisions are made by individuals, allowed to be products of unplanned activity, or allowed to happen as opposed to being decided. At the next staff meeting, the nurse manager discusses the need to come up with a strategy to promote nurse-physician collaboration. Jim shares his readings on the new wave nursing delivery models, product lines and case managed care. No decision is reached, but after the meeting Erika decides that the majority of the group favored product lines and writes the decision up in the minutes.

Change Features

In garbage can models, the decision is implemented incidentally with no plan or routine. Jim reads the minutes and organizes a task force to implement product lines with the acute psychiatric patient representing one line, the eating disorders patient a second line, and geriatric mental health patient a third line. Results are incidental and may tend to be repetitions of errors committed in the past. In organizing the unit to accommodate the product lines, Jim turns to the nurse manager for more staff. He forgot why they decided to change the geographic location of patients in the past to accommodate shortages of psychiatric technicians for patients requiring closer supervision. The decision choice may or may not solve the problem. No specific evidence of increased nurse-physician collaboration is noted on the geriatric mental health patient wing, which has been implemented as a product line. Feedback is characterized by new problems, solutions, and actors arriving on the scene. The nurse shortage is placed on the next nursing staff meeting agenda for resolution.

Other Components

Key players involved in this model would be actors that may perceive an opportunity to focus attention on their values by proffering potential solutions. Jim was definitely a key player in the psychiatric unit by advocating product lines as a solution to promote nurse-physician collaboration. The leadership in this model is weak and tends to negotiate decisions among the concerned parties. This definitely describes the nurse manager for the psychiatric unit.

The organizational structure would probably be an organized anarchy, adhocracy, or matrix as opposed to a bureaucratic structure. The structure would be characterized by little central coordination or control. The psychiatric unit is an adhocracy with little centralized control and decentralized decision making. If the decisions made supported the general organizational goals, it would be due to chance. In the psychiatric unit situation, the chosen alternative did not support any unit or decision goals. In the garbage can model, the information available for making the decision depends on the actors' ability to creatively generate lists of problems with solutions that may fit the current situation. Jim, in an example, recommended two creative solutions, but the solution list was not exhaustive in terms of solving the problem.

The timing for the entire decision-making process would occur by accident with no preplanned timeline for each step. On the psychiatric unit, there was no preplanned time for the decision-making process, and in reality the unit probably could have used another meeting to consider the alternatives more carefully. The decision may be implemented in time to save the organization from unfavorable consequences. The timeframe may be characterized by streams of free-floating problems, decisions, and decision makers that rearrange themselves over time, causing the timeframe to be continuous versus limited to one situation or problem (Cohen and March, 1974). This description definitely fits the psychiatric unit, with the alternatives chosen to solve one situation turning into a new situation requiring further decision making.

Pros and Cons

Disadvantages and advantages are relatively equal for this model. A major disadvantage is the potential to repeat errors committed in the past by having no overall goal or criteria for evaluating the alternatives generated. A major advantage for use of the model is that creative alternatives may be generated by allowing free-flowing lists of problems and solutions to be considered.

CYBERNETIC MODEL

Oftentimes programs are implemented within nursing departments that may require evaluation. These programs may be administrative, such as a new performance evaluation system or a different governance structure. Clinical program examples might include case management for congestive heart failure or education of the newly diagnosed diabetic patient. Veney and Kaluzny (1991) have suggested a **cybernetic model** for the evaluation of health care programs. In the cybernetic model, decisions are based on information about the problem that the program has been designed to address and information about the effect of the program on the problem (Veney and Kaluzny, 1991). This information is provided through continuous feedback so that program evaluation and modifications may be completed on an ongoing basis. Thus, the cybernetic model may be applied at any time during a program timeline, which includes three phases:

- Needs assessment
- Implementation
- Results assessment

Veney and Kaluzny (1991) define cybernetic decision making as control based on communication of information or feedback within a system. The system includes inputs, processes, and outputs or desired goals. Thus, feedback is used to modify inputs or processes whenever expected outcomes are not attained.

The cybernetic model for program evaluation (Table 2-6) may be applied through a series of sequential steps (Veney and Kaluzny, 1991), which are explored from the beginning to the end of a program timeline for the initiation of a new program.

Table 2-6 • Cybernetic Model

Program Phase I:	**Needs Assessment**
Step 1.	Determine the desired outputs or goals for the program.
Step 2.	Determine the nature of the problem and the level of goal accomplishment expected.
Step 3.	Determine program strategies.
Step 4.	Specify goal accomplishment criteria.
Step 5.	Construct a causal chain for program processes and desired outcomes.
Program Phase II: Program Implementation	
Step 6.	Determine if the program is in place and proceeding according to the original time plan.
Program Phase III: Results Assessment	
Step 7.	Determine if the program objectives were met.
Step 8.	Determine if program outputs are sufficient to justify costs.
Step 9.	Determine long-term impact on improvement in health and quality of life.

Adapted from J.E. Veney and A.D. Kaluzny, Evaluation and Decision Making for Health Services *(Ann Arbor, MI: Health Administration Press, 1991).*

Phase I

During the first stage of program implementation, a needs assessment is conducted. Goals for the program are determined as *Step 1* in this phase. In a case example, nursing staff at a 600-bed medical center voiced concerns over their present nursing documentation system as time consuming, duplicative, and in non-compliance with the Joint Commission standards. A task force of nurses from the Clinical Practice committee were called together to determine revisions needed for the system and to develop goals for the documentation system revision process. The committee developed four goals for the revision process:

1. To provide a single recommended documentation system that would decrease repetition and streamline the process
2. To provide an integrated consistent system that incorporated daily care planning
3. To meet standards defined by professional and regulating agencies
4. To posture the department for computerization in the future

Step 2 involves determining the nature of the problem that the program will address and the level of accomplishment for the goals which might actually be reached. In this case example, the nature of the problem was further defined by conducting a literature search to determine what aspects of a nursing documentation system should be included in a study. The committee chose four variables: nurse satisfaction with the documentation system, physician satisfaction with the documentation system, length and content of the documentation entries, and compliance and quality of the documentation for standards addressing each aspect of the nursing process. A study to determine baseline levels for the four variables was conducted. Specific levels of improvement were not established for each baseline variable; however, some improvement was expected for all variables.

Step 3 involves determining program strategies. For the case example, program strategies involved hiring a nursing consultant to further assist with specific revisions needed to the forms used to document each aspect of the nursing process. Then a task force for each nursing specialty area was called together under the direction of a project coordinator to review baseline data, system goals, and the consultant's report. The task forces decided to revise the history and physical assessment form, flowsheet, and nurse's progress note form, and adopt the focus charting format for progress notes as strategies to address the goals for the documentation system.

Step 4 is specifying criteria to assess goal accomplishment. *Step 5* is to construct a causal chain that describes the program process for influencing the desired outcome. The causal chain would consist of a diagram, including program interventions that lead to specific outcomes. This step helps to assure a logical causal link between program processes and desired outcomes. A timeline for the development, printing, inservicing, and implementation of the new forms was developed by the project director. Program goals and data for the baseline variables were linked to each element of the timeline so that a causal chain could be constructed and accomplishment of goals more easily evaluated in Phase III of the program evaluation process.

Phase II

The second stage of a program timeline involves program implementation. During this stage, *Step 6,* determining if the program is in place and proceeding according to the original time plan, is completed. Cybernetic decision making at this step would include checking to see if all resources or inputs needed to conduct the program were available, determining if pre-established program processes were being implemented, and assessing if outputs were being produced by the program. In the case example, program implementation consisted of oversight of the program by the director of nursing education and monthly meetings for the director of education, project director, and involved participants to keep the project moving according to the projected timeline. Problem areas were addressed along the way and changes made to the forms, policies and procedures, inservices, and pilot plans and times as needed.

Phase III

The last stage of a program timeline involves results assessment, which is aimed at determining the effectiveness, efficiency, and impact of the program. Effectiveness is determined in *Step 7* by assessing if the program objectives have been met. This was an easy step for the participants in this case example, as the goals for the revision process were already directly linked to specific interventions on the timeline and baseline data had been collected. Post-implementation data were collected from all pilot units on nurse and physician satisfaction, length and content of documentation entries, and compliance and quality of documentation for standards addressing each aspect of the nursing process. Revised forms were reviewed for repetition and redundancy in documenting various aspects of the nursing process

(Goal 1), care planning was incorporated into daily activities with the use of focus charting (Goal 2), data for standards indicated improvement in documenting all aspects of the nursing process (Goal 3), and the final form format could be adapted to individual computer screens when the nursing department decided to automate patient records (Goal 4). Additionally, satisfaction levels with the documentation system had improved for both nurses and physicians. The length of time spent on documentation was not significantly different. However, nurses felt that since some of the new forms were being completed at the patient's bedside, more time was being spent to involve the patient and family in the plan of care.

Efficiency is determined in *Step 8* by assessing if the program outputs are sufficient to justify the costs. When the costs for the consultant, project director, participants' time, and form duplication were compared to achievement of objectives, improvement in staff satisfaction, compliance, and quality of standards for documentation, and time available to spend involving the patient and his or her family in the care process, these nonmonetary benefits outweighed the costs. Staff felt that the new documentation system was definitely more efficient when reviewing the cost-to-benefit ratio.

In *Step 9,* long-term impact is assessed on improvements in administrative processes or health and quality of life for clinical programs designed to improve patient outcomes. Veney and Kaluzny (1991) admit that this step may be better accomplished by historians and academicians than program evaluators. In our case example, the nursing documentation system is part of a critical objective for the department that is reviewed annually during the strategic planning process. Thus, new documentation system problems may arise and precipitate reimplementation of the cybernetic model.

SUMMARY

Organizational-level decision-making processes using rational, political, collegial, bureaucratic, garbage can, and cybernetic models have been reviewed. A model for program evaluation was presented. Although individuals may follow the same processes and models that we described in Chapter 1, the organizational models help one to better understand how individuals might behave collectively within the organization. Case examples were included to illustrate how these models may be used to describe the decision-making process in daily nursing situations. Now, the reader has a larger inventory of processes to choose from for the next decision that he or she must make.

REFERENCES

Baldridge, J.V., Curtis, D.V., Ecker, G.P., & Riley, G.L. (1977). Alternative models of governance in higher education. In J.V. Baldridge & T.E. Deal (Eds.), *Governing academic organizations.* Berkeley, CA: McCutchan.

Chaffee, E.E. (1983). *Rational decisionmaking in higher education.* Boulder, CO: National Center for Higher Education Management Systems.

Cohen, M.D., & March, J.G. (1974). *Leadership and ambiguity: The American college president.* New York: McGraw-Hill Book Company.

Safire, W., & Safir, L. (1990). *Leadership.* New York: Simon & Schuster, Inc.

Veney, J.E., & Kaluzny, A.D. (1991). *Evaluation and decision making for health services.* Ann Arbor, MI: Health Administration Press.

Webster's New Collegiate Dictionary. (1977). Springfield, MA: G. & C. Merriam Co.

Sharon E. Beck

CHAPTER 3

Strategies

Know when to hold them, when to fold them, know when to walk away and know when to run.
—*The Gambler* (Schlitz, 1978)

INTRODUCTION

Nurses at all levels of practice find that there is an ongoing need to make decisions. Some of these decisions are made so automatically that the nurse is unaware that a decision-making process was used, or in some cases that a decision was even made. Usually it is when a decision is difficult or perplexing that the nurse becomes aware that she is in the process of making a decision. In the rapid pace of the hospital environment, on-the-spot crisis decision making is often used. This involves quickly assessing the situation, and based on experience, making and acting on a rapid decision. This is in contrast to more long-range decisions that require planning, and in many cases political savvy. Rowland and Rowland (1992) categorize these decisions into "considered decisions, operational decisions, swallow-hard decisions and ten-second decisions" (p. 57–58). The **considered decisions** are the complicated decisions that require a great deal of thought. The nurse may need to use more than one strategy to make this decision and often needs to get outside input. The **operational decisions** are those that are made daily and are usually based on knowledge of the situation and experience. The **swallow-hard decisions** are those that are unpleasant and hard to make, while the **ten-second decisions** are the ones that are made very quickly as a part of daily operations.

Russo and Schoemaker (1989) describe the key elements of all decision making: framing, gathering intelligence, coming to conclusions, and learning or failing to learn from feedback. **Framing** is defined as structuring the question. This also includes thinking about how others look at the question. **Gathering intelligence** seeks to estimate what is known and what is not known. Seeking all available information is important. **Coming to conclusions** forces the decisionmaker to weigh all aspects. Looking back and **evaluating the results** of the decision is the last step, an important step because it helps one to see whether the decision and/or the process was a good one. It is a way of learning from past experiences.

According to Stevens (1985), decision-making strategies can be divided into quantitative approaches and psychological approaches. The **quantitative approach,** according to Stevens, examines rational laws and rules and uses mathematical techniques, whereas the **psychological approach** concentrates on human behavior and the processes of the decisionmaker.

Quantitative approaches use such tools as computer programs, decision-making trees, and Gantt charts. According to Stevens, the following criteria need to be met for a decision to be made using a quantitative method:

- The problem must be stated in quantitative terms
- Relations among all significant variables must allow mathematical manipulations
- Results of actions must be predictable and measurable (p. 178)

Stevens further discusses the notion that **reductionism,** or a breaking down to simple parts, must be the focus, rather than looking at the whole. The objective is to come to a decision that offers the least possible risk.

The psychological approach, according to Stevens (1985), looks more at the intentions and personality of the decisionmaker, while the quantitative approach attempts to be more objective. Mintzberg (1976) offers three managerial strategies that are psychological in nature. The **entrepreneurial strategy** focuses on the manager's search for new opportunities within each decision-making area. This is a proactive approach. In the **adaptive approach,** the manager looks for remedial actions or ways in which to reduce conflict. This is a reactive approach. The third approach is a **planning approach.** This approach can use quantitative measures as well, and it involves setting goals and having a systematic plan for reaching the goals.

This chapter will examine a variety of strategies and will offer examples, advantages, and disadvantages for each.

QUANTITATIVE STRATEGIES

According to Marriner-Tomey (1992), quantitative strategies are useful for systematic approaches that can be expressed mathematically. It encourages organized thinking and allows for any number of variables to be considered. Marriner-Tomey also points out that the mathematical expressions are based on assumptions that if not true, render the tool useless.

Decision Tree

A **decision tree** is "a graphical model that displays the sequence of decision and the events that comprise a sequential decision situation" (Huber, 1980, p. 118). It is used when there are at least two possible alternatives. Standard symbols are used in the diagram. A square represents a decision node, and a round symbol represents a possible outcome or a state of nature. The lines connecting the symbols indicate alternatives (Strasen, 1987). Together it resembles a tree, thus its name.

Decision trees consist of the following steps:

- List the alternatives
- List events that might possibly occur
- Arrange choices in chronological order
- Decide the payoff from each choice
- Decide what the possibility is for the event to occur (Anderson, 1984)

Decision trees are useful in that they allow a person to go through the process of looking at alternatives and deciding, based on established goals, what is absolutely necessary and what is nice to have, but not necessary. The drawback is that the decision tree is only as good as the thought process that goes into it: Advantages or disadvantages have the potential to be left out accidentally or not considered; weights that are given to the options may not be realistic. Scenario 3-1 represents the use of a decision tree.

Scenario 3-1

A nurse has been working for five years. She believes it may be time to go back to school to get a masters degree in nursing in order to be eligible for promotion. She decides that she has three options: go to school full time, go to school part-time, or do not go to school at all this year. (See Figure 3-1.)

Option 1

If she goes to school full time she can finish quickly. She will, however, have to pay for her own tuition, and she will not necessarily have a job when she graduates. However, because of her experience and increased education, she could possibly obtain a better job then she has now.

Option 2

If she goes to school part-time, she will have a job and will receive some tuition assistance. It will, however, take her more time to complete the program, and she will have to give up her time for herself, friends and family.

Option 3

If she chooses to not go to school at all, she will have more free time, but she may not get promoted and may not feel fulfilled.

Gantt Charts

A **Gantt chart,** according to Strasen (1987), is a "project-or-program-scheduling technique that outlines the work and time relationships of steps to meet a specific goal" (p. 251). It is constructed on two axes. On the vertical axis, the activities or steps are identified, while the horizontal axis is used to identify the timeframes, which may be minutes, hours, days, weeks, months, years, or even decades, depending on the length of the project. When the task is complete, a line is drawn through the timeframe. These charts can be done very simply or can be quite complex,

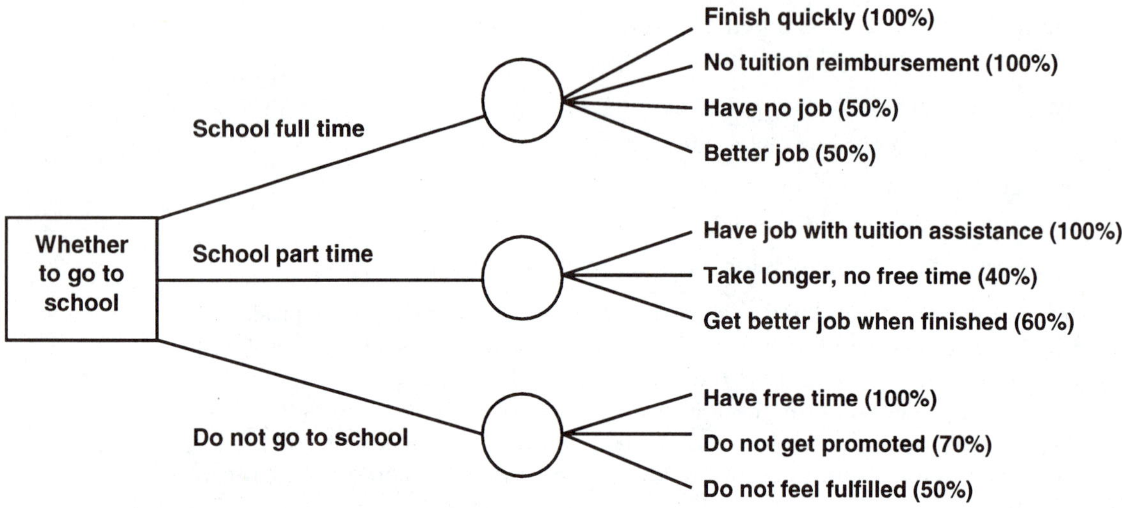

KEY Numbers represent percentage of possibility that event will occur

Figure 3-1 Decision Tree for Choosing Whether to Go Back to School.

based on the identified need or project. Gantt charts can be very useful for the manager in identifying the needed steps to be taken, evaluating the project, as well as being able to see whether the project is staying on track and meeting the timetable established. It has the advantage of being very easy to read. Timetables need to be set realistically or they are not useful. The disadvantage to using this strategy is that it is limited to simple projects. Scenario 3-2 shows the use of a Ganntt chart.

PERT Charts

PERT stands for Program Evaluation and Review Techniques. These charts were developed in the 1950s by the Navy to keep track of the multitude of tasks in the Polaris project (Strasen, 1987). The PERT chart is more complicated than the Gantt chart. It is, according to Marriner-Tomey (1992), a "network system model for planning and control under certain conditions" (p. 31). It is used to identify important activities, put them in a sequence, and assign them timeframes that can be monitored. Because in complex projects certain tasks must be completed before others, and subtasks may need to be completed first, this chart allows tracking of these events. As time is crucial to certain projects, projected timeframes are utilized. To understand how to construct a PERT chart, it is necessary to understand the critical parts:

- **Activities** describe the action steps to be taken between individual events
- **Events** are the points in which the activities are completed
- **Float** is the amount of extra time that could occur in an activity—it is possible that if there is no float time, the activity could be completed in a shorter period of time
- A **predecessor event** is one that must precede another event

Scenario 3-2

A nurse manager has agreed to have her unit pilot a new care delivery system on her unit within six months. The Gantt chart can be used to plan the progression of the project.

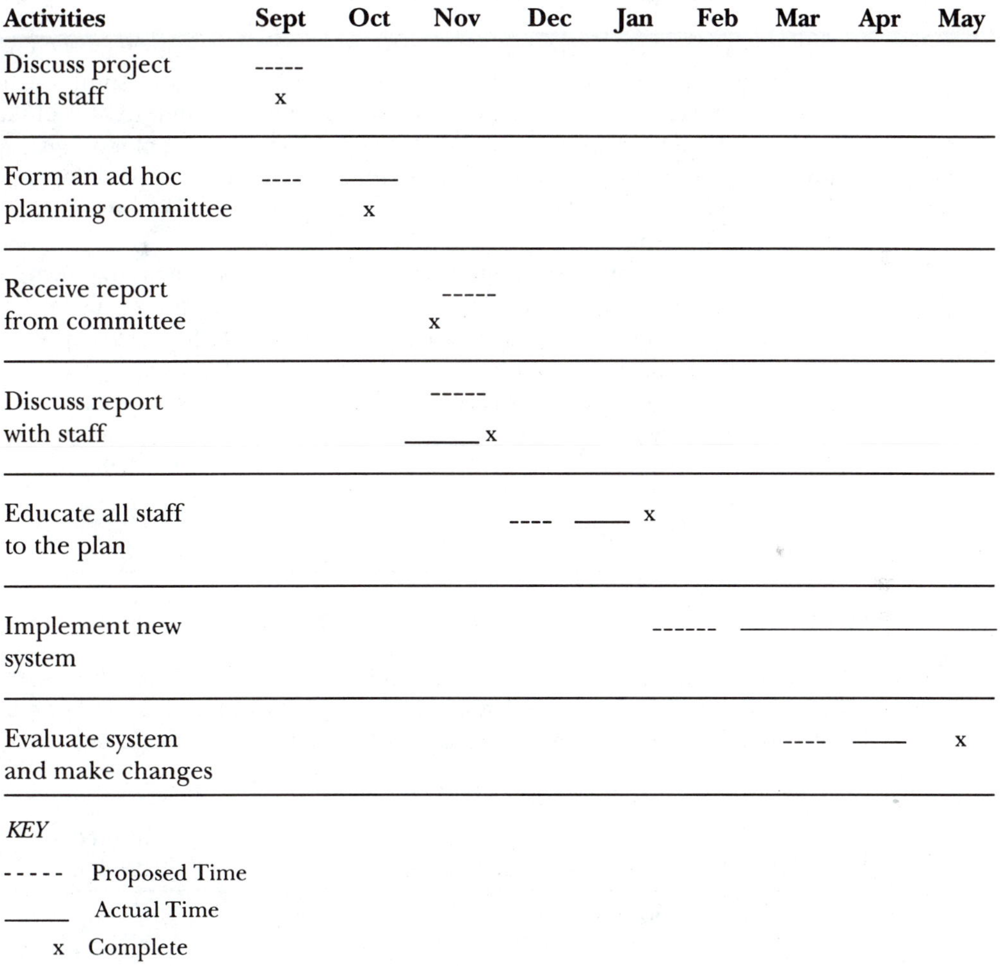

Activities	Sept	Oct	Nov	Dec	Jan	Feb	Mar	Apr	May
Discuss project with staff	----- x								
Form an ad hoc planning committee	----	____ x							
Receive report from committee			----- x						
Discuss report with staff			----- ______ x						
Educate all staff to the plan				---- ____	x				
Implement new system					------	____	____	____	____
Evaluate system and make changes							----	____	x

KEY

- - - - - Proposed Time
______ Actual Time
x Complete

Figure 3-2 Gantt Chart: Implementation of Care Delivery System.

- A **goal** is the primary objective of the project and is always the last event
- The **first event** is the starting point of the project.
- **Critical path** is the longest path from the start to the finish or goal attainment on the PERT chart
- A **milestone** is an event that lets the manager evaluate the progress toward the goal

- A **merge event** has two or more immediate predecessor activities constraining it
- A **burst event** is a predecessor for two or more activities
- A **dummy activity** requires no time but must be taken into account before another activity can occur
- **Expected time** is the time required to complete an activity or action step; it is written on the opposite side of the letter (Strasen, 1987)

Depending on the project and critical nature of the time, approximate times can be assigned to various activities based on past experiences with similar activities. This type of decision-making method can be very time-consuming. It is often used in projects where time is critical and computer support is available. Because length of time is an issue of cost, the shorter the time for the project, the lower the cost. Cost can actually be placed on the chart so that decisions could be made about possible cost-saving steps.

The biggest problem, according to Anderson (1984), is estimating times correctly. It is also important that each activity be sequenced in the appropriate order. It is possible that activities will be accomplished simultaneously, particularly if more than one subcommittee is working on different parts of the project. Strasen (1987) points out that if more personnel are used in order to finish the project early, costs may actually rise. (See Scenario 3-3 and Figure 3-3 for use and illustration of a PERT chart.)

Scenario 3-3

The vice president for nursing plans to change all units to include case managers. She believes that this can be accomplished within a year and one half. In order for this to be achieved the following activities and events have to occur:

Activity Symbol	Activity Description	Immediate Predecessor
A.	Form a multidisciplinary advisory group	None
B.	Agree upon definitions	A
C.	Notify members of subcommittees	B
D.	Write job descriptions	C
E.	Advertise for candidates for case manager	D
F.	Review qualifications of candidates	E
G.	Select candidates for case manager	F
H.	Review patient charts	None
I.	Write patient care maps	H
J.	Meet with case managers	None
K.	Orient case managers	J
L.	Orient unit and hospital staff	K
M.	Utilize case management process	L

Events

1.	Project begins
2.	Meeting of multidisciplinary committee
3.	Formation of subcommittees
4.	Subcommittee for job description meets
5.	Subcommittee for patient care maps meets
6.	Candidates for case managers are interviewed
7.	Candidates are hired
8.	Subcommittee for patient care maps meets to finalize maps
9.	Orientation begins
10.	Implementation begins
11.	Project is evaluated

Expected Time Calculations

Activity	*Duration*
A	.5 month
B	1 month
C	.5 month
D	1 month
E	1 month
F	2 months
G	1 month
H	1 month
I	2 months
J	1 month
K&L	1 month
M	3 months

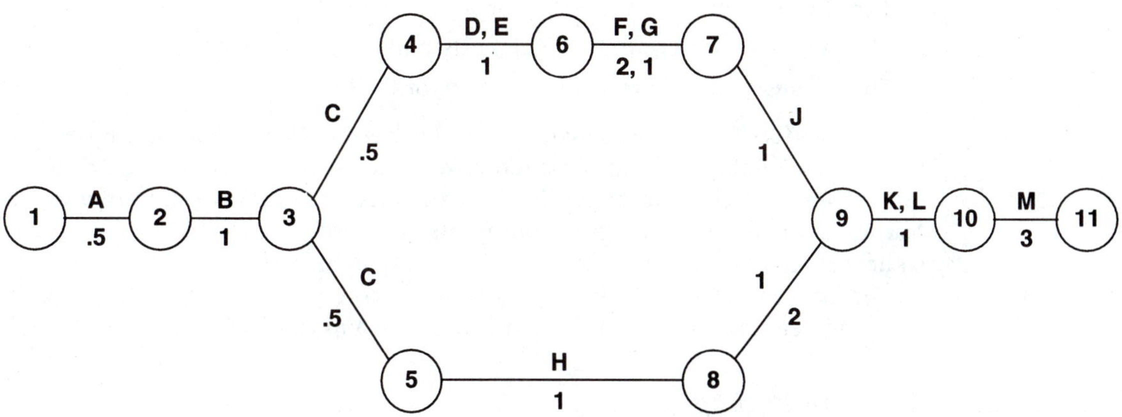

Figure 3-3 PERT Chart with Critical Path for Implementation of Case Management.

Critical Path Method (CPM)

The **critical path method (CPM)** is similar to the PERT chart. In addition to the PERT chart information, it adds a cost estimate for normal and **"crash"** operating conditions. Crash refers to conditions in less than normal time. The concept is particularly useful when cost is a factor: schedules can be crashed manually or on the computer. CPM allows the manager to monitor the critical paths, determine the interrelationships between the parts, and compare progress (Marriner-Tomey, 1992). A modification of this strategy is being used in case management, where critical paths are developed to plan the patient's course of treatment throughout his or her hospital stay. CPM allows the case manager to monitor the patient's care and to intervene as necessary in order to ensure cost-effective, quality care and appropriate discharge.

Cost-Benefit Analysis

Cost-benefit analysis, also called **cost-utility analysis,** is used to weigh the cost of a given program with the advantages, and is important to nursing administration because of the growing need to maximize limited resources. The decisionmaker must consider who benefits and at what cost. The individual benefiting may not be the one paying. For example, a hospital may provide tuition assistance for its employees. It can be argued that the employees benefit by becoming more skilled and perhaps more marketable.

The hospital may benefit by the employees' increased skill, as well as perhaps by their increased loyalty to the hospital, thus saving money in recruitment costs. Tuition assistance may also be viewed as a recruitment tool. However, the high cost of this benefit must be weighed against the ultimate benefit to the hospital. Lohman (1980) points out that not all benefits of human services activities can be measured in dollars. "Cost benefit analysis is largely a matter of determining the mathematical function that brings equilibrium to the cost-benefit equation" (Lohman, 1980, p. 246). Strasen (1987) lists assumptions that should be considered when doing a cost-benefit analysis:

- The quality of the product that is being produced
- The efficiency of the alternative that is being considered
- The potential for downtime, repair costs, and other essential costs, and
- The adequacy of the alternative selected for the job

Strasen (1987) also suggests constraints that need to be taken into consideration when putting dollar amounts on alternatives. These constraints may be difficult to quantify but can certainly affect the ultimate decision. Legal constraints, administrative constraints, technological constraints, resources constraints, and social constraints all may be influential in the decision-making process.

Cost-benefit analysis is only as good as the person or persons who are listing the costs and benefits. This in itself is a judgment call and can be biased.

Decision Packages

Decision packages are used for budgeting, and consist of several basic elements: "a listing of all current and proposed objectives or activities of a given team, nursing unit or department; alternative ways of carrying out these activities; the different costs of each alternative; the advantages of continuing the activity; and the consequences of discontinuing the activity" (Tappen, 1989).

Scenario 3-4

The obstetrical department would like to start a class for expectant families to learn more about the department and facilities.

Objective: Teach families about the department.

Advantages: Help families feel more comfortable about the department. May increase number of families using the hospital for delivery.

Disadvantages: Need to pay a professional to lead the class. Cost for refreshments.

Alternative 1: Have a volunteer teach the class.

Major Advantage: No salary cost.

Disadvantage: Volunteers would have to be trained and may not be able to answer all the questions in a professional manner.

Alternative 2: Teach the class on a Saturday when the unit tends to be less busy and use a member of the staff.

Major Advantage: No salary cost and more professional expertise.

Disadvantage: Floor could unexpectantly get busy.

PSYCHOLOGICAL STRATEGIES

Psychological strategies can be divided into individual and group strategies. Satisficing, optimizing, elimination by aspects, incrementalism, mixed scanning, and decisional balance sheet are all individual strategies. Delphi is a group strategy, while scenario development and mind mapping can be used both individually and with a group.

Individual Strategies

Staff nurses and managers are always faced with making decisions in their practice. These decisions can be personal or professional. The following individual strategies give the nurse some options. Before an option is chosen, the nurse needs to decide the importance of the decision and how much time can be allotted to the decision-making process. These factors will help in choosing which decision-making option is best for any given situation.

SATISFICING

According to Simon (1976), the individual making a decision often looks for a course of action that is "good enough," meets their minimal standards, or **satisfices.**

More than one criterion can be used. It is seen as settling. Simon points out that all decisions have an element of compromise. The selected alternative is never the accomplishment of all goals, but rather is the best solution under the circumstances. The environment in which the decision is being made limits the alternatives that are available. A nurse manager, for example, might be willing to accept a lateral move because no other job presents itself and she wants to stay within the organization. The job is not ultimately what she wants, but she is willing to take it for now. It is often seen as a way of playing it safe. Janis and Mann (1977) find that four variables are involved in satisficing:

- Number of requirements met—In this strategy only a small number of requirements are selected to be met
- Number of alternatives generated—The decisionmaker will limit the number of alternative options
- Ordering and retesting alternatives—Typically in this strategy the decisionmaker will only test the alternatives once
- Type of testing model used—The decisionmaker will set minimal criteria, and if the alternative does not fall above or below the minimum, then the option may be chosen

The advantage of this type of decision making is that it is relatively simple and can be accomplished quickly. The disadvantage is that although you believe at the time that you will be satisfied with the decision, in reality, by compromising, it may not be the best decision.

OPTIMIZING

Optimizing is used when the decisionmaker decides to look at all possible alternatives and select the alternative that will offer the maximum benefit. This depends on whether the decisionmaker has all the information and the information is accurate. In many cases, this strategy becomes satisficing when the decision actually is made (Gillies, 1989). Optimizing can also be very time consuming and may delay the decision-making process. The decisionmaker needs to determine a time limit in terms of information gathering, otherwise an important decision may not be made in a timely fashion.

ELIMINATION BY ASPECTS

Elimination by aspects is a strategy of satisficing described by Tversky (1972) in which decision makers use a set of decision rules that can be used to rapidly select from a number of alternatives, each of which meets the minimal standards. It is a narrowing down process. In this technique all the possible options are listed, then each is reviewed and a decision is made as to its feasibility. Cost, risk, time, effectiveness, and rewards may all be factors that could eliminate or not eliminate an alternative. Once this is accomplished, the list is again reviewed and the options that were not eliminated are reconsidered. This process can be repeated a number of times until one or two options remain. These options are then reconsidered and a decision can be made. This, too, can become very time consuming and can delay the final decision.

INCREMENTALISM

Incrementalism often comes about after a series of satisficing decisions (Miller and Starr, 1967). It is geared to alleviate concrete shortcomings in a present policy or to put out fires, rather than to make the best decision. The means are often chosen too quickly to accomplish the ends. This form of decision making does not take into account major goals, but is simply used to deal with a pressing situation quickly. It often results in a change or new policy.

While the advantage to this process is that it can be done quickly, the disadvantage is that it is often reactive and not proactive. Thus, decisions are made to meet the immediate crisis, but do not necessarily deal with the long-term implications of the problem. For example, a nurse manager becomes angry because too much overtime is being used. Rather than sit and discuss the problems that are causing the overtime with the staff, the manager unilaterally makes a policy that no more overtime will be allowed. Life decisions also are often incremental in that they are based on a series of smaller decisions that have been made over time without looking at long term goals.

MIXED SCANNING

Mixed scanning, developed by Etzioni (1967), has two main components:

- Optimizing combined with the elimination-by-aspects approach
- An incremental process based on the elements of satisficing

Scanning refers to the search, collection, processing, evaluation, and weighing of information. The decisionmaker scans intensively only those choices that are troublesome (Janis and Mann, 1977).

The process is as follows:

- List all relevant alternatives
- Examine all alternatives and reject ones not useful or objectionable
- For all alternatives not rejected, reevaluate
- Continue this process until only one alternative is left
- When possible, divide the implementation into several steps, allowing for additional information seeking, scanning, and possible change

DECISIONAL BALANCE SHEET

The **decisional balance sheet** was developed by Janis and Mann (1977) and consists of four aspects to consider in making a personal decision: utilitarian gains or losses for self, utilitarian gains or losses for significant others, self-approval or disapproval, and social approval or disapproval. Each alternative course of action is weighed against this criteria and plotted on the grid.

For example, in the case of the nurse manager who has to decide whether to accept a lateral move, she would first look at the gains or losses for herself. The gains might include such things as enhancing her clinical expertise, the challenge of developing a new staff and unit, and recognition from administration for being willing to be a team player. The losses may include such issues as no increase in pay or boredom with a similar job. For her significant others, the gains or losses might include more or less stress, and more or less time for them. The manager would have to decide whether taking this new position made a difference in how she felt about herself, and how it would be viewed in the hospital among peers and other departments. Once all of these issues were weighed against each other and plotted on the grid, a decision could be made that would serve the best interests of the manager. This strategy has the advantage of weighing the alternatives from a number of important perspectives. It can, however, be very time consuming.

Group Strategies

DECISION GROUPS OR COMMITTEES

According to Huber (1980), managers use **group decision making** for two major reasons: limited personal resources that a manager can bring to the decision, and to involve the persons most influential in implementing the decision in the decision-making process in order to gain support. By involving members in the group decision-making process, members feel a personal commitment to the decision and are thus more likely to support it, as well as to generate support from others. There are, however, disadvantages for using a group: Groups are time consuming; groups may make decisions not in keeping with organizational goals; group members may feel that they should be involved in all decisions; disagreements among members may cause the group to be unable to come to a decision (Huber, 1980). These problems can be overcome with good planning and leadership. The choice of group members may make an important difference in the outcome. Members who can work well together and yet provide different points of view are ideal. It is also useful to choose members who can compliment each other's talents and abilities.

DELPHI METHOD

The **delphi method** is used to forecast future trends in a particular area. It is an advanced form of an opinion poll. It has three features: (1) anonymity, (2) opportunity for opinion revision, and (3) summary feedback (Huber, 1980). In this procedure, a panel of experts in the field to be studied is identified. In the first round, the participants are asked to either respond to a questionnaire or to identify a list of trends in a given area. Subsequent rounds use a compilation of all responses and ask the panel to again respond. After several rounds, a summary of responses is mailed to the participants for their added comments. This strategy allows for maximum feedback from experts in the field, but can be quite time consuming, sometimes taking as long as one to two years, which can be a disadvantage, particularly in fields such as computers where technology changes so rapidly. On the other hand, it has been used successfully in areas of nursing, where it is important to look at the past and then project the future. Nursing education research priorities is one such area. It is important that recognized experts are chosen for the panel, and that consideration is given to diverse geographical areas, specialities, and other differences as appropriate.

BRAINSTORMING

Brainstorming is used to generate ideas. It can take place at an informal meeting in which ideas for a given problem are simply discussed, or it can take a more formal structure. It works best, according to Marriner-Tomey (1992), for simple and specific problems. The group needs to have some understanding of the problems. The atmosphere in the group should be one in which everyone feels that his or her ideas are welcomed and important and that they will not be criticized. The group leader will inform the group that this is an opportunity to be creative and to discuss new ideas. All group members are encouraged to participate in this permissive environment. Ideas are recorded on a blackboard or easel. No ideas are discussed until the brainstorming is concluded. Then each idea can be discussed individually for its advantages and disadvantages. The advantage of this group method is that it allows for a free flow of ideas from all members and has the potential to generate ideas not previously considered. The key to the success of this method is that all members of the group feel that their ideas are important and that no idea is too silly, stupid, or unworthy of discussion. This requires a certain amount of trust among group members and trust of the leader. When all ideas are treated seriously by the leader, the group members feel valued and empowered.

BRAINWRITING

Brainwriting is a form of brainstorming, discussed by Marriner-Tomey (1992), that involves writing ideas individually first and then passing these papers to another group member to read. That group member adds his or her ideas to the paper and passes it on to the next group member. This continues until the group feels that they have exhausted their ideas. The group shares ideas and a decision is reached. This strategy gives members the opportunity to put down their ideas succinctly in writing and allows them to see what other people are thinking. In some group situations, even though all are encouraged to participate, some may feel uncomfortable in doing so. This strategy gives everyone the opportunity to have his or her ideas considered.

NOMINAL GROUP TECHNIQUE

Nominal group technique was developed in the late 1960s by Andre Delbecq and Andrew Van de Ven, and involves a structured group meeting with a specific format. This strategy is useful for gaining input from a group involved in a particular situation. It is focused on one situation only. The process starts with members each writing ideas on a pad of paper. After five to ten minutes, each shares his or her ideas with no discussion. A recorder writes all the ideas as given on a flip chart or blackboard. After all group members have contributed ideas, comments and ideas about each of the contributions is sequentially elicited. When this process is completed, each member privately rank-orders the alternatives. The results are then tallied and discussed with the group for further feedback. This strategy has the advantage of concentrating on the issues and not on the social and psychological processes within the group. The disadvantage is that its structure may limit spontaneity and creativity (Huber, 1980).

Nursing manager groups may find this strategy particularly useful when trying to discuss an issue that would lead to a new policy. For example, if the managers wanted to set new policies on the use of supplemental staffing, the nominal method could be used to allow all the managers to express their opinions and then determine a mutually satisfactory policy. The nominal technique has the advantage of allowing for the opinions and private ranking of all the managers as opposed to a more vocal few making the decision for all.

Individual or Group Strategies

SCENARIO DEVELOPMENT

Scenario development is a forecasting strategy in which the manager, group, or individual staff members create possible stories about what might happen. Schwartz (1991) points out that this is not predicting the future, but attempting to perceive the future in the present. Each story includes various alternative scenarios that could occur with possible solutions. This strategy could be very useful to managers or staff in planning a project that might run into political difficulties. It gives the manager or staff the ability to anticipate what might happen and to plan proactive responses or strategies. It can actually function as a role play or a written response. It is useful to share the stories with others who may be able to add alternative scenarios or alternative solutions. Scenario 3-5 demonstrates the use of scenario development.

Scenario 3-5

A group of nurse managers is asked to submit plans for a new, more cost-effective patient care delivery system. They meet together to discuss their various viewpoints and realize that they have very different ideas.

They decide that the best way to proceed is to identify various possible systems based on a review of the literature. In their second meeting, they are able to identify three possible approaches to the delivery of care. They then divide into three teams, each charged with developing a complete scenario describing how its approach would work in the hospital setting. They are told to consider how the approach would affect other disciplines, as well as the staff that deliver the care and the patients who receive the care. In addition, they must identify the key players in the system and what possible resistances they may encounter. Once this is completed, they are asked to consider how future trends in healthcare will effect their particular choice and what possible vulnerabilities or pitfalls they are likely to encounter. They are then asked to discuss which of their choices is most likely to be accepted, implemented easily, and represents the best choice for the patient, staff, and hospital. Based on this process, the nurse managers feel confident in their decision and are able to proceed to the next step of presenting it to the whole management team.

Schwartz (1991) defines a process by which scenarios are developed. It is important that more than one scenario is developed at a time. The process includes:

- Identifying focal issues or decisions
- Looking for people or events that are key forces in the local environment
- Identifying driving forces
- Ranking by importance or uncertainty
- Selecting the specific scenarios

- Deciding on particular details of the scenarios
- Deciding on specific implications for each scenario
- Selecting leading indicators and signposts

Schwartz (1991) suggests that you have a good scenario when "they are both plausible and surprising; when they have the power to break old stereotypes, and when the makers assume ownership and put them to work" (p. 234).

MIND MAPPING

Mind mapping utilizes the right part of the brain, which deals with "rhythm, music, images, geometry, imagination, daydreaming, color, dimension, parallel processing, face recognition, and pattern or map recognition" (Manthey and Miller, 1991, p. 20). The strategy involves placing a central theme or concept in the middle of the paper and then writing key ideas related to the concept on lines around the theme. From those lines, other connecting ideas or details can be written on the map. Pictures and images can replace words, and there should be only one word per line. Every line is then connected to another. This method, according to Manthey and Miller (1991), can be used any time notetaking is appropriate. The advantage of this strategy is that it allows for the creative process to be stimulated and yet also helps to make and readily see the connections between ideas. The benefits of mind mapping include:

- Helping the group to focus on issues rather than individual personalities
- Being able to decide on solutions for correcting the problem
- The ability for the group to share their concerns and understand the concerns of others (Manthey and Miller, 1991)

SUMMARY

Nurses are called upon to make decisions every day. Some of these decisions are very complex, while others can be made rather easily. The strategies discussed in this chapter offer a full range, from simple to complex. Some complex decisions require quantitative analysis while others can use a more psychological analysis approach. In some situations more than one strategy might be useful. It is important for the individual to have a repertoire of strategies readily available so that an appropriate choice is made as to which decision approach would produce the best results. Evaluating the decision process used and its effectiveness gives the decision-maker experience and feedback and leads to making better future decisions.

REFERENCES

Anderson, C. (1984). *Management skills, functions and organization performance.* Dubuque, IA: Wm C. Brown.

Etzioni, A. (1989). Humble decision making, *Harvard Business Review,* July-August, 122–126.

Gillies, D. (1989). *Nursing management: A systems approach,* 2nd ed. Philadelphia: W.B. Saunders.

Huber, G. (1980). *Managerial decision making.* Glenview, IL: Scott Foresman.

Janis, I., & Mann, L. (1977). *Decision making.* New York: Macmillan.

Lohman, R. (1980). *Breaking even.* Philadelphia: Temple University Press.

Manthey, M., & Miller, D. (1991) Tools for leaders . . . Tools for managers. *Nursing Management, 22,* 20–23.

Marriner-Tomey, A. (1992) *Guide to nursing management,* 4th ed. St. Louis, MO: Mosby.

Miller, D.W., & Starr, M.K. (1967) *The structure of human decisions.* Englewood Cliffs, NJ: Prentice Hall.

Mintzberg, H. (1976). *The structuring of organizations.* Englewood Cliffs, NJ: Prentice Hall.

Rowland, H., & Rowland, B. (1992). *Nursing administration,* 3rd ed. Gaithersburg, MD: Aspen.

Russo, J.E., & Schoemaker, P. (1989). *Decision traps: The ten barriers to brilliant decision making and how to overcome them.* New York: Simon & Schuster.

Schlitz, D. (1978). "The Gambler", recorded by K. Rogers. On *The Gambler* (cassette). Hollywood, CA: Liberty Records.

Schwartz, P. (1991). *The art of the long view: The path to strategic insights for yourself or your company.* New York: Doubleday.

Simon, H. (1976). *Administrative behavior: A study of decision-making processes in administrative organization,* 3rd ed. New York: Free Press.

Stevens, B. (1985). *The nurse as executive,* 3rd ed. Rockville, MD: Aspen.

Strasen, L. (1987). *Key business skills for nurse managers.* Philadelphia: J.B. Lippincott.

Tappen, R. (1989). *Nursing leadership and management: Concepts and practice,* 2nd ed. Philadelphia: F.A. Davis.

Tversky, A. (1972). Elimination by aspects: A theory of choice. *Psychological Review, 79,* 281–99.

Alice Donahue
Suzanne G. Martin

CHAPTER 4

Individual Decision Making

Accept rigorous debate, and then make a decision. You're the one who has to do it; you can't just hope it will evolve by some mystical group process.

—*Abraham Zalenick (cited in Safire and Safir, 1990)*

INTRODUCTION

The purpose of this chapter is to examine the significant factors related to individual decision making, including what factors influence an individual's decision-making process, when individual decision making may be more advantageous than a group process, and how to evaluate decision outcomes and rebound if the outcome is poor.

Deciding on what specific situation needs your attention first is probably the most frequent decision you will make during your career. Although the scenario described on the following page requires a decision to be made in a short period of time, you may be faced with other situations where you have an already identified problem and now you must make a decision about what to do with the information.

This nursing example illustrates three important characteristics of decision making:

- A decision can be made by an individual
- Even a brief decision-making process can be both logical and complex
- Information is an indispensable element

In order to be a good decisionmaker, you need to have the skills necessary to assess both your own abilities and the nature of the external environment (Kaye, 1992).

Scenario 4-1

It is 6:00 AM, one hour before the end of your shift, you are making rounds, and Mrs. Smith in Room 279 requests pain medication. As you return to the medication room, you hear a loud noise down the hall, the phone is ringing at the nurses' station, and the intercom linking your unit to the operating room alerts you to prepare your patient, Mr. Brown in Room 283, for surgery. From experience, you know the operating room technician will arrive in ten minutes to pick up Mr. Brown. How do you decide what to do first?

As a nurse trying to decide what to do first in the above situation, you need to gather all the information. The crash at the end of the hallway may need to be explored first; however, you know that this area is not accessible to anyone and you had just been in there putting away supplies next to the bedpans. The sound was consistent with a bedpan falling from a shelf.

The patient going to the operating room is another situation. This will be a decision based on the rules and regulations of the hospital. The patient needs to be in the operating room holding suite at 6:30 AM, so you have one half-hour to prepare him. In order to make an intelligent decision about what to do first, you need adequate information. Answering the phone would be essential in order to gather the information.

Mrs. Smith's request for pain medication must be addressed. What type of pain is she experiencing? Is it new pain? Is it related to her present condition?

Although you are aware of the impact of delaying Mr. Brown's transfer to the operating room, you decide to further assess Mrs. Smith's pain. During the information-gathering stage, you realize that Mrs. Smith's pain is new and is associated with symptoms related to cardiac involvement.

WHAT IS DECISION MAKING?

Individual decision making can be defined as the process of generating an outcome based on a variety of cognitive, social, and contextual influences. Outcomes may vary, and include affective states of the decisionmaker (such as satisfaction, frustration, etc.) as well as behavior and implementation actions (MacPhail-Wilcox and Bryant, 1988). However, it is probably safe to say that most individuals are probably unaware of their processes while they are making the decision. Generally, theories of decision making have been dominated by models from mathematical, philosophical, and economic sources (Hastie, 1991).

THE ROLE OF THE NURSE

Decision making is an integral component of the role of the professional nurse; effective decision making is necessary if a hospital administration expects to function efficiently. As the nurse's role expands and complexity of care increases, meeting this challenge becomes more difficult. The decisions the nurse will face can range from routine to life-and-death situations.

Decision making in nursing takes place in a rich social context. Decisionsmakers frequently rely upon information supplied by others, and disagreements can lead to conflict. Nurses must have an understanding of the most appropriate manner in which to approach the decisional process. Factors that determine what type of pattern to use are:

- The seriousness of the risks resulting from the decision
- The possibility of finding a better solution
- How much time is available to find a solution

Individual factors, such as experience, also influence the process. Cassel (1973) suggests that decision making is a competency and can be improved. Experience enhances knowledge, thus increasing the cognitive resources available for processing information.

Benner (1982) describes experience as a refinement of preconceived notions and theory by encountering many actual practical situations that add nuances or shape of differences to theory. She describes how different levels of experience influence the care and the planning and decision making of the nurse. For example, a new nurse is guided by rules and lacks any discretionary judgment. A seasoned nurse or expert nurse considers far fewer options when analyzing a problem, and generally gets straight to the facts. This limits the number of alternatives that must be evaluated and reduces the complexity of the decisional process. Although there are a variety of models, at least three major stages appear with some consistency in the literature. These stages consist of:

- Perception and information gathering
- Information processing
- Choice (MacPhail-Wilcox and Bryant, 1988)

DECISION STAGES

The **perception and information gathering stage** involves recognizing an opportunity (or necessity) for a decision and gathering the required data to clarify the issue and make an informed choice. Individual personality style and attitude will influence this stage (MacPhail-Wilcox and Bryant, 1988). The decision opportunity may result from a demand from one's manager, a request from a staff member, or one's own initiative.

Information processing requires the decisionmaker to understand the concept(s) involved, collect information by asking questions, analyze information, and make judgments about the relative value of different concepts. Asking the right questions is critical at this stage. Information must be interpreted, integrated with existing knowledge, and evaluated. While interpretation may be a matter of pattern recognition (for instance, Has this happened before, and if so, what were the circumstances?), integration makes use of a variety of problem-solving strategies, including algorithms, heuristics, and intuition. **Algorithms** are calculations for which there are definite, proven solutions. An example of an algorithm might be the administration of disciplinary action based on a well-defined human resource policy to address a specific infraction. In contrast, **heuristics** are general guidelines about how things usually behave. Heuristics are calculated risks based on an educated guess about what the consequences of each action might be. Heuristics are essentially shortcutting strategies. In the case example given in the introduction, the nurse uses a heuristic when the assessment is made that the noise at the end of the hall is *probably* the result of a bedpan falling off the shelf. Finally, **intuition** involves working from one's "gut," that is, decisions are made based on what feels right to the decisionmaker. It is not based on any objective potential outcome evaluation, but may in fact be a valid and effective problem solving strategy for some individuals. Integration of information is a critical stage in influencing judgment accuracy (MacPhail-Wilcox and Bryant, 1988).

Once this process is complete, the **choice** of the best alternative should be fairly obvious. Choice is the critical decision stage where the decisionmaker selects a course of action after having progressed through the previous stages. The entire process may take as little as ten seconds or as long as several months. Healthcare reform is an example of a decision that must take an enormous effort of fact-finding and consideration of options before this final stage can be reached. Naturally, the urgency of the situation will determine the timeline.

The decisionmaker should not misuse this stage as a form of procrastination (Kaye, 1992). The challenge is to be able to identify when the point of diminished return has been reached and a decision needs to be made.

THE INDIVIDUAL DECISIONMAKER

Decision making is choosing one alternative from several. A decisionmaker's actions are guided by goals. Courses of action are generally linked to various outcomes. Information is available regarding the alternatives, the likelihood that each outcome will occur, and the value of each outcome relative to the goal. On the basis of his or her evaluation of the information, the decisionmaker chooses one alternative. **Context frequency** describes how often a particular decision recurs, and **information conditions** describe how much information about the predictability of various outcomes is available. The **frequency of recurrence** determines whether a decision is programmed or nonprogrammed.

A **programmed decision** recurs often enough for a decision rule (or algorithm) to be developed. Programmed decisions or routine decisions constitute the majority of daily decisions. (Evans, 1990). A **decision rule** tells the decisionmaker what alternative to choose once he or she has information about the decision situation. Whenever the situation is encountered, all that is often required is the implementation of a previously specified course of action or standard operating procedure. An example of a programmed decision in nursing would be the determination of how many nurses are required to cover a shift, based on nursing care hours per patient day. A manager, facing the recurring decision of how many nurses to schedule per day, simply feeds census information into a formula to determine the appropriate number of nurses to schedule.

However, when a problem or decision situation has not been encountered before, the **nonprogrammed decisions** occur. These decisions cannot be made based on a previously established decision rule. This decision requires problem solving because the issue is usually unique, requiring development and evaluation of alternatives without the aid of a programmed decision rule. Since non-programmed decisions are usually poorly structured, with vague information available, and generally associated with high risks, the decisionmaker must exercise sound judgment and creativity when selecting alternatives. The use of heuristics and intuition is not uncommon in this type of decision.

Information conditions describe how much information about the predictability of various outcomes is available. The range of available information can be depicted as a continuum whose endpoints represent complete certainty and complete uncertainty. At a point between the two extremes, the decisionmaker has some information about the possible outcomes and may be able to estimate the probability of their occurrence. Stoner, Collins, and Yetton (1985) suggest that when decisions are made under conditions of certainty, the decisionmaker knows what will happen in the future. Under risk conditions, the probabilities of each possible outcome can be estimated, but under conditions of uncertainty, the probabilities, and even the possible outcomes, are not known, due to a lack of information. When a decisionmaker faces complete uncertainty, he or she may wait for more information to reduce uncertainty or rely on judgment, experience, and intuition to make the decision.

MYERS-BRIGGS TYPE INDICATOR

The choice or decision action is strongly correlated to the decisionmaker's beliefs, values, and style. A highly respected instrument for measuring decision-making styles is the **Myers-Briggs Type Indicator**. The Myers-Briggs is essentially a personality test based on Carl Jung's theory of personality type. The tool provides a way of measuring people's tendency to perceive and judge situations in different ways (Davis, Grove, and Knowles, 1990).

According to Jung (1968), behavior differences between individuals is a function of the way an individual prefers to approach life. Based on this theory, four different indices of personality can be identified in the Myers-Briggs Type Indicator. The indices are extroverted-introverted, sensing-intuiting, thinking-feeling, and judgment-perception. These indices represent one's innate orientation toward life, and ways of perceiving the world, arriving at a decision, and dealing with the outside world (Davis et al., 1990). The sensing-intuiting and thinking-feeling indices are particularly applicable to individual decision making.

Sensing-Intuiting Index

The **sensing-intuiting index** essentially classifies individuals based on their style of information gathering and processing (MacPhail-Wilcox and Bryant, 1988). The sensing or analytic individual concentrates on detail and breaking problems into component parts. Individuals using sensing styles prefer hard objective facts. They are data sensitive. In contrast, the intuitive individual operates holistically and filters data. Intuiting individuals prefer insight in analyzing a problem. In a way, intuition involves processing information by means other than the senses, that is, through the unconscious (Davis et al., 1990). Sensing individuals prefer structured situations, while intuitive individuals prefer unstructured situations. In making a decision, sensing types tend to focus on cognitive method, while intuitives will consider the decision in terms of fit or how well the decision accommodates to others (Hunt, Krzystofiak, Meindl, and Yousry, 1989).

Malley and Davis (1988) suggest that the intuiting individual is a problem generator, while the sensing type is a problem solver, and that with increased practice, problem-solving styles seem to change. What works best early in one's career may change over time from an intuiting style to a sensing style. Therefore, one changes from a problem generator to a problem solver as a normal progression with experience.

The problem here is that sensing individuals are real-time-oriented, and strategic planning, which is generally considered necessary for an organization's survival, is future-oriented, a characteristic of intuiting individuals. If a person is told that he or she tends to create problems where none exist, this trait might be a strength! Maybe the individual is a problem generator, and his or her future orientation, if presented in the appropriate forum, can be an asset to his or her career development and assist the institution in the strategic planning process.

Unfortunately, high-level managers tend to prefer problem solving to the detriment of the strategic planning process. Problem generation may be enhanced by advanced education, suggesting that upper-level managers should be encouraged to acquire additional education, or at a minimum attend executive educational programs to correct problem generation deficits and thereby become more successful in strategic planning.

Thinking-Feeling Index

The **thinking-feeling index** of the Myers-Briggs indicates how one obtains and uses information, and is related to the information processing stage. Individuals with feeling styles focus more on subjective values and affective information. Thinking individuals focus more on objective criteria and factual information, a logical process that is both rational and impersonal (MacPhail-Wilcox and Bryant, 1988; Davis et al., 1990); they are coolly analytical in applying decision rules and models.

Davis et. al (1990) identified four decision-making styles by arranging sensing-thinking (ST), intuiting-thinking (NT), sensing-feeling (SF), and intuiting-feeling (NF) together. They hypothesized that individuals with an ST decision style would perform best on a decision-making task, followed in order by NT, SF, and NF styles. Instead, the data indicated a performance order (from best to worst) of SF, ST, NF, NT.

What does this all this information mean? Basically, that individuals with a sensing-feeling decision perspective seem to be able to make better decisions within a relatively well-structured environment than intuiting decisionmakers (Davis et al., 1990). It is possible of course that within a less structured environment, another decision-making style might prove to be more effective, but within the patient care arena most frequently encountered by professional nurses, it would seem that sensing individuals will outperform their intuiting counterparts. Specifically, those nurses who can combine a preference for hard facts with a humanistic approach will perform best of all—a position that is consistent with the philosophy that nursing is both an art and a science.

RATIONAL DECISION MAKING

If the individual is to improve on his or her decision-making abilities, it is imperative to have an understanding of the process. Several models offer insights into the decision-making process. The rational model often used in business organizations is appealing because of its logic and economy. This model outlines a systematic step-by-step approach. The rational model is generally applied in individual decision making. However, this model ignores the reality of questionable emotional priorities in decisions (Kahneman, 1991). The current bias is to treat irrationality as a failure of reasoning. However, emotional and social factors are a facet of the decision process. Even the most controlled individuals stand to have their decisions colored by their affective states and past experiences.

According to Harbison (1991), the various schools that maintain a rationalist perspective for decision making in nursing believe that an analysis of the situation should be carried out, subsequent actions should be rational and logical, and the nurse should be able to make his or her knowledge and judgment explicit. This position accords well with the current trend in nursing toward research/rationale-based nursing and accountability.

Decision Analysis

The approach that best exemplifies this perspective is **decision analysis.** In decision analysis, a model of the problem is constructed, showing the available options that are to be considered and the consequences of following each. An attempt is made to assign a probability to each outcome. The analysis is often depicted as a decision tree. A common nursing decision of whether to use side rails can be depicted using this method (Table 4-1).

In this example, the decision to keep the cot sides up is supported by the higher overall value of this option (54 versus 22). The overall value is the summation of the expected values. Expected values are derived from the probability of each occurrence (fall, safe, psychologically threatened) multiplied by the utility value of each probability.

Unfortunately, the majority of decisions encountered by the individual nurse cannot fit into the rigid assumptions common to the rational model and decision analysis. Nor does this approach lend itself to the type of prompt decisions that are characteristic of nursing. The amount of information available is usually limited, and most decisionmakers have limited ability to process information about alternatives. Moreover, not all alternatives lend themselves to quantification in terms that will allow for easy comparison (Harrison, 1981). However, since individual decision making is often not a rational process, the very features of this model have been questioned.

Table 4-1 • **Decision Tree: The Use of Cot Sides**

Option		Outcome	Probability of Outcome	Utility (Value)	Expected Value	Overall Value
Option	Cot Sides Up	Fall	0.5	0	0	54
		Safe	0.5	80	40	
		Psychologically threatened	0.7	20	14	
	Cot Sides Down	Fall	0.5	20	10	22
		Safe	0.5	20	10	
		Psychologically threatened	0.1	20	2	
			Scale 0–1	Scale 0–100		

MODIFIED RATIONAL APPROACH

The authors, Donahue and Martin, suggest using a modified rational approach to decision making. This approach consists of the framework of the rational model, but recognizing the limitations of time, available information, and the decision-maker's ability to process all information and select the single best solution. This model takes into account the behavioral characteristics that influence decision making and provides a more realistic approach, taking into account the constraints of time and resources. This model is referred to as a **practical model of decision making** in business organizations. This process is conceptually similar to the decision tree, but without the quantitative analysis. It involves the following steps:

1. Identify the goal
2. Identify the alternatives
3. Consider each alternative in terms of: Does it meet the criteria? Is it feasible? Do you have the power to implement or do others need to be consulted or approve? What is the potential impact on others? Are there resources available to implement? Get the facts!
4. Select the alternative that best meets the criteria

Scenario 4-2

Consider the example of a new assistant nurse manager confronted by a staff member who refuses an assignment. The goal is to ensure that safe and quality patient care is given and that staff assignments are equitably distributed. The staff nurse's refusal clearly places this goal in jeopardy and undermines the authority of the assistant.

What are the options? The assistant can choose to ignore the insubordination (not recommended!), she can sit down with the staff nurse and discuss the situation, she can dump the problem on her nurse manager, or she can review the institution's disciplinary policy and recommend the appropriate action.

Let's say that she considers all the alternatives and decides to recommend disciplinary action. Now she is faced with another decision: Does she verbally counsel? Issue a written warning? Suspend? Or terminate? Again, it is necessary to consider her own level of authority. Is she empowered to discipline staff or simply to advise? Does she have all the facts? Did she consult the personnel policy? Has the employee done this before? Check out the employee's personnel file. The more resources consulted in this case the better. Having evaluated all information available, the assistant is now in a good position to make a low-risk decision.

RISK AND DECISION MAKING

Personality and risk tolerance are also important factors influencing an individual's decision-making style. At one end of the continuum is the impulsive decisionmaker who moves quickly without much consideration of possible drawbacks. At the other end are those decisionmakers who slowly and carefully consider the advantages and disadvantages of each choice before making their decisions. Certainly, the greater the risk involved, the greater the probability that the decisionmaker will behave nonimpulsively. By nature, risk-created conflict may induce possible gains, which are blocked by possible losses. The frustration that this engenders creates anxiety and guilt. The greater the amount of perceived risk, the more unpleasant the emotions for the decisionmaker. Individuals with a higher threshold for conflict will tend to be able to take greater risks than those who react more negatively (Dahlback, 1990).

Fear of making a mistake usually occurs at work when a difficult decision has to be made. Regardless of how much research is done or how may times one has weighed the pros and cons, sometimes one must face the possibility that a wrong decision will be made.

Rectifying a mistake, or changing directions, may take a bit of time and energy, but it is not the anxiety-producing situation one anticipates. Making difficult decisions and a few mistakes along the way is really critical to professional growth. In risking failure, one learns something from every decision made, regardless of whether it turns out to be right or wrong. Improving decision making reduces the chances of making mistakes. In order to improve decision making, one must have an understanding of the process.

Identify the problem. Make sure the decision addresses the problem. List the options and have a contingency plan. Recognize that the solution arrived at initially may not be the final one implemented.

CONFLICT AND DECISIONS

Decisional conflict arises as a result of the differing roles of a nurse. According to Huckabay (1986), the nurse has two roles: a professional role that deals with loyalty to the profession, maintenance of high standards, and responsibility to patients in his or her care; and an employee role that emphasizes loyalty to the institution and following its rules and regulations. Decisions that threaten the integrity of one of these roles may result in conflict and uncertainty for the individual (Evans, 1990). Conflict may also develop if the decision does not meet the expectations of a particular group or department.

Decisions often involve conflict. Conflict develops when an individual is caught between pros and cons. It may be as significant a decision as initiating an emergency response, or as insignificant as deciding on when to go to lunch. Conflict as a situation choice involves affirming one option at the expense of another. It is complicated by the risk of uncertainty about the consequences. In a rational model, the decisionmaker selects the option with the highest value. However, conflict impedes this process, and if severe, may lead an individual to indefinitely defer the decision and continue to seek other options. Maybe you can have your cake and eat it, too. This delay does not occur when the added options present no conflict, but can occur in situations where conflict needs to be resolved (Tversky and Shafir, 1992).

THE ROLE OF STRESS

Psychological stress occurring during the decisional conflict can emanate from at least two sources (Janis and Mann, 1982): first, the decisionmaker's concern about material and social losses as a result of the decision; second, from the recognition that his or her reputation and self-esteem as a competent decisionmaker is also at risk. The greater the perceived losses, the greater the stress will be. This stress can adversely affect the decision. Janis and Mann (1977) suggest that different patterns will emerge as a means of coping with decisional conflict and stress (Figure 4-1).

Depending on the circumstances surrounding the decision, the following patterns could develop: vigilance, complacency, defensive avoidance, and hypervigilance. It has been argued that stress reduces the quality of decisions. Certainly, any crisis situation will create stress for the decisionmaker. The key is to maintain perspective and avoid maladaptive choices that may be caused by cognitive distortions under pressure.

Why does this occur? Fink (1986) suggests several possibilities. It could be that the decisionmaker is swamped with too much information that he or she cannot process, and he or she is unable to extract the significant data from a maze of conflicting information, a condition of psychological overload. The danger is that the

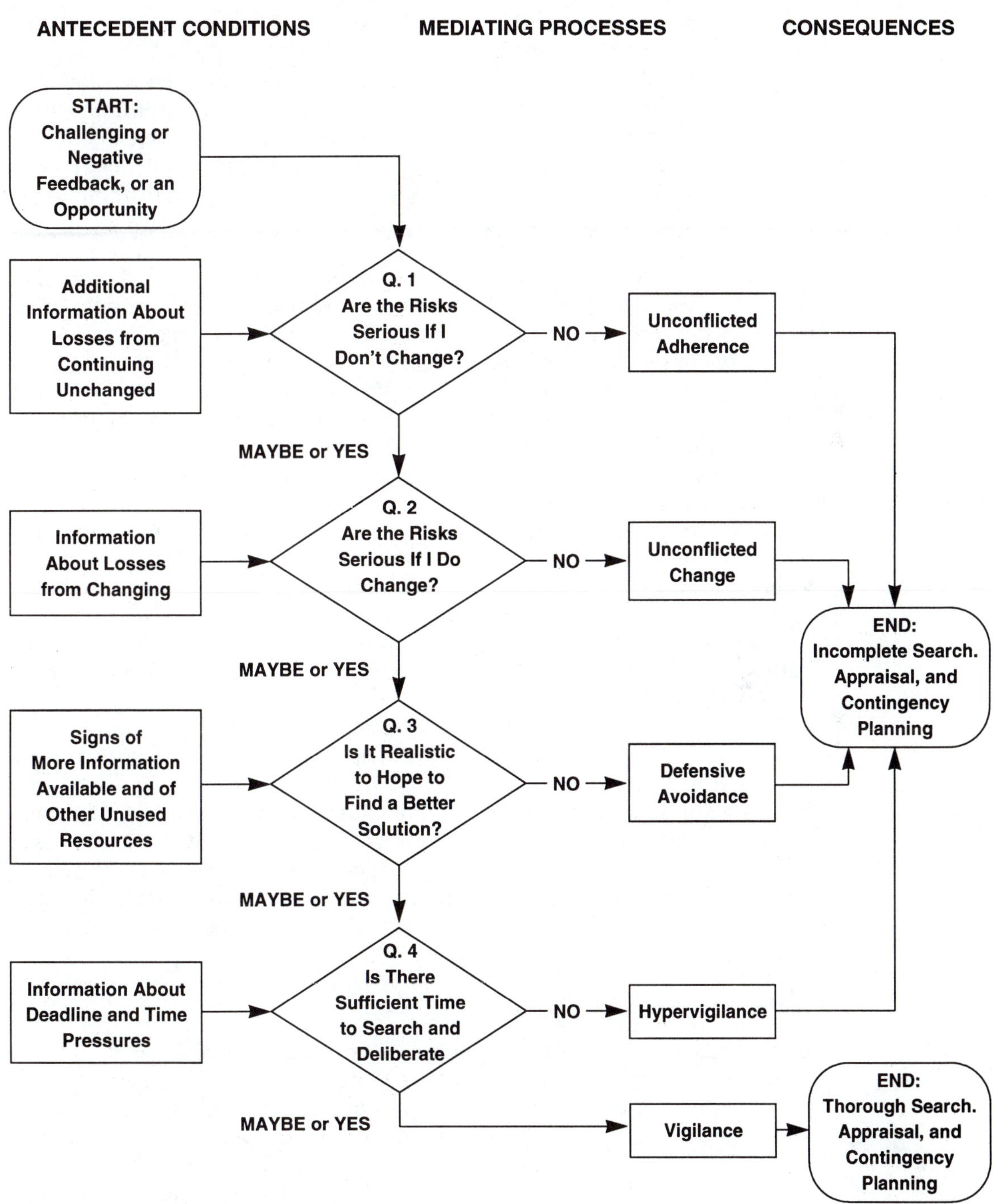

Figure 4-1 Janis-Mann Conflict Model of Decision Making. *From I.L. Janis and L. Mann,* Decision Making: A Psychological Analysis of Conflict, Choice, and Commitment *(New York: The Free Press, a division of Macmillan, Inc., 1977). Reprinted with permission.*

person will fail to make any decision, because he or she is convinced that there is no good choice among the possibilities.

Another consideration is that the decisionmaker may fear the possibility of looking foolish, and as a result lets anxiety get in the way of an appropriate decision. While a little anxiety will enhance decision making, too much anxiety will reduce cognitive functioning and decision-making skills. In a situation such as this, decisionmakers may regress and act on "gut feeling" rather than on a well-thought-out cognitive process.

Another cognitive error that may occur in a stressful situation is when the decisionmaker feels confronted with an either/or decision and loses perspective of other alternatives. This may result in a premature decision that fails to consider other options. In this case, the decisionmaker may be so anxious to bring closure to the crisis that he or she essentially stops dealing with it.

Naturally, the goal is to avoid having to make a crisis decision in the first place. This can often be accomplished by the equivalent of knowing where the fire exits are for every predictable scenario. As mentioned earlier, this knowledge will reduce the number of decisions to be made in a crisis. Have an emergency plan and know it. The manager needs to make sure that the staff also know the plan and test it periodically to see how well the plan will work if needed. But, if the unforeseen does occur, and it sometimes will, the manager should try to avoid making decisions in a vacuum. Check out the options with others, brainstorm where possible, and then *decide.* No decision is often the worst choice.

What's the good news? In an experiment investigating the aftereffects of stress (Schaeffer, 1987), increases in both the use of heuristics and confidence in decisions was noted.

Where there is a lot to lose, merely accepting satisfactory results may be unacceptable (Kleinmuntz, 1991). A simple transcription error may not seem like a big deal, but if that error costs someone's life because of an incorrect medication administration, the results are catastrophic. Research shows that individuals are frequently unaware of their decision errors. Interestingly, Wolfe and Grosch (1990) have demonstrated that correctness of decisions is not significantly related to the amount of confidence individuals place in them. Overconfidence in a person's own decision-making abilities leaves him or her vulnerable to unpleasant consequences.

Vigilant Decision Making

Vigilant decision making occurs when the individual is aware of the seriousness of the decision. In order for this pattern to emerge, the nurse must realize the seriousness of the identified issue, have the appropriate amount of time to analyze all the data, select the solution, and communicate the decision to the appropriate people.

Steven Fink (1986) identifies the concept of "vigilant decision making" (p. 143). Vigilant decision making assumes that the individual has gathered the necessary facts, considered the alternatives, weighed competing interests, and finally made a decision that can be defended. As an example of vigilant decision making, Fink cites President Harry Truman, who once the decision was made to drop the atomic bomb on Hiroshima and Nagasaki, is reported to have never once experienced any post-decisional regret. He had weighed the options and decided. Certainly it was a monumental decision, and whether one agrees or disagrees with the result, Truman obviously was able to make a decision that he could live with.

Unfortunately, vigilant decision making can be maladaptive in situations where split-second decisions are required. However, it does not equate to an obsessional decision-making style. Alternatives cannot be weighed indefinitely, and when the situation calls for a split-second decision, one will need to be able to fast forward the process and make the right decision quickly. A vigilant decision maker will always have a crisis management plan to deal with the unforeseen. The plan may not give the right decision, but, if effective, it will provide some of the answers (e.g., who to call), and therefore will help to reduce the number of decisions to be made and the amount of information needed to process and problem solve.

Complacency

Complacency emerges when the decisionmaker fails to see, or refuses to believe, the warning signs that serious risks are present. The decisionmaker continues with the present course of action, ignoring any information that may be relevant to the decision. An example of this occurs when the nurse fails to notice signs of deterioration in a patient's condition. Decisions are made without regard to information that may have otherwise altered his or her final choice (Wheeler and Janis, 1980).

Defensive Avoidance

Defensive avoidance is the decisionmaker's attempt to avoid or postpone the stress of making decisions. It is manifested by procrastination, shifting of responsibility, or rationalization (Evans, 1990). This type of behavior may be seen when a nurse has been asked by a family member the exact prognosis of a loved one's illness. The nurse may procrastinate and avoid the questions posed by the family or shift the responsibility to the physician. Use of either technique by the nurse solves her decisional dilemma. Procrastination generally reflects a person's unwillingness to make a decision, rather than an inability. Shifting of responsibility is usually followed by rationalization as to why they were unable to make the decision and why it was more appropriate that someone else take care of the problem.

Hypervigilance

Hypervigilance, or panic, represents a frantic search for a solution, and shifting back and forth between alternatives with a failure to see obvious faults in the possible solutions. Panic reactions are most often seen when an individual must make a personal decision after a crisis has passed. An example of this might be when a terrible medication error is made. The nurse must decide what course of action to take. In this situation, the emergence of panic may occur. The nurse, as a decisionmaker, may have impaired cognitive functioning and be unable to see serious faults in possible solutions (Evans, 1990).

Decisions associated with a high level of conflict, uncertainty, and stress are common in the practice of nursing. During their careers, nurses will experience the temptation to adopt avoidance behavior during decision making. Competency develops with experience that refines the decisionmaker's evaluation and interpretative skills. As this competency develops, the stress and conflict associated with decision making will decrease.

OTHER ISSUES

In general, research seems to support the belief that in most situations, groups of five to eleven will outperform individuals in decision-making tasks. However, some exceptions have been noted (Michaelson, Watson, and Black, 1989; Hinsz, 1991):

- Groups tend to be slower than individual decisionmakers
- Individuals tend to generate more creative ideas
- Individuals set more difficult goals than groups

In addition, two dangers exist in group decision processes: individual dominance and groupthink.

Dangers in Individual Decision Making

INDIVIDUAL DOMINANCE

In a group situation, one individual may be dominant because of personality, position, or social status. Typically, the presence **(individual dominance)** of a senior manager will tend to inhibit group discussion, and the advantage of group participation is lost. Group members may conform for the sake of approval and group participation will suffer.

GROUPTHINK

While group cohesiveness may improve group performance, when the desire for uniformity and consensus **(groupthink)** is stronger than the desire for accuracy and correctness, performance will suffer. As evidenced by the space shuttle Challenger disaster, the results can be devastating.

"Best Member"

Yetton and Bottger (1982) identified that an individual **"best member"** may perform as well as a group. In an experiment using the NASA moon survival problem, group members chose a colleague whose solution they agreed to accept as the group decision. This exercise required the group to reach a consensus in attempting to identify its best member. This best-member strategy can equal the performance of an interacting group. When an individual decisionmaker exhibits an expert knowledge base, a best-member strategy can outperform a group decision.

Strengths of Individual Decision Making

No matter how many other people are involved with a decision, eventually it is the individual who must process the information and ultimately make a choice. One strength of individual decision making is that when individual decisions precede a group effort, group performance is enhanced (Miner, 1984).

van Dissel (1986) demonstrated that individual decision making is enhanced when feedback is provided about the relative importance of other preferences of available choices. This finding would seem to suggest that when a decision is required, one would do best to get input from others regarding available options and potential concerns. This is not to suggest that decisions should be made by a committee, but rather that the quality of the decision will generally be superior with more input. There is a risk here, however, that if others are solicited for their opinions and preferences and a decision is made that does not reflect these contributions, great pains should be taken by the individual responsible to explain the reasons behind the final decision. The reality is that it will not always be possible to make a decision to please everyone, but the decisionmaker does have a responsibility to at least consider other opinions and balance the decision accordingly.

WRONG DECISIONS

Even the most carefully considered decision can go wrong. It is important for the decisionmaker to recognize that the particular decision is faulty and avoid the temptation to hang on to that decision. One must accept the losses, analyze the causes, and attempt to regroup. If a particular decision was the result of a multistep process, it is incumbent on the decisionmaker to reverse the process and attempt to identify any missteps. If the decision is completely off base, the decisionmaker may want to totally revise the plan. This may require consultations with others. However, the most important thing to remember is that when a decision goes wrong, one must analyze when, why, and how. This can teach a great deal. Remember, failure often triggers more knowledge than success. By learning from a poor decision, a person will develop the skills and basic trust in him- or herself that is essential for effective decision making.

In addition, there may be times that a decision that was initially well thought out will need to be reconsidered and possibly reversed by a change in circumstances. The change may be sudden or gradual, but it would be inappropriate to hang onto a poor decision in the face of new information because of a fear of "losing face." Consider, as an example, a nurse who initiates a code on an admission, only to be confronted with the information that the patient is a "no code." It would be unconscionable for the nurse to persist in her effort to resuscitate once this fact became known. Don't be afraid to reverse decisions. Remember that while reversing a decision carries a price, so does not reversing. Make the choice that best meets the needs of the situation. Effective decision making is also adaptive (Kaye, 1992).

MONITORING DECISIONS

Once you have made what you consider to be a good decision, remember to monitor the decision over time. You always need to be sensitive to change and new information. Don't assume that the staffing pattern or policy of 1984 will be right for 1995. Be proactive and sensitive to the environment. While you cannot predict the future or eliminate uncertainty, you can monitor your decisions to ensure that they are appropriate for the times. Make it a point to review significant decisions every year and evaluate the effectiveness of these decisions against current needs.

SUMMARY

In an era marked by the quest for continuous quality improvement at decreased cost, decisions will be required at both group and individual levels on an ongoing basis. As Kaye (1992) states: "Decisions simplify life by channeling energies and making you less divided" (p.37). The ability to make good decisions and be flexible when required is critical to the success of every nursing professional. Take the time to develop the necessary skills and courage to be an effective decisionmaker. Ask for advice, but do not feel compelled to accept it. A person needs to feel comfortable with the decision made because ultimately that person is the one who will be held accountable for the outcome.

REFERENCES

Benner, P. (1982, March). From novice to expert. *American Journal of Nursing,* 402–407.

Cassel, R.N. (1973). *The psychology of decision making.* Norwell, MA: The Christopher Publishing House.

Dahlback, O. (1990). Personality and risk-taking. *Personality and Individual Differences, 11*(12), 1235–1242.

Davis, D.L., Grove, S.J., & Knowles, P.A. (1990). An experimental application of personality type as an analogue for decision-making style. *Psychological Reports, 66*(1), 167–175.

Evans, D. (1990). Problems in the decision making process: A review. *Intensive Care Nursing,* 179–184.

Fink, S. (1986). *Crisis Management.* New York: American Management Association.

Harbison, J. (1991). Clinical decision making in nursing. *Journal of Advanced Nursing, 16,* 404–407.

Harrison, F. (1981). *Managerial decision making practices.* Boston: Houghton Mifflin.

Hastie, R. (1991). A review from a high place: The field of judgment and decision making as revealed in its current textbooks. *Psychological Science, 2*(3), 135–138.

Hinsz, V.B. (1991). Individual versus group decision making: Social comparison in goals for individual task performance. *Journal of Applied Social Psychology, 21*(12), 987–1003.

Huckabay, L.M.D. (1986, Spring). Ethical moral issues in nursing practice and decision making. *Nursing Administration Quarterly,* 61–67.

Hunt, R.G., Krzystofiak, F.J., Meindl, J.R., & Yousry, A.M. (1989). Cognitive style and decision making. *Organizational behavior and human decision processes, 44,* 436–453.

Janis, I.L., & Mann, L. (1982). Introduction: Theoretical models and research orientation. In I.L. Janis (Ed.), *Stress attitudes and decisions.* New York: Praeger Publishers.

Janis, I.L. & Mann, L. (1977). *Decision making: A psychological analysis of conflict, choice, and commitment.* New York: The Free Press, a division of Macmillan, Inc.

Jung, C. (1968). *Analytical psychology, its theory and practice.* New York: Vintage Books.

Kahneman, D. (1991). Judgement and decision making: A personal view. *Psychological Science, 2*(3), 142–145.

Kaye, H. (1992). *Decision power. How to make successful decisions with confidence.* Englewood Cliffs, NJ: Prentice Hall.

Kleinmuntz, D.N. (1991). Decision making for professional decision makers. *Psychological Science, 2*(3), 135–141.

MacPhail-Wilcox, B., & Bryant, H.D. (1988). A descriptive model of decision making: Review of idiographic influences. *Journal of Research and Development in Education, 22*(1), 7–22.

Malley, J.C., & Davis, D.L. (1988). Strategic decision making behavior: Aspects of the problem formulation phase. *Journal of Human Behavior and Learning, 5*(2), 44–52.

Michaelsen, L.K., Watson, W.E., & Black, R.H. (1989). A realistic test of individual versus group consensus decision making. *Journal of Applied Psychology, 74*(5), 834–839.

Miner, F.C. (1984). Group vs. individual decision making: An investigation of performance measures, decision strategies and process losses/gains. *Organizational Behavior and Human Performance, 33,* 112–124.

Safire, W., & Safir, L. (1990). Leadership. New York: Simon & Schuster.

Schaeffer, M.H. (1987). Effects of environmental stress on individual decision making [diss]. *DAI, 50,* 2332B.

Stoner, J.A.F., Collins, R.R., & Yetton, P.W. (1985). *Management in Australia.* Englewood Cliffs, NJ: Prentice Hall.

Tversky, A., & Shafir, E. (1992, November). Choice under conflict: The dynamics of deferred decision. *Psychological Science, 3*(6), 358–361.

van Dissel, B.J. (1987). Managing strategic decision processes: The effects of evaluations of interdependence on individual decision-making in organizations [diss]. *DAI, 47,* 3487A.

Wheeler, D.D., & Janis I.L. (1980). *A practical guide for making decisions.* New York: Macmillan.

Wolfe, R.N., & Grosch, J.W. (1990, September). Personality correlates of confidence in one's decisions. *Journal of Personality, 58*(3), 515–534.

Yetton, P.W., & Bottger, P.C. (1982). Individual versus group problem solving: An empirical test of a best member strategy. *Organizational Behavior and Human Performance, 29,* 307–321.

Sandra M. Gomberg
Teresa A. Long

CHAPTER 5

Group Decision Making

Two heads are better than one.
—*Old adage*

INTRODUCTION

A group is a set of two or more people who have come together with a common purpose. Groups use decision making as a vehicle to achieve their goals. The dynamics of group decision making differ from those of making a decision as an individual. These differences can translate into advantages and disadvantages to be considered when planning to form a group (Table 5-1).

Nurses are members of many kinds of groups. A group can be the nurse-patient dyad focusing on discharge teaching. A group is also the collection of nurses working on a particular shift, sharing the patient care needs so that safe care is provided. Or, a group can be nurses within a related specialty, such as cardiology, all of whom share an interest and expertise in caring for this special group of patients. Nurses are usually members of multiple groups.

Nurses are group members for a variety of reasons. Nurses join work groups:

- To obtain financial compensation
- To gain expertise in a given clinical specialty
- To practice theories and skills learned in school
- To provide a service to people in need

THE INDIVIDUAL AS A GROUP MEMBER

Individual members bring different life experiences to the group. Members experience ongoing personal changes as they move through stages of individual psycho-

Table 5-1 • **Advantages and Disadvantages of Groups**
Advantages
• Easy and inexpensive way to share information
• Opportunities for face-to-face communication
• Opportunity to become connected with a social unit
• Promotion of cohesiveness and loyalty
• Access to a larger resource base
• Forum for constructive problem solving
• Support group
• Facilitation of esprit d'corps
• Promotion of ownership of problems and solutions
Disadvantages
• Individual opinions influenced by others
• Individual identity obscured
• Formal and informal role and status positions evolve—hierarchies
• Dependency fostered
• Time consuming
• Inequity of time given to share individual information
• Existence of nonfunctional roles
• Personality conflicts

social growth and development. The developmental levels of individual group members color the overall personality of the group. Group members will assume different roles that are comfortable for their developmental levels as described in Scenario 5-1.

This group as a whole has taken on the predominant characteristics of its members. The majority of nurses in this work group are grappling with the professional developmental challenges associated with trust and autonomy. Using Erikson's

Scenario 5-1

A new 48-bed surgical unit opens at a large urban teaching hospital. At the end of its first year, 55 percent of the staff have graduated from nursing school within the last 18 months. Many of these newer professional nurses are just beginning to define their professional identities and roles. Many feel confused and indecisive in the face of challenges questioning their authority. For example, the patient still experiencing severe pain three days postoperatively may not have her pain medication adjusted if the nurse feels intimidated and does not appropriately approach the attending physician to question the treatment plan.

stages of human psychosocial development, parallels can be drawn between the nurses' behavior and their ability to make quality decisions on behalf of the patient.

New graduates demonstrate a taking-in phase consistent with Erikson's first two stages of development: trust versus mistrust, and autonomy versus shame and doubt. Scenario 5-2 describes the reactions of a new graduate. The first stage is concerned with acquiring a sense of basic trust while overcoming a sense of mistrust (Whaley and Wong, 1987). Acquiring this trust promotes a feeling of security that allows a person to experience unfamiliar situations with minimum fear. In Erikson's second stage, a toddler has the need for self-esteem and autonomy while overcoming a sense of shame and doubt (Whaley and Wong, 1987). He is relinquishing his dependence on others. Technical mastery of basic nursing tasks precedes psychosocial mastery over self-control, will power, and the ability to make independent, accurate decisions in the face of inconsistencies.

Scenario 5-2

A nurse on a busy inner-city postpartum unit feels confused and angry as she discharges newborn infants to adolescent mothers who have limited social support. She begins to offer her home phone number to those mothers with whom she relates best. The nurse is struggling with her feelings of concern for others and defining limits within professional relationships. She has not mastered these feelings or the sophistication of initiating the appropriate community referrals to best support these mothers and their new babies.

Young and middle adulthood, according to Erikson's generativity versus stagnation stage, focuses on creation and care of the next generation (Whaley and Wong, 1987). Nourishing and nurturing behaviors are key, as individuals keenly demonstrate concern for life. Frustration arises when a person is unable to separate personal cultural norms and healthy relationships from professional cultural norms and patient interactions, such as is demonstrated in the scenario above.

In any potential group of nurses, there are innumerable possible combinations of individual personalities and stages of development. Every group, then, will approach decision-making opportunities with different abilities and potentials. Successful group decision making is linked to the recognition of the group's identity and readiness to define its purpose, begin and complete its work, and evaluate the work before moving on.

GROUP PROCESS

Group process is making a dynamic series of decisions and it refers to the changes and decisions that occur within the group as the members work together to achieve goals. In order for the group to move forward productively, the following must be defined:

- How problems are identified
- How goals are met

- How work is accomplished
- How work is evaluated
- How feedback is shared (Walch and Bernhard, 1990)

Nurses experience this process as members interact, allowing group integrity and identity to unfold. This interaction occurs only as a result of the members' participation in a series of decisions consistent with the group's purpose and goals. Group process is often more quickly negotiated with a small group such as the nurse-patient dyad (Walch and Bernhard, 1990).

The nurse-patient dyad begins formally by assignment rather than by choice. Questions and answers characterize the early stages of this group development. The nurse utilizes expert assessment skills to direct clinical decisions, such as obtaining a blood pressure when the patient reports dizziness with a change in her position. Together the group members, the nurse and the patient, must come to agreement on a plan to assure this patient's safety. The joint decision is made that the patient will remain in bed and call the nurse for assistance when desiring to get out of bed. The patient has a call bell and will decide when to activate the plan. The nurse understands her role in the decided plan and responds promptly to the call bell.

Nurses face challenges when in larger groups with complex goals. Agreement on the purpose and goals of the group is a greater struggle when multiple members are involved. Even after the goal of the group is clear, other difficulties will emerge that do not have anything to do directly with the real work of the group. The issues that will surface are related to how members interact, communicate, and behave as individuals, and together as a group.

The group process is directly characterized by the developmental level obtained by the group as a whole. As individuals move through stages of growth and development, so do groups. The group's ability to make quality productive decisions is directly related to the group's stage of development. A variety of theories describe group development.

OERMANN'S MODEL

Oermann (1991) describes a model of group development that includes three stages: the orientation stage, the working stage, and the termination stage.

Orientation Stage

The orientation stage is an awkward period of introduction of the group members. There is uncertainty about expectations or norms. The choice of norms identified by the group leads to the success or failure of the group's work. The essential work of the group at this stage is deciding on the expectations for group membership. Decisions made during times of stress and uncertainty are often inconsistent and in the best interest of a few, not all, group members.

The orientation stage progresses until norms are defined. The norms adopted by the group can be supportive to the achievement of the goals of the group. Conversely, the chosen norms could serve as restrictions that will delay group decision making (Loomis, 1979). The leadership within the group must offer guidance to assure group norms enable the group to meet its goals (Oermann, 1991).

Scenario 5-3

Two nurses who formerly worked on an adult surgical unit are hired to work on the pediatrics unit. The two new nurses are buddied with two senior nurses for their orientation. The new nurses are nervous about caring for this different patient population. During their first two weeks of orientation, they seem tentative while giving physical care and medications to their patients.

In the next two weeks, the senior nurses develop an action plan to help the new nurses become more comfortable with the "norms" for these patients. Written nursing care standards for each patient's diagnosis are shared with the new nurses and reviewed immediately after shift change report is received, before they begin their work for the day. Proper medication dosages are reviewed before administration.

Working Stage

In the working stage, group process intensifies. Relationships between group members are solidified and cooperation results. The group is now able to articulate its goals and form smaller work groups to get the work done. Differences in ideas and opinions of group participants can spark conflict. Decision making is directed at conflict resolution. Conflict can develop between members as the work group delegates and evaluates assigned work projects. Additionally, decisions made may not be the choice of all, but will be the choice of the majority or by consensus. Most of the group's work will be done in this stage.

Scenario 5-4

In the second month of orientation, after each shift change report, the new nurses verbally share their plan of care for the day with the senior nurse, outlining specific short- and long-term goals for their patients. Before administering each medication, the new nurses also state the purpose and normal dosage for each drug. The new nurses are no longer working in a "buddy system" where they are totally dependent on the senior nurses. Instead, the patient assignment is altered to value the contribution of the new nurses. Each new nurse will have three patients, and the senior nurse will have two patients, but will lend guidance as necessary. This shift in assignment will maximize the autonomy of the new nurses while recognizing the support that they still need.

Termination Stage

As the group reaches the termination stage, trust, cooperation, and respect are maximized (Oermann, 1991). The group comes together to acknowledge the completion of its assigned task and, at times, allows for evaluation of its efforts. Oermann (1991) notes that the termination stage is managed differently by each individual experiencing the transition. The opportunity to fully process the closure of group relationships provides the reinforcement needed by members as they move on to other groups.

Scenario 5-5

At the end of the two-month orientation, the new nurses are independently giving physical care and medications to a district of five patients. The senior nurses recognize the successful assimilation of the new nurses into the work group. Orientation is formally completed after the nurse manager meets in conference with each new nurse and senior nurse. At this time, closure is brought to the orientee-preceptor relationship. During the conference, future goals are identified and plans are made for the new nurses to move to night shift where they will begin to find places in a new work group.

TUCHMAN AND JENSEN'S MODEL

Gillies (1989) summarizes Tuchman and Jensen's five stages of group development: forming, storming, norming, performing, and adjourning.

Forming

The forming stage is characterized by the members' entrance into the group and the realization of what contributions group membership demands and what rewards are available (Gillies, 1989).

Scenario 5-6

As two new professional nurses are hired to the night shift, the work group will take on a new appearance. The new staff members have ten years' prior experience in adult surgical nursing, and have opted to move into the pediatric specialty. The manager tells her staff how lucky they are to add such mature staff to their shift group. The night shift was anxious to have the vacancies filled, yet reluctantly welcomed these two new nurses.

Storming

The storming stage signals imbalance as members move to gain position and power among a variety of interpersonal styles. These intragroup challenges force emotions to surge. During this stage, the integrity of the work group is in chaos.

Scenario 5-7

Silently threatened by the past experience of their new colleagues, the night shift nurse members begin to vie for position as shift leader and expert. Hostility runs high and the new staff report to the manager that they are being unfairly tested. During this time, even common decisions, such as assigning admissions, often end in conflict. The new staff hesitate to ask questions for fear of reprisal. The original staff hesitate to include the new staff in problem-solving sessions, since "they aren't pediatric nurses anyway."

Norming

Resolution demands that the group move into the norming stage. In this stage, members recognize that cooperation is essential for the welfare of the patients and for the success of the work group. Rules are defined and understandings are reached by members. Individuals begin to abandon selfish disagreements in the best interest of the group at large. Order is obtained and decisions are made and supported by the group members.

Scenario 5-8

The manager seeks out her longevity night shift staff. She shares her perception of poor cohesion among the night shift and offers her support to resolve the conflicts. The staff minimizes the manager's concerns and assures her that all is well. Together, though, they realize that the disruption within the group is impacting on the unit as a whole and on patient care.

The two new nurses complete orientation and, surprisingly, the night shift hosts a small party for them. The staff begin to joke and laugh while sharing in the festivities. During the next few weeks, the clinical decisions reflect cohesion and cooperation. The decision to identify to whom admissions would be assigned occurs without conflict. The night shift staff is now perceived as a connected group able to make productive decisions and provide quality patient care.

Performing

Once cooperation is achieved, the group must be able to channel its efforts to assure the work output is completed properly. The performing stage boasts collective efforts to solve problems and complete the workload (Gillies, 1989). Peer-to-peer support is evident as the group undertakes its work with a sense of mission and purpose (Gillies, 1989). Group members who make decisions in the performing stage are now able to fully execute these decisions to achieve the group's desired goal.

Scenario 5-9

The pediatric unit has begun to admit pediatric oncology patients. While many of the senior pediatric nurses have been certified to administer the chemotherapy medications, there is high anxiety about using central venous lines. The two new nurses, though, have had extensive experience with central venous lines in the adult population. Together, this group decides to pool their collective skills to assure these special patients receive expert care. They are then able to share their efforts with the nursing staff from the other shifts. The decision-making ability of the group has strengthened the standard of care for the pediatric oncology patients who require the placement of a central line.

Adjournment

The final stage is adjournment, where group members recognize that their task is completed. Members begin to separate psychologically from each other and begin to seek other opportunities for relationships (Gillies, 1989). In nursing, true adjournment is not realized consistently. More often, group members proceed through these stages at various points in the group's existence.

Nursing groups constantly gain and lose members, so groups may experience one or possibly all five stages of group development. However, as the integrity of the group changes, the group may not experience the stages in the exact order as described above.

In the case of the nurse-patient dyad, nurses regularly bring closure to this relationship when the patient is discharged. Nurses often participate in many dyad relationships at one time, all of which are at different stages of development. The decisions made during the nurse-patient relationship are oftentimes sensitive. The nurse-patient group will ideally move through these stages so that the performing stage is reached prior to discharge and a forced adjournment. Failure to do so leaves both group members frustrated and less willing or able to reenter a similar relationship.

The nurse's larger professional group memberships, such as the nursing unit or shift, do not realize true adjournment unless they leave the unit for an alternative position. Within the larger group, smaller subsets of colleagues will connect for a special purpose, such as developing standards of care or serving in a preceptor-orientee relationship. When these special tasks are completed, members return to the aggregate until a new purpose is identified and a new subset of group members connect.

Success in moving through these stages of group development reinforces the power of cohesive decision making. Positive decision-making outcomes facilitate timely adjournment of a work group, whether a dyad or larger. Feedback about well-made decisions supports individuals to promptly seek out new collaborative opportunities with fresh energy and intention. The experience of successful decision making facilitates future movement through the early stages of group formation.

THE COMMITTEE AS A GROUP

A **committee** is a type of group that comes together solely to achieve a predetermined goal. Usually membership is voluntary and participation is compelled by personal interest in achieving a goal. Committees vary greatly in size and longevity. Committees take many different names. The type of committee, goal, structure, and purpose is related to its type of membership and anticipated duration.

The decision-making tasks of the committee can appear overwhelming. A planned approach for discussion can be helpful as group leaders guide members through the agenda. Groups will choose an approach best suited to the nature of their pending tasks and timeframe for completion.

Loomis (1979) notes that the decision-making work of the group will be accomplished through either a content-focused or process-focused approach. In the **content-focus alternative,** the group centers on the specific detail of the topic under discussion. A group of fifty staff nurses attempting to choose a method for requesting schedule changes and a holiday rotation plan may utilize a content-focused approach. The group's discussions would be characterized by listing the major facts related to the topic. Issues such as seniority status, the number of holidays in question, and past practices that worked and did not work would be reviewed. By utilizing this approach, the group would try to reveal the issues of greatest concern to the members. Open forums, impromptu gatherings, and brainstorming sessions would be common. Numerous staff would verbalize their opinions before a decision was finally reached.

A **process approach** emphasizes how the topic will be discussed. The same group of nurses could opt for a more process-oriented approach. Discussion would then center around the manner in which the points of concern would be addressed. Agendas would be clear at scheduled meetings. Leaders would surface as they planned, presented, and supported ideas. Separate task forces would evolve with the charge to refine the options that will be brought before the group as a whole.

SUMMARY

Groups are dynamic subsets of people that move through developmental stages similar to those of the individual members. Groups exist to maximize resources and strengths to achieve outcomes. Decision making is the vehicle that individuals and groups use to narrow down options and make choices. Successful decision making is dependent on the group's ability to perform together in a productive way. The type and quality of decision making is related to the developmental level of the group as a whole.

Nurses are members of many different types of groups simultaneously. Each nurse brings a unique perspective to each group in which she participates simply by virtue of her life experiences and personal developmental level.

Nurses need to recognize that there are advantages and disadvantages to decision making in groups. Failure as well as success in decision making must be recognized and examined in the context of group development. Implementing a variety of approaches to decision making leads to productive group work efforts and to personal growth. These experiences set the foundation for nurses to feel motivated to enter groups and to utilize creative decision-making strategies in the future.

REFERENCES

Gillies, D.A. (1989). *Nursing management, a systems approach* (pp. 196–197). Philadelphia: W.B. Saunders Co.

Loomis, M. (1979). *Group process for nurses.* St. Louis: C.V. Mosby.

Oermann, M.H. (1991). *Professional nursing practice: A conceptual approach* (pp. 77–85). Philadelphia: J.B. Lippincott Co.

Walch, M., & Bernhard, L.A. (1990). *Leadership—the key to professional nursing* (pp. 23–31). St. Louis: C.V. Mosby.

Whaley, L.F., & Wong, D.L. (1987). *Nursing care of infants and children* (p. 114). St. Louis: C.V. Mosby.

Ellie Mack

CHAPTER 6

The Effects of Cultural Factors

It's O.K. to be different.

—*Anonymous*

INTRODUCTION

Anthropology has not historically been emphasized in professional nurse prepara tion programs. As a science, anthropology assesses the origin of mankind; its physical, moral, and intellectual development; varieties of cultures; and customs and beliefs. Anthropologists "use the term culture as a broad, integrating rubric to cover values, techniques, life plans, ways of doing. . ., and other basic beliefs, practices, goals and concerns of a social group" (Jameton, 1990, p. 443). People gradually learn of their culture as infants and children, consistently growing to reveal it in a variety of ways. An individual's culture can be readily revealed in conduct, gestures, and preferred terminology of expression. An individual's culturalization represents his or her ethnicity, geographical location, gender, and morality. This chapter will cover the pertinence of issues associating culturalism to nursing practice, in general, and decision making specifically.

The process models described in Chapter 1 (Table 1-1) are adaptable to all situations associated with the diversities of culturalism in nursing decision making at management, unit staff, and patient levels.

The need for the integration of a transcultural component into nursing practice has been recognized as cultural diversity has increased. Certainly, the relationship of cultural and ethnic differences within nursing practice is without dispute. The way we interpret events and issues is central to our culturalization. "Culture goes beyond beliefs and values to include the nature of relationships among those in the culture" (Jameton, 1990, p. 445). Many people void of cultural association with one another share like beliefs. Sometimes the similar beliefs are characteristic of unidentified current or historical social relationships shared in common.

The focus of decision making in nursing integrates the appropriate action in a particular situation to the role and realm of responsibility of the professional nurse. Reference to the code of ethics for nurses states "The nurse provides services with respect for human dignity and the uniqueness of the client, unrestricted by consideration of social or economic status, personal attributes, or the nature of the health problems" (American Nurses Association, 1989, p. 2).

As the proliferation of cultural diversity continues in the United States, nurses must accept the challenge to accelerate all efforts toward the achievement of the goals written into the Code of Ethics for Nurses. Culturalization, a common characteristic in many encounters with patients and families, ultimately affects the treatment plan and overall care. Thus, nurses must remember to invite patients and families to openly communicate any culturally associated needs they may have.

In response to the nursing shortage of the 1980s, many hospital nursing departments expanded their recruitment efforts nationally and abroad. As a result, applicants from all backgrounds applied for the numerous positions, and a multicultured nursing staff was created, particularly in the larger cities. An awareness and appreciation of culturally associated beliefs and practices within a nursing community can serve to strengthen the community's collaborative efforts. The knowledge of cultural variables stands to positively influence working relationships. Job satisfaction and effective care delivery through cooperative team efforts are outcomes. Conversely, a lack of cultural awareness may undermine the ability of the nursing community to assert the group process so vital to some situations in nursing. Consider an American nurse serving as orientation mentor to a newly hired nurse of Asian descent. Direct eye contact in the Asian culture represents a sign of disrespect. The American nurse, unaware of this cultural phenomena, may interpret the nurse's looking in another direction as a sign of disinterest.

GENDER AS A CULTURE

Our assessment of the variety of cultures interacting within the field of nursing begins with gender itself as a culture as described in Scenario 6-1. In every known society, **gender** is a fundamental criterion for assigning tasks considered necessary for the well-being and continuity of the individual, family, and community. Some tasks are assigned primarily on the basis of sex-linked physiological differences, for example, only females can nurse the young; only males are strong enough to perform certain kinds of heavy work. Norms pertinent to the roles and status of the two sexes penetrate every sector of life and may well outlast other types of social differentiation more thoroughly explored by sociologists.

In consideration of interactions between male and female nurses of western cultures, there is a potential for conflict without attention devoted to accepted male-female strategies for successful negotiations. Women due to their intuitive nature are viewed as better listeners and far more sympathetic than men. Generally, women begin their socialization as sympathizers and care providers from birth. They are presented with dolls to "care for," and are told "don't fight with your brother or friends, it's not ladylike." Compromise is fostered and rewarded. Women learn to approach negotiations with minimal combative confrontation. They search for middle-ground solutions agreeable to all individuals involved. Over time, a **"win-win" strategy** evolves. Women are socialized to compromise with the goal to satisfy all parties as much as possible.

Conversely, men are socialized to behave like men. That behavior includes "fighting back," "standing up for themselves," and not backing down. Over time, they develop a competition-oriented approach to negotiations, and a **"win-lose" strategy** evolves. There exists no visible middle ground. You either win or you lose.

Nursing requires a negotiated compromise in many instances. Initially, there may exist an advantage for women in the profession; however, an awareness of the gender culture can foster the necessary adjustments in male attitudes and behavior to enhance female nurse–male nurse cooperative interaction(s).

Scenario 6-1

I recall a situation occurring in an orthopedic unit where a very long-term patient had progressed to wheelchair transportation when it became necessary for him to go to other departments for X-rays or other services. This patient asked a female nurse, not his usual nurse, to see if he could get permission to sit with his wife outside on the hospital lawn for lunch. The hospital policy did not encourage this activity on a daily basis. However, the nurse, empathizing with the patient's situation, went through the appropriate channels of administration and obtained physician's orders to honor the patient's request. The patient and his wife were very appreciative and enjoyed the experience immensely. However, the covering nurse was not aware that this patient's usual nurse, a male, had informed the patient on two previous occasions that hospital policy did not permit hospitalized patients on the grounds. When the male nurse, on his return, heard his patient applaud the covering nurse's efforts, he become very angry and conflict between the two nurses ensued.

In this situation, both nurses behaved in a professional manner with the patient; however, the female nurse demonstrated empathy of greater depth and responded accordingly. The two nurses were able to eventually resolve their conflict; however, it did require extensive intervention from nursing management.

THE INFLUENCE OF CULTURALISM ON COMMUNICATION STYLE

An individual's cultural norms strongly influence consideration of personal as opposed to group interest in decision making. In a study of the cross-cultural differences in the use of decision rules, Mann and Radford (1985) define **collectivism** and **individualism** in societies. Collectivistic societies promote group harmony, in contrast to individualistic societies where greater interest is placed on individual rights, contributions, and compensation. Achievement, self-sufficiency, competition, and autonomy are meaningful to people of individualistic societies, whereas interpersonal harmony dominates in a collectivistic society.

Leung and Lind (1986) found that Asian and South American countries have collectivistic cultures, whereas English-speaking and European countries have individualistic cultures. In an example of decision making for the purpose of patient assignments, Jein and Harris (1989) noted that American nurse managers frequently assigned the more difficult patients to international nurses. Jein and Harris concluded that American nurse managers perceived international nurses as more cooperative and loyal than American nurses. The international nurse resents being given the heavier assignment; however, she will not demand fair treatment because of her collectivistic orientation. Yet, the perception of unfair treatment may contribute to a high turnover rate.

In Table 6-1, high turnover rate, decreased communication, and international

***Table 6-1* • Process Outline Relating to Problem of Increased Nursing Unit Turnover Rate**

Step I Problem Identification	a. High turnover rate of nursing staff b. Minimal management ⟷ staff communication c. Minimal staff ⟷ staff communication d. International nurses' resentment of assignment pattern
Step II Seeking Alternatives	1. a. Promotion of management ⟷ staff communication b. Promotion of staff ⟷ staff communication c. Management assessment of nursing staff job satisfaction d. Assess nursing staff input to balancing assignments 2. a. Maintain status quo of high turnover rate
Step III Selecting Workable Alternatives	1. a., b., c., d. (from seeking alternatives *Step II*)
Step IV Implement Selected Alternatives	Occurs almost simultaneously with *Step III*
Step V Solution Evaluation	Success determined by: a. Reduced nursing turnover rate b. Increasing nurse job satisfaction

nurse resentment represent Step I, problem identification for the decision-making process.

Table 6-1 highlights potential and selected alternatives with the potential solution of reduced nursing turnover. In this instance, a lack of cultural sensitivity to the international nurses' collectivistic socialization promoted an inappropriate decision of patient assignment. Collectivistic behavior is driven by environmental and personal harmony. Nurses socialized and trained in this manner may refrain from potential conflictive situations, even if the purpose is geared toward the resolution of conflict. While some individualistic American nurses will thrive on environments of challenge, achievement, and autonomy, the collectivistic international nurse will endure situations even though he or she may feel personally offended by them. Educating nurse managers to individual cross-cultural norms could facilitate eradication of this common scenario.

Kohls (1987) identified education, training, orientation, and briefing as the key factors associated with intercultural relationship preparedness. The key element in the process would be identifying the cultural variations associated with behaviors of cultural diversities by communicating with the constituents.

Situations are managed differently with consideration to cultural orientations. A professional nurse of western culture, driven by achievement orientation, may clinically work harder, volunteer for extra duties and advance educationally with a goal of promotion from a staff nursing level position to a position in management or advanced clinical practice. A nurse of eastern culture may derive satisfaction in a primary nurse position for an extended time period without assertion towards procuring a position of advancement.

There also exists a culturally oriented difference in the context level of language. A knowledge of language context has been identified to strengthen communications between nurses at all levels. Becker (1986) expressed high-context communications as originating from stable communities that have basically remained identical over many generations. Within these communities, much of the nonverbal (high-context) communication is a result of a type of intuition of a telepathic nature (Becker, 1986). In contrast, the low-context communication style utilizes far more words with very detailed explanation of meaning. Western cultures use low-context communication, Easterners high-context. Understanding the differences in communication styles could possibly prevent the conflict of misunderstandings that result from the migration of low-context individuals, western cultures, to high-context communities, eastern cultures, and vice versa.

Conflicts may occur when nurses speaking in a high-context language unknowingly fail to express themselves clearly enough to nurses speaking in low-context language. Consider a low-context nurse, following the change of shift report, deciding her district patient care assignment and prioritizing her initial patient care activities based on an insufficient information exchange. A nursing staff with a mix of high- and low-context communicators would stand to benefit from an orientation on:

- The components of both communication styles
- An introduction to realistic methods of adaptation to promote unit harmony

Understandably, this training could benefit nurse-to-patient interactions as well.

THE CULTURE OF NURSING

Joyce Fitzpatrick, a nurse, reflects on the culture of nursing. She states

> . . . my nursing concern for the whole person led me to be concerned about all people in all situations . . . human issues and concerns have been dominant factors in all aspects of my decision making . . . How can we possibly measure tangible outcomes of what we do and experience in our professional nurses' roles? (Fitzpatrick, 1991, p. 1).

The decision to spend additional time with the frightened child being prepared for surgery, the decision to embrace the young woman following another failed invitro fertilization attempt, the decision to sit silently with the young man recently informed of a cancer diagnosis are all inherent to who we are as nurses. Though we all have personal issues to deal with, the culture of nursing adopts a caring, empathetic, sharing, and resourcefulness beyond the capacity of many other professions.

CULTURALISM AND NURSING ADMINISTRATION

Transcultural knowledge enhances the provision of nursing care and building of unit nursing staffs in our multicultural society. The nurse manager's awareness of his or her staff's cultural concepts will facilitate more efficient management of cultural diversities within a unit. The recognition of cultural diversities will prepare nurse managers to acknowledge and intercept ensuing conflict prior to its snowballing into major disputes.

Nursing administrators at all levels should be knowledgeable about concepts of culturalism and also alternative methods of dispute resolution based on the cultural preparedness of involved staff members.

Felstiner, Abel, and Austin (1981) identify a mechanism to assess the dispute process in involved individuals. They propose the existence of a process of transformation, naming four steps in this process. The first step is **naming**—a recognition that an experience is injurious; the second step is **blaming**—the placing of the fault of the injury on another person; and the third step is **claiming**—when the perceived injured individual(s) asks for an action of remediation; the fourth step is **transformation**—the rejection of a claim resulting in probable legal action. Perhaps, cultural training can facilitate conflict resolution prior to progression through the fourth step of transformation (Felstiner et al., 1981).

The dispute process steps outlined in Table 6-2 are evident in the following scenario.

Staff involvement in the problem-solving process would have strengthened the unity of staff, expanded the base of creative ideas, and improved morale.

Table 6-2 • Organized Steps in Dispute Process Resulting from Change in Assignment

Step I	
Naming	Unintentional heavier assignments to Latino nursing assistants
Step II	
Blaming	Assignment of perceived "discrimination" to the practice
Step III	
Claiming	Developing conflict between nursing administration and nursing assistants with LPN's caught in center of the dispute
Step IV	
Transformation	Nursing assistants resorting to legal action

Adapted from W.L.F. Felstiner, R.L. Abel, & S. Austin, The Emergence and Transformation of Disputes: Naming, Blaming, Claiming. *Law Soc Revised, 15(3–4), 631–654.*

Scenario 6-2

A small private suburban nursing home had clients from middle-class professional backgrounds ranging in age from 65 to 103. The care providers were predominantly Latino nursing assistants with a few Anglo licensed practical nurses (LPNs). Nursing administration was aware of the inability of some younger residents to understand the Latino-Americans because of their accents. Nursing administration made the decision to redirect assignments of the younger residents to the LPNs and the older, less communicative residents to the nursing assistants. Understandably, the older residents required far more physical care then the younger residents. The Latino assistants interpreted the action as a practice of discrimination against them and sought legal action through their union representation.

Of course, as negotiations progressed, the rationale behind the change in assignment surfaced. Consider some possible alternative administrative approaches to this conflict. A less complicated approach may have been to inform the nursing assistants and LPNs of the problem and to invite their involvement in the solution. A simple solution may have been to direct the nursing assistants to speak slower: They were fluent in speaking English and the problem in understanding only occurred when they spoke rapidly.

HOSPITAL CULTURE

Hospitals as institutions also develop a culture. Individuals draw conclusions and expectations about an organization from an understanding gained from prior personal or learned experiences. In general, a society perceives hospitals to be places where people go when ill to get better, with the role of hospital personnel to facilitate patients' recovery. Multiple cultural factors will dictate the occurrences within a hospital.

The culture of surrounding communities will considerably influence patient care, for example, in western culture, hospital personnel, particularly nurses, are expected to provide the major part of overall patient care, even in instances where family members are present and have experience providing care for the patient in the home environment. In contrast, many eastern cultures hold expectations that family members will significantly share in the physical care of patients within the constraints of their ability to do so. Migrating nurses, oriented within an eastern culture without proper orientation to the western-style hospital culture, will consistently have conflicts with family members, who will perceive them as being neglectful and uncaring of a hospitalized family member's physical needs.

A patient's and family's understanding of health and illness strongly influences their health beliefs and associated behavior. A study was conducted to evaluate the importance of a family assessment for hospitalized immigrants with the following findings:

- Italian families perceived the hospital as a place to die and expressed mistrust of healthcare providers while maintaining a vigil around hospitalized relative(s)
- Greek families viewed illness requiring hospitalization as a "punishment," particularly if the family member had a cancer diagnosis, with expectations for healthcare professionals to provide immediate relief from illness
- Chinese families viewed health as holistic without separation of the physical, psychological, and social entities of being (Boston, 1992)

Nursing knowledge of a patient's cultural beliefs, values, and systems of support relative to hospitalization will ultimately result in a care plan that is culturally sensitive and relative to the patients and family members.

Physician-patient-family interrelationships can also be culturally driven. Western-style doctors, from experience, are generally expected to spend minimal time explaining treatment plans and answering questions. They prescribe treatments, multiple medications, and rely on surgery and highly sophisticated technology to facilitate care. In contrast, eastern-style doctors are known to spend extended time periods with patients, explaining the origin of illness and treatment regime rationale, answering questions, and prescribing herbs and dietary change regimes. Physicians become aware of patients' expectations and tend to respond accordingly. The clinical reality this negotiates between physicians, patients, and families has been well documented in numerous societies (Kleinman, 1975).

The social implication of diversities within the multicultural mix of U.S. society impacts on nursing in general, and nurse-nurse and patient-nurse interactions specifically. The challenge of providing culturally sensitive nursing requires awareness of the culturally diverse issues. Effective strategies must be developed to provide care and accomplish the goal of maximized health and wellness and illness prevention in client populations. A careful observation of culture can prepare nurses to make intelligent decisions and propose new solutions to the many issues that we face.

As hospital nursing departments and patient populations continue to represent diversity, nursing must aim to improve the preparation process by teaching and fostering the understanding of multicentric variations, including the lifestyles of involved ethnic groups. Awareness of the differences and increased communication skills can serve to enhance cooperative nursing care decisions.

An interesting approach has been documented to amplify awareness of cultural diversity and experiences. Some nursing programs have included international and transcultural experiences within program curricula (MacAvoy, 1988; Macey and Morgan, 1988). Some of these programs are successful because they allow students to recognize their individual tendencies toward ethnocentrism. Once the student has developed an awareness of his or her ethnocentrism, then exposure to international cultures is provided. Students are afforded the opportunity to compare multivariant beliefs and attitudes from the various cultures.

Recognizing the potential benefit of a transcultural experience in nursing, students from the University of Delaware were provided the opportunity to participate in a program to "acquire first hand knowledge of another health care system, and also to observe the significant difference between nursing in the United States in comparison to nursing in other countries" (Beeman, 1991). The students articulated a greater understanding of what cultural associations existed in nursing. Students gained an expanded acceptance of themselves as nurse professionals (Beeman, 1991).

SUMMARY

The influence of culture on decision making in nursing, traditionally not addressed, must become more integrated on campus and throughout the nurse's professional experience. The diversity of a student body stands indicative of alternative approaches to building an effective community of education and experience.

REFERENCES

American Nurses Association. (1989). *Code for nurses with interpretive statements.* Kansas City: Author.

Beeman, P.B. (1991, February). Nursing education, practice and professional identity: A transcultural course in England. *Journal of Nursing Education, 30*(2), 63–68.

Becker, C.B. (1986). Reasons for the lack of argumentation and debate in the Far East. *International Journal of Intercultural Relations,* 75–92.

Boston, P. (1992). Understanding cultural differences through family assessment. *Journal of Cancer Education, 4*(3), 261–266.

Felstiner, W.L.F., Abel, R.L., & Austin, S. (1981). The emergence and transformation of disputes: Naming, blaming, claiming. *Law Soc Revised, 15*(3–4), 631–654.

Fitzpatrick, J. (1991). The culture of nursing. *Applied Nursing Research, 4*(1), 1.

Jameton, A. (1990, September). Culture, morality and ethics: Twirling the spindle. *Critical Care Nursing Clinics of North America, 2*(3), 443–451.

Jein, R.F., & Harris, B.L. (1989, June). Cross-cultural conflict: The American nurse manager and a culturally mixed staff. *Journal of the New York State Nurses Association, 20*(2), 16–19.

Kleinman, A.M. (1975). Explanatory models in health care relationships. *Health of the Family.* National Council for International Health Symposium. Washington, DC: NCIH, 159–172.

Kohls, L.R. (1987). Four traditional approaches to developing cross-cultural preparedness in adults: Education, training, orientation and briefing. *International Journal of Intercultural Relations, 11*(1), 89–106.

Leung, K., & Lind, E.A. (1986). Procedural justice and culture: Effects of culture, gender, and investigator status on procedural preferences. *Journal of Personality and Social Psychology, 50*(6), 1134–1140.

MacAvoy, S. (1988). A transcultural learning opportunity: USSR 1985. *The Journal of Continuing Education in Nursing, 19,* 196–200.

Macey, J.C., & Morgan, S.A. (1988). Learning on the road: Nursing in the British Isles and Ireland. *Nursing Outlook, 36,* 40–41.

Mann, L., & Radford, M. (1985). Cross-culture differences in children's use of decision rules: A comparison. *Journal of Personalized and Social Psychology, 49,* 1557–1564.

Patricia Hentz Becker

CHAPTER 7

Ethical Decision Making: The Morally Reflective Practitioner

What is the right thing to do?
–*Anonymous*

INTRODUCTION

Ethical decision making is the *process* of decision making, including the knowledge sphere, ethics. This process is comprised of resolving a problematic area, a situation of major concern, and/or a dilemma at hand. Thus, the decision-making process is a common one, found in any problematic situation. However, the difference lies in which details are important. Ethical situations are guided by knowledge of ethics, just as medical decisions are guided by medical knowledge. Determining which knowledge domain to draw upon requires sensitivity to the situation. Moral sensitivity is a sensitivity to the details of a situation, raising such questions as: What is right and good? Just and fair? Are we respecting this individual's human dignity? What are the benefits and burdens in this situation?

By its very nature, ethical decision making is a complex and multifaceted process nested within a social context. Factors included in the ethical analysis include: ethics, social/interactional aspects, and situational/contextual factors. The morally reflective practitioner needs to be aware how each of these areas impacts on decision making. Figure 7-1 is an illustration of the awareness spheres relevant in ethical decision making. The morally reflective practitioner attends to these awareness spheres when analyzing ethical situations. These spheres represent content areas that impact on the ethical decision-making process, and will be explored in more depth.

This chapter will provide an overview of ethical theories and principles; moral development theory and nursing theory and how both theories guide ethical deci-

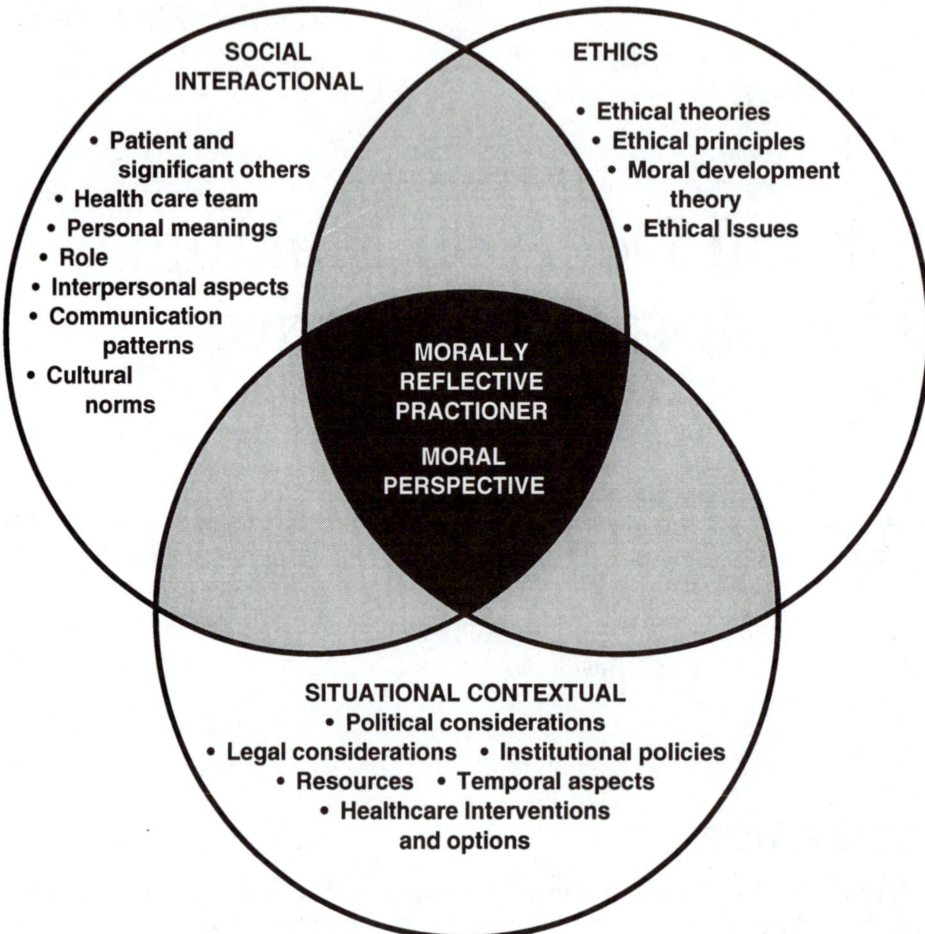

Figure 7-1 Awareness Spheres for Ethical Decision Making. ©*Patricia Hentz Becker.*

sion making; the social and interactional aspects involved in ethical situations; the influence of situational and contextual aspects; and finally, a guide for ethical decision making for the morally reflective practitioner.

Ethical decision making is more than a debate over ethical principles. Ethical situations do not exist solely in the sphere of ethics. For example, the "right to die" issue often involves a conflict of ethical principles, however; issues surrounding death and dying have become much more complex. Legal implications, technological advances, and allocation of resources often enter into the decision-making process. Patients' wishes and family concerns also impact on decisions. For nurses, ethical situations may also include conflicts involving their duties and obligations. Nurses are faced with the duty of meeting the needs of patients, while at the same time, they have an obligation to follow hospital policy, comply with doctor's orders, and take into consideration the legal implications of various actions and interventions (Becker, 1991a and 1991b).

The benefits and burdens of medical interventions and the allocation of scarce resources, like other ethical dilemmas, are human dilemmas within a social reality. As such, individuals involved often hold very different values and points of view. Ethical decision making, as a collaborative activity, requires an awareness and understanding of the moral perspectives of those involved in the ethical situation. Therefore, one needs to be aware of the social and interactional aspects of the situation, as well as the contextual and situational factors.

Ethical decision making is more than a process of balancing ethical principles. It involves the sphere of ethics; however, because it exists within the context of human experience, it overlaps with the social/interactional and situational/contextual spheres. Anyone who has ever been involved in an ethical dilemma in his or her practice knows that it is much more difficult to resolve than a case study from a textbook. Case studies present flat pictures, frozen in time. In reality, ethical situations are ever-evolving and changing, and are rich with contextual details.

SPHERE OF ETHICS: ETHICAL THEORY

A foundation for ethical decision making includes a basic understanding of ethics and ethical theory. **Ethics** can be described as the sphere of knowledge concerned with what is right and good, just and fair. Ethics, derived from the Greek term *ethos*, originally meant customs, habitual uses, conduct, character. **Moral** refers to culturally based standards of what is good and right, just and fair. The word moral is derived from the Latin, *mores*, meaning customs or habit. Moral standards are those that are commonly accepted as good and right, just and fair, and are *culturally* bound.

Views change over time in response to changing problems and conditions. Many of the ethical dilemmas we are facing today were beyond imagination fifty years ago. Changes in social conditions and technological advances have spurred many of our present-day ethical dilemmas, such as allocation of scarce resources and the right to die. Change in the conditions of health care (contextual and situational factors), have forced us to reexamine our views of what is right and good. Relying on customs, or "moral habit," without critical moral reflection as to what is right and good has led to some of our current ethical dilemmas. Moral habit refers to a way of setting situations that is grounded in a person's values and beliefs. It is termed habit because it is automatic in nature and usually accepted without question. For example, fifty years ago if a physician asked a family, "Do you want me to do everything possible to save your mother's life?" the answer would be fairly uncomplicated. Today, this question is not so easy, and the moral habit do everything possible to preserve life needs to be reexamined. Questions such as Life at what price? and What quality of life? enter into this reexamination.

Ethical theories and theories of moral development describe how a person uses details and facts of an ethical situation to determine ethical outcomes. It is important to note that there is little agreement among experts about which theory is best, and thus decisions may vary depending on the theory applied.

Deontological Theories

The **deontological approach,** derived from the Greek term *deon,* meaning "duty," focuses on actions or rules as morally right or wrong. As a guide for decision making, the deontological approach maintains that it is the action or rule itself that determines what is right and good rather than the outcome. To illustrate how this theory guides decision making, study the following scenario.

Scenario 7-1

Mr. Jones is a 30-year-old white male admitted to the emergency room with extreme respiratory distress and impending respiratory failure. He was brought to the emergency room by his significant other, Mr. White, following an episode of respiratory distress while at home. Mr. Jones is currently under treatment for AIDS and has become increasingly more symptomatic in the last year, requiring several hospitalizations. He has been unable to work for the last year, and has for the most part been homebound. Mr. Jones has seen many of his close friends die from AIDS, and has expressed his wishes not to have his life prolonged if his condition becomes extreme.

Using *rule deontology,* one type of deontological approach, a healthcare provider might subscribe to the rule, "Always try to save a life." Using a pure rule deontological approach, the ethical decision would be in favor of intubating Mr. Jones. The consequences would not be the focus. In addition, using such an approach, there would be little attention to the contextual details or social aspects of the situation because decision making is grounded in ethical rules.

Act deontology is similar in that the morality of the situation lies in the act itself and not in the consequences. Given an ethical situation of whether to intubate a patient in respiratory arrest admitted to the Emergency Room, using an act deontological perspective, the moral act would be "Try to save a life." Act deontologists judge the action itself as good or bad. Rules are viewed only as guides, not absolutes, and sometimes there are good actions that may be exceptions to the rules.

Using a pure deontological approach, whether rule or act, limits the focus for decision making to the immediate situation. The consequences, situational and contextual details, and the social and interactional aspects are not the primary focus. An exception to this would be a *mixed deontological approach,* which gives some consideration to the outcomes when making a decision. In general, this approach places emphasis in the sphere of ethics.

Utilitarian Theories

A **utilitarian (teleological) approach** differs from the deontologic in that consequences of one's interventions become the focus. Teleological theories are derived from the Greek term *telos,* meaning end, and thus are referred to as **consequentialist theories.** The goal is to maximize the good with the least amount of harm, thus one's moral obligation is always to perform good over evil. What is moral lies in the outcome of one's actions, and one is obligated to choose the path that creates the most net good.

However, one area remains problematic for the utilitarian—whether the greatest good must also include the greatest number. The following illustrates how the two utilitarian views differ regarding good outcomes. There are ten units of good (whatever it is) divided among five people. In the first case, everyone would get some good, but it would not be distributed equally among them. This is referred to as *limited utilitarianism,* which takes a narrow scope in what is good outcome. *Universal utilitarianism,* on the other hand, looks at the situation more broadly and the ten units would be divided equally.

A striking example can be seen in how decisions are made regarding scarce resources. The first, the limited utilitarian, might ask, Who should receive bone marrow transplants? Here the focus is on a small segment of the population needing such a procedure. The second, the universal utilitarian, might ask, How can we provide basic health care to all? This approach takes into consideration equal distribution of good. The latter view may determine that some form of distribution of scarce expensive resources is not feasible because it could not provide "the greater good for the greatest number."

Returning to the example of Mr. Jones, a utilitarian would focus on the consequences of a person's actions. What would produce the best outcome? If Mr. Jones had made it explicit that he did not want to be maintained on a respirator, the benefits and burdens would need to be assessed. The rule utilitarian would ask, What rules, if followed by everyone all the time, will maximize the good in the world? If the general rule "Honor an individual's wishes and respect human dignity is applied," the utilitarian position that would follow might be, What would happen if everyone were to deny or ignore patients' wishes? (Boyce and Jensen, 1978, p.39). The act utilitarian relies on the general rule and more on what actions will produce the most good. The common phrase "The ends justify the means" reflects this philosophy, and temporal factors are in focus using this approach. If I take this action now, how will it impact on the future good?

Situational Ethics

A **situational perspective** is one that takes into consideration the unique context of the situation. Such an approach does not use a set of ethical rules or actions. Given the case of Mr. Jones, many more details are needed to make an ethical decision. The three awareness spheres and the interactions among them come into focus using this perspective.

Philosophers have not come to any general agreement on which ethical theory is "best," but rather acknowledge that each offers a different point of view. Relative to the decision-making process, each point of view brings different aspects of the ethical situation into focus. The deontological approach might be described as a close-up lens, with the social/interactional and contextual/situational details out of focus. The utilitarian perspective would be more like a normal lens letting us see beyond the immediate situation but lacking contextual depth. The situational perspective could be described as a wide-angle view, allowing one to see the contextual richness. Thus, as Frankena (1973) points out, it is possible to have conflicting but equally valid moral judgments about precisely the same situation. What becomes problematic in the decision-making process is when one view claims to represent moral reality.

ETHICAL PRINCIPLES AS GUIDES IN DECISION MAKING

Moral outrage and distress are common when conflicting perspectives exist, and the question of what is right and good is often a matter of perspective. The major ethical principles which act as guides for decision making include **beneficence, non-maleficence, justice,** and **autonomy** as defined in Table 7-1. As abstract concepts they alert one to examine the situation in light of benefits and potential burdens; however, they do not define such benefits and burdens. Because ethical situations are not "objective realities," and attitudes and values influence how a situation is viewed, one needs to take "subjective meanings" into consideration. And, since ethical situations are also social in nature, conflicts among points of view will occur. One's "moral point of view" refers to how one defines "right and good" in an ethical situation.

Becker (1991a) identified a common theme among nurses regarding situations where conflicting points of view existed. Nurses stated, "Why do I have to fight so hard for what is right and good?" Conflicts stemming from different moral points of view, or what can be termed "moral perspective," has led to high levels of moral distress in nursing. Each different perspective defines right and good for different outcomes. Thus, it is imperative that nurses become morally reflective about their own definitions of right and good, as well as become aware of others' definitions, especially those with whom they work. It is not enough to be able to analyze ethical situations and find "right answers," because there are few absolutes, given the social

Table 7-1 • **Ethical Principles**

Beneficence: "The doing of good or the active promotion of good, kindness and charity" (Frankena, 1973, p. 47). According to Frankena, this principle includes the following four elements:

1. One ought not to inflict evil or harm (*Nonmaleficence*)
2. One ought to prevent evil or harm
3. One ought to remove evil or harm
4. One ought to do or to promote good (Frankena, 1973)

Autonomy: The most general ideal of personal autonomy is that of self-governance. "One should be one's own person unconstrained by another's actions or by psychological limitations" (Beauchamp and Childress, 1983, p. 59).

Justice: According to Rawls, resources should be allocated according to two basic principles: liberty and equality. He further qualifies that inequality is acceptable only when it is to the benefit of the least well off (Veatch and Fry, 1987).

Scenario 7-2

Mr. Ren is a 32-year-old white male with a malignant brain tumor. He is unresponsive to pain and is currently on a respirator. Without surgery, the prognosis is that he may survive a day. With surgery, Mr. Ren has a 1 percent chance of survival, although the surgeon is unable to say what survival actually means.

Response 1: I believe that it is important to do the surgery; he will die without it. (Act deontology with good defined in terms of medical outcomes, sanctity of life)

Response 2: It is our duty to do whatever we can to save life. (Rule deontology, medical outcomes)

Response 3: I think that we need to talk to the family about the prognosis and discuss what Mr. Ren would want. He may have a living will and not want to live. (Act utilitarian, quality of life concerns, person focused)

Response 4: I think it is the patient's and his family's decision whether the surgery is performed. We have to consider their rights. We have to have respect for human dignity and self-determination. (Rule utilitarian, autonomy rights, person focused)

nature of such situations. Scenario 7-2 above illustrates how different perspectives influence decision making.

MORAL DEVELOPMENTAL THEORY

Ethical principles that are used to analyze ethical situations are "abstract concepts." They are actually social values that have stood the test of time. Principles such as autonomy, beneficence, nonmaleficence, and justice are probably the most familiar. However, how does one decide which principle is most important in ethical situations; and, as illustrated above, how does one define right and good?

Justice Perspective

A large body of research in nursing has focused on ethical decision making and moral reasoning based on Kohlberg's theory of moral development. Kohlberg's theory, derived from Piaget and Dewey, uses the principle of justice as the ultimate factor for resolving ethical dilemmas. His model involves six stages with each stage reflecting a more advanced social perspective based on the principle of justice (Kohlberg, 1976). Actions or interventions are determined by analyzing the ethical problem as one of conflicting rights and obligations. The contextual or situational variables are often neglected. Becker and Burke (1988) cited the example of a pregnant woman addicted to cocaine. Using a justice perspective, the mother's rights are in conflict with the fetus's rights. Thus, one needs to balance the mother's interest in freedom, autonomy, and bodily integrity against her offspring's interest in being born healthy. The justice perspective examines the principles of autonomy, beneficence, and justice in light of the two separate claims of the mother and the infant.

Care Perspective

There has been much skepticism as to whether Kohlberg's model can be generalized to women (Ford and Lowery, 1986; Gilligan, 1988) Kohlberg follows the deontological tradition in defining "morality of an action by its intent rather than its consequence" (Aaron, 1977, p. 102).

It is not surprising that an alternative moral developmental approach, a care perspective, has developed to express a different voice for dealing with ethical situations. Noddings (1984, 1987) and Gilligan (1987, 1988) focus more on producing good outcomes that share some of the characteristics of the teleological approaches. However, this perspective places emphasis on relationships and the process of responding to needs. According to Noddings (1984), moral problems are more than problems of principle, reasoning, and judgment. Concern is placed on meeting needs while emphasizing pre-act consciousness and awareness of the one caring (Noddings, 1984).

Lyons (1987) argued that while women are able to use a detached approach, they feel conflicted in doing so because of a need to understand the situation in the context of human relationships. In essence, "In order to understand others they seemed to step into, not back from, situations to see and respond to others in their own particular situation and context" (Lyons, 1987, p.41). With a care approach, the focus shifts from one of right to one of needs. Coming back to the example of the cocaine-addicted mother, focus would be on the needs and the interrelationships involved. The fetus and mother are viewed as connected rather than separate, and thus understanding and responding to the mother's needs will have the potential for meeting the needs of the fetus. Contextual and relational detail are in focus. The relevant details could include the following: Pregnant women who abuse drugs are faced with burdens of poor health and malnutrition; they often are single parents or lack support from their husbands, have low self-esteem, lack close interpersonal relationships, and frequently have a history of sexual abuse. In addition, the female addict is often lacking in the quality of motherliness because of her own inadequate experience as a child (Kantor, 1978). The care perspective shifts the focus from principle-based decision making to one that examines a complex web of interrelated needs.

NURSING THEORY: HUMAN CONNECTION

Understanding of the human condition and respect for human dignity are at the core of a humanistic ethic of human care (Becker, 1991a and 1991b). Ethical dilemmas as human dilemmas place the person in the foreground. A comment by a staff nurse seems to capture this perspective. There are some nurses who titrate the morphine drip of the dying patient, and there are other nurses who hold the hand of the person on the morphine drip. Attention and focus is on the patient as a person. In addition, attention to cues that facilitate human connection are essential for the morally reflective practitioner. Some examples of such cues that draw focus to the person(social/interactional sphere) are: "he reminds me of my grandfather"; and a letter to a newborn taped to her isolette reminding us that this tiny infant is a member of a family, and has a brother at home waiting. Each of these cues helps to give the patient an identity beyond his or her medical condition. A striking example of how cues can help the nurse shift his or her view of the patient from a medical condition to a person with a medical condition can be seen in the following nurse's experience.

Scenario 7-3

While caring for a female patient who was unconscious after a stroke, and thinking of all the tasks that had to be done, I opened her bedside table. Inside was a red purse and matching pair of red shoes. And it hit me: This woman was an individual who probably liked getting dressed up and took pride in her appearance. I could picture her walking down the street with her red shoes and her red purse. This changed how I looked at the patient. Since then I have tried to see beyond the illness and focus on the person.

This nurse was able to broaden her awareness beyond the situational and contextual aspects of the patient's medical condition to include the social aspects of the patient as a person. The perspective above is an example of a humanistic approach, a moral perspective that places the person at the foreground, or focus, of care.

Becker (1991a and 1991b) identified three perspectives of ethical care, a **reductionistic perspective,** a **humanistic perspective,** and a **humanistic contextual perspective**. While each exists in nursing, there is evidence that experience plays an important role in movement toward a humanistic perspective. The reductionistic perspective focuses attention on the biological being, and determines benefits and burdens in terms of medical outcomes. Using a reductionistic perspective, futility of treatment would be related to the illness and the potential for a cure. Using a humanistic perspective, the focus shifts toward the human being, with emphasis on human dignity and understanding the person with the physical illness. The humanistic contextual perspective focuses on respect for human dignity and self-determination, with an awareness of multiple perspectives and their impact on care.

The reductionistic and humanistic perspectives represent very different ways of understanding ethical situations. When these two perspectives meet, it is often in conflict, rather than harmony. In essence, each attends to different details of the same picture. According to Schon (1987), individuals with different views or different ways of framing may pay attention to different facts and make different sense of the facts they notice. Figure 7-2 illustrates this point. What do you see? What details are in focus? How have you organized the details to determine what you see? Are you able to shift your point of view? Do you see two faces or a vase? The point to be emphasized is that while the details remain constant, the understanding and organization of the details can be very different, depending on the perspective of the viewer.

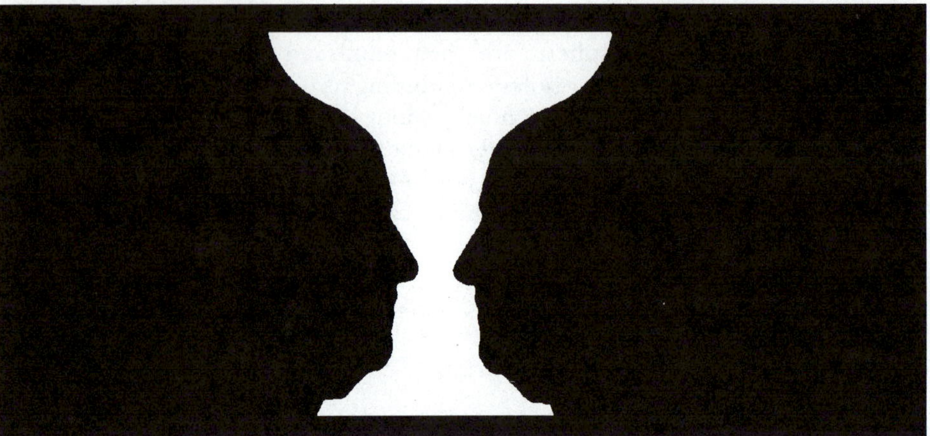

Figure 7-2 Methods of Viewing or Framing a Situation.

The third perspective described by Becker (1991a and 1991b), the humanistic contextual perspective, involves a focus on human dignity, with an awareness of multiple perspectives and how each impacts on healthcare decisions. This individual is able to shift focus to see the ethical situation from different points of view, or ethical perspectives, just as one can shift focus from seeing the two faces or the vase. As Becker (1991a and 1991b) stated, it is not enough to understand one's own point of view; when one is able to understand multiple perspectives, one is able to see the contrasting details and understand the situation more fully. In essence, no one perspective represents reality, but rather is an interpretation or understanding of reality.

THE SOCIAL/INTERACTIONAL SPHERE AND NURSING

Ethical decision making is a social act. Thus, the nurse may find it difficult to achieve moral autonomy within the healthcare environment. As stated by Dallery (1986), "moral dimensions are social and collective in nature. The moral dilemma is not what is my duty or obligation or which value has priority, but to whom or what am I loyal, and to whom or what am I advancing though this decision?" By shifting the focus from ethical theories and principles as guides for ethical decision making to a focus on social interaction, and loyalties and commitments within a social environment, the question shifts from What are the ethical principles relevant to this situation? to, To whom are we responsible, and who should be involved in the decision-making process?

Nursing today has many loyalties including loyalty to clients, to institutions, to colleagues and coworkers, to the nursing profession, and to society. Balancing loyalties requires the nurse to set priorities. Interfacing loyalties with one's ethical perspective leads one to examine situations more closely: "Good for whom and for what ends?" Loyalties need to be based on a conscious, reflective choice. Indeed, frustrations regarding moral autonomy and having a nursing moral voice may result.

***Table 7-2* • The Social/Interactional Sphere**

1. Are channels of communication among healthcare professionals open and clear regarding the patient's needs and choices?
2. Once channels of communication are open, are efforts to maintain communication established?
3. Are members of the healthcare team clear regarding the obligations and responsibilities of the members involved?
4. Has trust been established and maintained in the nurse-patient relationship?
5. What role in the decision-making process does the nurse have (i.e., degree of moral autonomy)?
6. What role do significant others play in the decision making regarding the patient?
7. What role expectations do the patient and family have of the nurse and the other members of the healthcare team?
8. What information and knowledge must the nurse have to support and inform the patient? (i.e., legal rights and healthcare options) What are the legal and ethical implications involved in assuming the advocate role in this situation?

From P.H. Becker, Advocacy in Nursing: Perils and Possibilities, *Holistic Nursing Practice, 1(1) (1986), 54–63.*

The Nurse and Patient Advocacy

Patient advocacy from a philosophical perspective is a conscious state of concern and support for the patient, where the nurses' actions are focused on assisting patients "to authentically exercise their freedom of self-determination" (Gadow, 1980, p. 85). Due to conflicting loyalties, nurses need to evaluate the personal risk involved and take measures to minimize such risk. The considerations in Table 7-2 above will help the nurse assess the interpersonal aspects of the ethical situation.

THE PATIENT'S ROLE

Healthcare has had a history of strong paternalism. **Paternalism** is defined as making a decision for another, based on what one believes to be the other's best interest. This condition is most commonly seen in situations where a parent decides what is in a child's best interest. While paternalism has been a traditional perspective in healthcare, it has the potential for interfering with a patient's autonomous rights. It also leaves the patient without a voice regarding his or her care. **Parentalism** has come to replace the outdated term paternalism, and refers to the process of choosing for another in his or her best interest. Since ethical situations are interactional in nature, it is important to be cognizant of traditions and whether such traditions are in keeping with the values of the day. Increasing interest and concern for patient rights and the patients' need to have a voice in decision making has spurred the development of living wills and advanced directives.

THE CONTEXUAL/SITUATIONAL SPHERE

Although there is not a set list of contextual or situational factors, general categories include healthcare interventions and options, temporal aspects, resources available, and institutional policies. For example, a patient being cared for in the home who voices his wish to die without any extraordinary measures will present different questions and concerns than the patient in the surgical intensive care unit who makes the same request.

GUIDE FOR ETHICAL DECISION MAKING

Ethical decision making may be thought of as a moral process involving the following steps:

1. Identifying an ethical situation (Moral sensitivity)
2. Awareness and analysis of relevant information using the awareness as a guide (Moral reflection)
3. Developing a moral point of view (Moral perspective)
4. Awareness and understanding of different perspectives by those involved in the case (Plurality of perspective)
5. Decision-making process applied (Table 7-3)

Table 7-3 • **Ethical Decision-Making Process**

Moral Sensitivity: The awareness that an ethical situation exists. Ethical dilemmas are human dilemmas and therefore elicit emotional responses. The emotional response moves an individual to explore and examine the details of the ethical situation.

Moral Reflection: The conscious process involving awareness spheres for ethical decision making (ethics, social/interactional, and situational/contextual). The process of reflection involves attending to details in each sphere.

Moral Perspective: The organization of the details of the ethical situation and the development of a moral point of view. Moral perspective also requires one to be able to articulate and explain one's moral point of view.

Plurality of Perspective: The ability to understand how details of an ethical situation can be organized to form different moral perspectives.

Moral Decision Making: A social process that involves a dialogue reflecting multiple moral perspectives. Through dialogue and understanding there can be movement toward responsible collaborative action.

Adapted from P.H. Becker, Perspectives of Ethical Care. *(Doctoral Dissertation) Teacher's College, Columbia University 1991a. and* Ethical Practice in Nursing: Nursing's Moral Voice. *PLN Visions, 3(2): 4–5 1991b.*

Moral Sensitivity

Moral sensitivity alerts one that there is a problem. It may begin as a sense that something is just not right. Ethical dilemmas as human dilemmas alert us that there is a need to take a closer look at a situation. And, although historically emotion in moral decision making has been frowned upon, ethicists have come to realize that emotion creates moral drive and is critical for moral sensitivity. Emotions and reason should coexist and "should be mutually correct resources in moral reflection" (Callahan, 1988, p. 9). In reality, even choices of details to consider in resolving an ethical issue reflects a subjective judgment (Becker, 1991a and 1991b). John Dewey captured the essence of the rational and emotional aspects of moral decision making in his *Theory of the Moral Life.* As stated by Dewey (1960), ethical principles are guides for decision making but not ends in themselves. He described sympathy, which in essence prevents outcomes from being products of mere calculation, as a critical aspect in decision making.

Moral Reflection

Moral reflection is the conscious process involving awareness of and the analysis of the ethical, social/interactional and situational/contextual components of the ethical situation. It involves attending to details in each sphere.

Moral Perspective

Moral perspective involves developing a moral point of view based on an analysis of the relevant details. It also requires the ability to articulate and explain one's position. As stated earlier, there is not a singular ethical perspective; therefore, the morally reflective practitioner needs to be able to logically determine his or her position.

Plurality of Perspective

Which lens does one choose in coming to ethical decisions? Does one always use the same approach, or does it vary from situation to situation? Moral reflection requires one to examine how details of an ethical situation are analyzed. With moral reflection, one comes to understand one's own moral perspective, as well as how others develop their moral points of view. While each awareness sphere impacts on how an ethical dilemma is appraised, individuals vary on how they derive meaning from the details. "It is important for nurses to understand that priorities in resolving ethical dilemmas vary among those involved in the decision-making process. Harmony among the voices will not always be the case" (Becker, 1991(a), p. 2). For example, the benefits and burdens assessed by a surgeon may be based on the biological aspects; an administrator using an economic perspective may focus on the scarce resources; and the nurse using a humanistic perspective may focus on respect for human dignity and the wishes of the patient and family.

Moral Decision Making

Although moral reflection is a personal activity, ethical dilemmas are social in nature. Nurses are responsible participants in the decision-making process; however, this responsibility is shared. Thus, the process of decision making involves skill in conflict resolution, collaboration, and communication. The process must have a foundation of trust, and a willingness to express and work through differences. Rather than debating whose perspective is better or more valid, open dialogue and reflection are needed by all involved, with each moral voice acknowledged.

SUMMARY

Ethical practice in nursing is a complex process which involves an understanding of the *content* of ethical situations as reflected in the awareness spheres for ethical decision making (Figure 7-1), as well as the *process* for making ethical decisions, discussed in the guide for ethical decision making section and outlined in Table 7-3. It is critical for nurses to take an active role in moral decision making and for nursing's moral voice to be heard. Once nurses have learned the content and process of ethical decision making they will develop ethical nursing practice as morally reflective practitioners.

REFERENCES

Aaron, I.E. (1977). Moral philosophy and moral education: A critique of Kohlberg's theory. *School Review,* February, 197–217.

Beauchamp, T.L., & Childress, J.F. (1983). *Principles of Biomedical Ethics,* 2nd ed. New York: Oxford Press.

Becker, P.H., & Burke, S. (1988). Neonatal drug addiction: an analysis from two moral orientations. *Holistic Nursing Practice, 2*(4): 20–27.

Becker, P.H. (1986). Advocacy in nursing: Perils and possibilities. *Holistic Nursing Practice, 1*(1): 54–63.

Becker, P.H. (1991a). *Perspectives of Ethical Care.* (Doctoral Dissertation) Teachers College, Columbia University.

Becker, P.H. (1991b). Ethical practice in nursing: Nursing's moral voice. *PLN Visions, 3*(2): 4–5.

Boyce, W.D., & Jensen, L.C. (1978). *Moral reasoning: A psychological-philosophical integration.* Omaha, NE: University of Nebraska Press.

Callahan, S. (1988, June/July). The role of emotion in ethical decision making. *Hastings Center Report,* 9–14.

Dallery, A.B. (1986). Professional loyalties. *Holistic Nursing Practice, 1*(1), 64–72.

Dewey, J. (1960). *Theory of the moral life.* Carbondale, IL: Arturus Books, Southern Illinois University Press.

Ford, M.R., & Lowery, C.R. (1986). Gender differences in moral reasoning: A comparison of the use of justice and care orientation. *Journal of Personality and Social Psychology, 30*(4), 777–783.

Frankena, W.K. (1973). *Ethics,* 2nd ed. Englewood Cliffs, NJ: Prentice-Hall.

Frankena, W.K. (1973). *Ethics,* 2nd ed. Englewood Cliffs, NJ: Prentice-Hall.

Gadow, S. (1980). Existential Advocacy. In S.F. Spilker & S. Gadow (Eds.), *Nursing images and ideals.* New York: Springer.

Gilligan, C. (1987). Moral orientation and moral development. In E.F. Kittay & D.T. Meyers (Eds.), *Women and moral theory* (pp. 19–33). Totowa, NJ: Rowman & Littlefield.

Gilligan, C. (1988). Remapping the moral domain: New images of self in relationship. In C. Gilligan, J.V. Ward & J.M. Taylor (Eds.), Mapping the moral domain, (pp. 3–19). Cambridge MA: Harvard University Press.

Kohlberg, L. (1976). Moral stages and moralization. In T. Lickona (Ed.), *Moral development and behavior: Theory, research and social issues,* New York: Holt, Rinehart & Winston.

Kantor, G.K. (1978). Addicted mother addicted baby—A challenge to health care providers. *Maternal Child Nursing, 3,* 283.

Lyons, N. (1987). Ways of knowing, learning and making moral choices. *Journal of Moral Education, 16*(3), 226–239.

Noddings, N. (1984). *Caring: A feminine approach to ethic and moral education.* Berkeley: University of California Press.

Noddings, N. (1987). Do we really want to produce good people? *Journal of Moral Education, 16* (3), 177–188.

Schon, D.A. (1987). Education of the reflective practitioner, San Francisco, CA: Jossey Bass Publishers.

Veatch, R.M., & Fry, S.T. (1987). *Case studies in nursing ethics.* Philadelphia: J.B. Lippincott Co.

Terry B. McGoldrick
Elisabeth T. Hallman

CHAPTER 8

Computer-Assisted Decision Support

Nurses have traditionally been the gatekeepers of information flow.
–Ozbolt, 1987

INTRODUCTION: THE PAST AND PRESENT

Information handling has always been a problem in healthcare in general and in nursing in particular. It frequently has kept practitioners from the bedside as they juggled care plans, kardexes, nurses' notes, test results, and multiple phone calls to coordinate and communicate the patient's care and studies (Scenario 8-1). But times are changing.

Remember the days when the most high-tech equipment used was a ballpoint pen? For many of us, those days have not yet passed (Schroeder, 1992). As technology advanced, society replaced the abacus with the adding machine, the adding machine with the tabletop calculator, the tabletop calculator with the hand-held calculator, the desktop computer with the laptop, the laptop with the notebook computer, and pens with light pens. By the late 1970s, microcomputers had been introduced, and in 1981, the IBM personal computer (PC) was being marketed. The PC brought the power of computers to the workplace.

Over the past twenty years, hospitals have introduced computerization into their information systems. Initially, they were automated versions of the manual systems and most often designed around the billing system needs. But today, hospitals have access to a wide range of applications, including word processing, database systems, clinical decision systems, automated medical records, and order entry. These applications offer nursing the opportunity to increase productivity, streamline decision making, contain costs, and, most importantly, the opportunity to return to the bedside to deliver quality care to the client as the nurse begins to relinquish the role of

Scenario 8-1: The Way We Were

You are working nights, your unit is short staffed, you have eight patients, and have just received a patient from the emergency room. Dr. Jones calls the floor to order a barium enema and intravenous pyelogram (IVP) for his patient, which need to be done first thing in the morning. Another nurse answers the phone, calls you to the desk, you discuss the order with Dr. Jones and he hangs up. You pull the patient's chart and write the verbal order. You addressograph the proper forms and complete the necessary information on two radiology request forms (because each study requires a separate form). You look up the procedure in the policy manual to see what supplies and prep the patient will need. You check the chart to see if the patient is allergic to anything that may be used during the studies. You call pharmacy and storeroom to order the necessary supplies. You stamp the appropriate forms so that the patient gets charged for the supplies you have ordered. You call the dietary department to hold the patient's breakfast. You call radiology to schedule the studies. Radiology refers you to the two departments where the studies will be performed. You call these areas to schedule the two tests. You call patient transportation to arrange to have the patient taken to radiology for the studies. You update the kardex, develop a care plan, and write a note in the chart. How long did this take? Now you can get back to your patients. You are halfway down the hall when one of your coworkers calls you back to the desk because Dr. Jones is on the phone. He has decided to cancel the barium enema and IVP. You pull the patient's chart and write the verbal order . . . .

"gatekeeper of information flow." As we move ahead, we need to understand what to expect from today's computers, determine what the strengths and weaknesses of computer technology are, and define its impact at the bedside.

COMPUTER MAGIC?

A highlight of computerization is the apparent "magic" inherent in the ability of the system to collect, store, and process large volumes of information in relatively short periods of time. All computer systems, regardless of size or functionality, consist of hardware and software components. **Hardware,** the things you can see and touch, consists of **input devices** (for example, keyboards, light pens, bar code readers, and voice receivers), **output devices** (terminals, printers, modems, connections to other computers), and most importantly, a **system unit** (the engine to make the system function).

The system unit is comprised of a **central processing unit, memory, power supply,** and an **internal clock.** Two kinds of memory are required:

- **ROM (read only memory)**—holding all instructions for internal processing
- **RAM (read and write memory)**—used to store and operate programs while the system is working

Hardware requirements and size are dependent upon the operations or activities to be completed by the system.

Software is the heart and mind of the system. Software defines the type of operations to be completed, carries all instructions for use of the system, holds and stores the data, and interprets and completes input and output commands. Software requirements must be carefully considered. Novices may wish to seek the advice of an experienced consultant when system selection criteria are being determined.

Does the clinical nurse need to understand all of this in the practice of daily computer use, or can it remain "magic"? A basic understanding of the current technology and a thorough review of the user (i.e., nursing staff) expectations and needs from the computer prior to system selection is a minimum requirement. More importantly, knowledge related to specific functionality, departmental interactions, and role of the computer in the completion of daily operations is necessary for successful implementation and use of the system.

COMPUTER APPLICATIONS FOR NURSING CARE

Today's computers play multiple roles in decision support and management. The blending of typical PC applications, such as word processing, spreadsheet design and analysis, database management, and graphics, lend powerful support to the day-to-day functioning of a clinical manager.

Computers are slowly being incorporated into care activities at the bedside. The imbalance between current price and undefined and unproven benefit realization of computer usage has made the implementation of bedside support systems slow but closely observed. To justify the cost, hospital administrators are waiting for proven response from bedside systems before launching into costly computer solutions.

How are computers incorporated into daily care activities? Ozbolt (1987) defines two distinct categories for the kinds of decisions nurses make. These fall under the umbrellas of either coordination of care or nursing process activities.

Decisions required in the coordination of patient care have been well supported by computer applications. These applications include order entry, result reporting, patient scheduling, and care planning types of nursing station software. At the nursing station or bedside, computers are effectively used to collect and store data, communicate rapidly with other departments, sort and set priorities for information, and suggest diagnostic and care alternatives.

The second type of decisions nurses practice define much more complex operations and involve attempting to replicate and define logistically the steps of the nursing process (Ozbolt, 1987). Although the procedure is well defined, the multitude of factors that support and foster decisions made by nurses have stifled the progression of computer support for this process. Major difficulties have been attributed to the lack of a consistent, well-defined body of nursing knowledge, and the variability inherent in multiple theoretical and structural conceptual frameworks currently in use that fail to consistently support computer applications (Ozbolt, 1987). To date, many existing computer systems have done little more than replicate manual documentation systems. A "good" replica will actually improve the quality of documentation by providing prompts, reminders, and required fields that dictate entries. Nauert, Lower, and Cox (1993), through data analysis of computer nursing entries, state "introduction of an automated system will not improve the quality of documentation unless the information is prompted or is inserted automatically via default" (p. 114). Effort, however, is still needed to define and streamline nursing documentation standards. The computerization of a manual, time-intensive, lengthy documentation process will not facilitate nurses' work.

Bedside or point of care terminals have become the envy of nursing informatics specialists. Indeed, the concept of immediate access to data entry and retrieval sounds appealing. As described by the Peat Marwick (1988) bedside study, the use of a full-function terminal at the bedside results in a decrease in errors of omission, reduced numbers of medication errors, and greater accuracy and completeness of documentation. However, the value and cost of bedside availability versus any access to automation, in general, is only just being tested. Marr and colleagues (1993), in addressing the effect of bedside terminals on the quality of nursing documentation, compared the timeliness and completeness of data entry at the bedside versus other locations. The hypothesis of a positive relationship between quality and bedside entry was not substantiated. This finding suggests the need for additional studies to determine the cultural and structural components required to support the nurse in the delivery of care in the acute setting, as well as a clearer definition for the usefulness of computerization as a documentation tool.

A flip side to the automated charting requirement is the need for system expertise. Thompson, Ryan, and Kitzman (1990) interpret the current problems related to expert system development as difficulties in defining "process," or the nature of expertise. An additional stumbling block identifies the lack of a consistent vocabulary or database. Indeed, the Nursing Minimum Data Set (NMDS) (Werley, Lang, and Westlake, 1986) has begun the task of defining reliable, standard, uniform data elements as a basis for the description, study, and reporting of nursing. Leske and Werley (1992) report use and implementation of the Nursing Minimum Data Set in an infancy state and stress the need for nursing to define a computerized, stored, and standardized documentation database, and a role for nurses in "promoting, implementing, and testing the NMDS in the interest of advancing both the improvement of patient care and nursing as a research-based profession" (p. 263).

COORDINATION OF CARE

Early entries as *clinical* computer solutions have centered around communication- and charge-capture-related information. Order entry capabilities have been designed to meet both of these needs. Results reporting, and the ability to quickly locate test and procedure data, is an added, undeniable benefit of early computer implementations.

Clinical system vendors have gradually developed nursing systems, highly proclaimed to decrease nursing time and streamline the nursing documentation process. Because these systems have been developed independently, or often as an afterthought to a departmental system, many bedside systems lack integration or interface capabilities required to provide data accessibility.

To be truly functional, communication-based systems must be integrated or interfaced with other departmental systems. Integration means one-time entry with multiple activities or communications in the same software system resulting from the initial entry. **Interface** involves the sharing of data between two or more software systems. A properly interfaced system will allow for the same flexibility and ease of communication as an integrated option.

Explore this concept of integration in the example of completion of the physician orders for a barium enema and an IVP. A truly integrated, or properly interfaced, system will allow single entry of the order by the physician, nurse, or clerk. The system would then automatically confirm the patient schedule, prioritize the order of complction—for example IVP followed by BE—notify the pharmacy or storeroom to send the required prep, hold meal trays as defined by radiology protocol, check for allergies and provide the appropriate warnings, provide pertinent clinical data, patient history, and reasons for study to the radiologist, schedule and send the escort, update the patient care plan, post the charges to the patient's bill, and eventually store the result on the patient's medical record for retrieval and review. This method of one-time entry with predefined data analysis and communication routes supports nursing by eliminating much of the busywork required in coordination of care activities.

Due to the excessive expense of system development, purchase, and implementation, most hospitals have developed a patchwork plan for automation or have adopted a single vendor solution for all departments. Single vendors do not necessarily allow for the best solution for each department using the software. Interface requires specific documentation and nomenclature to allow for data transfer. This requires standards and rule definitions, and vendors are now slowly coming to consensus with national computer groups to support, develop, and foster efforts toward standardization. Neither option is without cost and compromise to provide true integration and the functionality required at the bedside.

Integration is critical even when considering a stand-alone nursing system software. The ideal system will capture workload and patient acuity definitions from a single entry in flow sheets, care plans, or nursing orders, and care delivery documentation. One of the goals when selecting a system is to take these standard, routine decisions away from the nurse by embedding them naturally in the software, thus freeing the nurse for more patient-outcome-oriented activities. The move toward the computerized patient record (CPR) will provide opportunities for enhanced integration and promote clinical system standard development. From the hardware perspective, the advancement of **open architecture systems**—that is, communication channels capable of transmitting and sharing data—is a prerequisite for the integration required in an ideal clinical support system.

BEDSIDE DECISION MAKING: ARTIFICIAL INTELLIGENCE OR EXPERT SYSTEM?

How does the nurse make a decision at the bedside? One of the major difficulties is the lack of definition for the steps in this process (Sinclair, 1990; Ozbolt, 1987; Woolery, 1990). Using the Carnevali and Thomas (1984, 1993) model for decision making, the complexity of clinical judgment and decision processing is apparent. (See Figure 1-1 in Chapter 1.) Imagine the following example.

Scenario 8-2

The nurse answers a call bell. The patient asks for "something for pain." Using the Carnevali model, the nurse first draws upon the *preencounter* information she knows about the patient, that is, data gleaned from shift report and the patient chart. Knowing that the patient is a 40-year-old female, post-op day two, and NPO since surgery, the nurse's first assumption is incision discomfort. However, the nurse will not stop here. Phase two, *entry into the patient situation,* requires the gathering of additional cues. Assessment and questioning reveals complaint of generalized discomfort, a feeling of fullness, slight abdominal tenderness, some nausea, and difficulty voiding since foley catheter removal eight hours earlier. The nurse will synthesize these clues into *clusters* or *chunks,* and now begins to hypothesize:

- Incision pain
- Urinary retention
- GI tract immobility

Continuously searching the data fields will prompt the nurse to ask more detailed questions, to clarify the symptoms already defined and move to *testing a goodness of fit* for the various diagnoses hypothesized. After repeating the loop, clustering data, testing hypotheses several times, the nurse concludes that the patient requires intermittent bladder catheterization and mild sedation provided by the previously prescribed pain medication regime. The *assignment of a diagnosis* only remotely resembles the initial preencounter mind set of the reason for the request for "something for pain" for this patient. Herein lies the major difficulty with computerized clinical support systems. Where is human interaction and thought processing absolutely required to facilitate decision making and where does the computer excel?

HOW COMPUTERS MAKE DECISIONS

The simplest explanation of computer processing mimics the decision tree model. The logic flow travels through a series of preprogrammed paths, making turns and taking direction at yes/no decision points along the way. When multiple pieces of data must be examined at a decision point, the program directs the computer into loops to repeat the decision multiple times until the data is exhausted or a best choice decision is determined. As you can see, this somewhat parallels the Carnevali and Thomas (1984, 1993) model in that data gathering, decision points, and repeated decision loops lead to a diagnosis and re-evaluation mode.

There are two types of recognized computer decision assistance and support systems: those that directly make decisions and those that support the decision-making process by assisting in making a decision faster, cheaper, or "more correctly" than a nurse alone could make (Brennan, 1988).

The decision-making systems are appropriate only for specific, well defined, logistically based types of decisions. Brennan (1988) describes the characteristics of these systems:

- Clearly and fully defined data and information
- A finite and small number of problems
- All necessary information is objectively defined and available at the time the decision is to be made
- The data compiled must point to only one possible diagnosis
- The intervention defined must be entirely determined on the basis of the diagnosis generated

This logic is illustrated by the concept of computer-controlled medication administration. For example, a predetermined algorithm defines parameters for monitoring arterial blood pressure. Guidelines define increase and decrease in micrograms per kilogram per minute volumes of medication according to fluctuations in systolic and diastolic pressure changes. The computer monitors pressures, maintains corrected drip rates, and records both pressure and medication volumes at preset intervals. Alarm systems are specified to alert the nurse to extreme variations or exceptions to the algorithm. As discussed earlier, these systems have gained limited usage due to the expense and the inability of the various component systems to communicate information. The need for standardization and interface capability is again apparent.

In contrast, clinical decision support systems are designed to support and improve, but not replace, clinical decision making for the nurse. This type of software is described as either **modeling or expert system solutions.** Modeling systems assist the nurse in breaking down the problem into component parts and organizing these to point to options that identify the best possible solutions and outcomes. Such a system would provide data *clues* as an adjunct or reminder to the nurse. For example, while preparing to give a medication, the nurse would display the order on the terminal. In processing the request to display, the system would automatically check lab values, intake and output recordings, time of last dose, and potential interaction with other drugs and treatments. It would then display reminders such as "urine output decreased and below expected volumes for this patient." Such a message would provide information to the nurse for determining the appropriateness of dispensing medication at this time.

Expert systems function to improve the quality of the nurse's decision-making activities. With this type of system, quality is measured by reduction in the length of time required to complete the decision-making process, access to better information, better conceptualization and organization of the problem, and ideally, an increase in correct, optimal decisions effecting patient care.

Generally, the components of an expert system include the **knowledge base** and the **inference engine.** The knowledge base, made up of thousands of facts, formulates rules known as heuristics. These rules are manipulated by the inference engine to make associations, determining answers to a series of if/then, yes/no questions.

As does a nurse at the bedside, the system will gather a series of data clues and begin to sort through the series of predetermined questions to prioritize and rule in possible decisions. The rules are stated in an *if/then* or *and* format and define pathways through the decision tree. To accommodate potential uncertainty or multiple solutions, expert systems build in weighted certainty factors at decision points. For example, an expert might define a particular conclusion as absolute certainty and assign a weight of 1. Other less sure conclusions would be weighted smaller, and a mathematical calculation of probability would then direct the logic flow. In our medication example, the expert system would have been preprogrammed with rules such as "do not give medication when urine output is below 30 cc per hour and if the potassium level is less than 3.8, or if the BUN and creatinine values are 2 standard deviation units below the normal values as defined for this patient." When selecting the order for review, the system would complete the if/or/and loops, determine if the patient should receive the drug and issue a message to the nurse "hold medication as prescribed, urine output is less than 30 cc per hour." The decision, made based upon the rules embedded in the software, is made for the nurse.

These expert systems require the experience and defined proficiency of a nurse expert and a knowledge engineer to define data elements, rules, and pathways. Pieces of information are stored in the computer memory via techniques such as **semantic nets** and **data frames. Hierarchical relationships** are then assigned to data elements. The working premise is an item will inherit all of the qualities of the data elements above it on a hierarchical scale. For example, the item "pregnant" would assume the qualities of female sex and age range definition. This allows faster interpretation of clues or data elements since each item serves as a pointer to other items via analogy or heuristic properties.

More recent computer applications are designed as **learning systems.** With this concept, the computer is programmed with the initial knowledge base, heuristics, and coded information related to storage of information. The knowledge base grows as the computer is fed information and completes the predetermined tasks, analogies, interpretations, and applications. As time passes and with extensive use of the system, the software learns the hidden, implied rules built into making a good decision. In the example above, the nurse may decide that the urine output is sufficient and overrides the computer prompt. The learning system would remember this information and either not prompt or prompt with a caveat when this situation occurred again. Regardless of the type of system, the accuracy of the outcome decision is only as good as the data input at each step in the process.

THE PROBLEMS WITH EXPERTISE

The logic becomes more complicated as the decisions become more complex. **Artificial intelligence,** or computer-based decision support systems, require programming specifications approved by known experts in the field. Woolery (1990) denounces current expert systems for relying heavily upon nursing faculty and textbooks as their sources of expertise. Relying upon the works of Benner (1984) and others, Woolery (1990) cites two distinct types of knowledge utilized by experts:

- Knowledge used to explain or define the problem
- Knowledge used to actually perform the task

At an expert level, the nurse has a difficult time defining or reconstructing the problem-solving steps utilized. The value and amount of input gained from experience and intuition is not definable and is often missing from verbal or written descriptions, that is, steps leading to a particular decision. The novice, however, is more likely to base a decision on data and thoeretical, analytical heuristics.

Should the expert systems then, be designed for the beginning practitioner or truly expert practitioner? Since most human thinking involves second kind thinking or recognizing and reasoning about patterns, making snap judgments, associations, generalizations, and analogies, computers may not be able to handle these *fuzzy concepts* that lack precise and constant meaning (Time-Life Books, 1987).

Sinclair (1990) has described the distinction between expert systems and decision support systems. Using Brennan's (1988) definition, decision modeling systems are designed to structure clinical problems, consider risk and uncertainty, and select courses of action consistent with a set of objectives. In contrast, the expert system recommends solutions by providing extensive memory support through rapid analysis of quantitative data. The invaluable role of the nurse, either beginner or expert, is qualitative in nature. The balance must be achieved through human expert judgment supported by vast and extensive knowledge data analysis by the computer.

The movement towards integrated clinical support systems is still evolving. The prototypes for development of a centralized data repository that can be accessed, manipulated, displayed, and organized to meet the needs of the requester are being developed and tested. The technology is rapidly developing to make these wishes a reality.

MAKING THE DECISION TO AUTOMATE

Is there a system that meets the needs of the nurse today? Childs (1992) stated: "Unlike the line from the movie *Field of Dreams*—'If you build it, they will come'—I'm afraid the perfect system for the near future is still a dream. And if by chance someone could build it, it might be very difficult to sell" (p. 4). Difficulties, as described above, contribute significantly to the impossibility of developing the perfect system. And, once such a system existed, its market value in meeting the needs of all hospitals and in all clinical situations would be negligible. The decision to automate in the clinical areas is an extraordinarily individualistic exercise in finding the right software match.

It is imperative that nurses be involved in the selection of computer systems within the hospital, and that staff nurses be an integral part of a team effort to complete the decision-making process. A thorough understanding of the day-to-day activities of the nurse is required to optimize the work of the computer while minimizing the workload for the nurse. If available, the expertise of a systems engineer as well as information systems staff who can relate to the vocabulary and activities detailed in the day-to-day operations of the nursing station and bedside should be included in the decision task force.

Initially, a complete and intensive study of daily shift-to-shift activities as well as a review of existing systems, policies, procedures, and internal data flow should occur. Although some work flow may need to change, the implementation of an informatics system should not totally redesign the nurse's work. Some prepurchase and even predecision activities also need attention, such as a review and definition of the reasons to automate, including the development of a list of expected benefits. Benefits that may be expected from the purchase of an automated system include:

- Quality of care
- Time management
- Fiscal savings

The next step involves establishing a *wish list* of computer functions to support and enhance the operations of the staff. Free associate and allow your mind to wander and dream. This list will then be broken down into the following categories:

- Must have
- Would like to have
- Save for the future
- Can probably live without

These lists become the basis for a Request for Proposal (RFP) document that may be submitted to vendors.

What should be included in a wish list? Korpman (1990) lists five key points for patient care automation:

- New, open-style architecture
- Primary patient care optimization (nurses and doctors) as the central focus
- Elimination of the paper record
- Point of care data capture
- System-wide integration around the patient

Using these guiding principles, Korpman (1990) further defined nine attributes required of computer systems:

- Automated patient scheduling
- Individually customized work and information processing
- Data and departmental integration
- Automated data screening
- Automated data encoding
- Continuing professional feedback
- Appropriate data grouping and presentation
- Long-term data storage and retrieval
- Widespread data and terminal distribution

Computer systems that meet the criteria and demonstrate support of these attributes will optimize patient care and streamline nursing functions.

To fully understand the implications of these criteria for your institution, many factors must be considered when deciding to purchase, build, and implement clinical or bedside computer functions. Of prime importance is definition of the types of activities that may be automated. Of routine reflection are scheduling, order entry, result reporting and charge capture communication, documentation, and care planning. These baseline systems should have the capabilities of integration and/or interface to nursing information and other departmental systems for one-time entry of relevant data. Do a literature review and search for solutions that meet all the requirements of your *must have* list as well as your *would like to have* list. Search for vendors who have solutions to your needs, and investigate the company's short- and long-range research and development plans. Send an itemized RFP, asking specific questions requiring detailed, narrative answers accompanied by examples to preferred and alternate choice vendors. Most systems have the basics, and therefore vendors will answer "yes" to all typical questions asked on the RFP. Preparation of this document can be one of the most time-intensive steps in the decision process.

Once the RFPs are returned, narrow your decision process to three or four prime candidates. Now is the time to really scrutinize each system for the best fit for your organization. Delve into the details.

The routes of communications between nursing and the bedside with inter-departmental systems cannot be underestimated. This is where nursing involvement and input toward the overall plan for hospital-wide automation with movement towards an automated, permanent medical record is essential. Implementation of that plan on the nursing, bedside level will necessitate careful consideration and perhaps some compromise and negotiation to meet the needs of each party. Is the primary focus of the software the patient or the patient's bill?

Security and confidentiality issues cannot be overlooked. Patient data must be readily available, yet secure from tampering, unauthorized changes, and simply reading by non-essential persons. Systems to insure data security and equipment security are to be built into the design and remain a critical element of the purchase decision.

Who will manage the system and control the database—nursing, the institution, or the vendor—is an often-neglected question. Most vendor contracts will include a clause related to annual updates and criteria for training and help for your facility. Of equal importance, however, are answers to the questions, who will make database changes, how will corrections or additions to standard screens occur, and what are standard or typical allowances or charges for customization. Is the vendor help desk truly a help desk? Is help available twenty-four hours a day? Do the vendor's working hours coincide with your working hours? A suggested topic to pursue with the vendor is a discussion of the most recent requests for system enhancements or a review of the minutes from recent user group meetings as an example of recognized system needs or shortcomings. Talk to current users, both new and long-timers. Make site visits and observe the system, live. Ask for a list of customers before agreeing on a visit site. Don't allow the vendor to preselect a site.

Ask for help from your information systems specialists to calculate and determine system hardware specifications. Spend the time to prepare a projected plan for future growth and expansion. It is tempting to try to cut hardware costs as a means of bringing the price into a more reasonable range. However, five-year growth, at a bare minimum, should not be a compromise of your basic system requirements. Here is where system architecture, actual interface, and integration protocols and standards utilized will be critical.

Spend some time reviewing ergonomics. The following are questions to consider:

- Where will the terminals, printers, and other hardware be stored?
- What are the size restraints?
- Will patient care occur nearby?
- Can the hardware be cleaned, is it noisy, do light and glare affect the user or the patient?
- What are the wiring needs?
- Is the system available twenty-four hours per day?
- How many terminals are really needed?
- Is the system truly user-friendly?
- How easy is it to access the system?
- Does it require typing skills to operate effectively or are other input devices available?

Find out the typical training needs, both time and instructor requirements, for the various levels of staff. Are printed user documentation manuals and training tools available?

Careful consideration of data and system reliability and validity standards must occur. For example, consider the following questions:

- How does the system handle multiple updates to the patient record at the same time?
- What is the standard for downtime and system recoverability?
- What is the recovery process should the system fail or be unavailable for an update from an interfaced system?
- How does a nurse correct a mistake?
- What happens to the original record entry when a mistaken entry is corrected?
- What are the accountability and audit trails included in the system?

Assistance may be needed to interpret the answers, but ask these and other questions. Don't rely upon your computer experts to evaluate these areas without nursing involvement.

This is a small sampling of factors to consider during the decision-making process. The message, simply, is to involve the right people, spend the time, and evaluate all aspects of the system. There is no perfect system, but there can and should be a computer solution for every care facility.

Scenario 8-3

The year is 2001. You are working nights, you are short staffed, you have eight patients, and you are receiving a patient from the satellite emergency center on the other side of town. Dr. Jones voice activates his computer terminal from his home to enter his orders for the patient you are receiving from the emergency center. All patient history and data is retrieved from the national medical database and entered into the hospital's information system; the orders that Dr. Jones entered are automatically entered and communicated to the hospital system; all departments affected by the patient's admission (nursing, dietary, laboratory, radiology, housekeeping, patient accounting, etc.) are automatically notified within minutes of Dr. Jones's activating his home order system. All orders are automatically cued, according to acuity, so that services are triaged and scheduled based on the patient's condition. The patient's estimated time of admission and appropriate information to begin to develop a plan of care is displayed on the terminal at the patient's bedside. You will not leave the patient's room to admit, assess, develop a plan of care, and document it. You will spend quality time in the room at the bedside talking with the patient and providing the psychological and educational support needed. By the way, this patient will have a cardiac cath at 0900, a laser coronary bypass at 1100, and be discharged in twenty-four hours.

THE WAY WE NEED TO BE

As we prepare for the twenty-first century, it is evident that computers will be a part of everyday life, both at home and in business. Futurists agree that in all probability, approximately 75 percent to 80 percent of all homes will have computers.

"It happened again: the Joint Commission on Accreditation of Healthcare Organizations (JCAHO) had to order nurse participation in the technology management process. Why did an *outside authority* have to mandate this?" (Simpson, 1991, p. 26) Nursing's limited commitment to computerization stems from several problems: cost, overextended staff, and lack of knowledge. As the economics of healthcare change, so must nursing change to incorporate a leaner, meaner, more cost-effective approach to quality healthcare, utilizing resources that are becoming more and more limited. Nursing must commit itself to becoming computer literate, for computerization provides nurses with the opportunity to more efficiently utilize time and resources to provide quality patient outcomes.

But what are the necessary steps to prepare nurses at all levels for the changes to come? First and foremost, there must be a vision, commitment to the vision, and the ability to articulate that vision at all levels of staff. Commitment is required from senior management to develop and maintain these skills for all levels of staff.

The next step is to form a steering committee that will have the authority and responsibility for overseeing the development, implementation, and ongoing evaluation of the informatics program. From the steering committee, task forces and work groups must be developed. These groups are charged with the in-depth study and definition of computer needs, and the detailed deliberation of available systems and vendor offerings. Once the task force groups have made their recommendations, the steering committee should select a system that will support the institution's needs around the clock and the vendor who can service such a system. Post-implementation ongoing maintenance and continuing education are essential to maintain a state-of-the-art system. This state-of-the-art system must also have ongoing evaluations to assess its impact on the productivity of the care providers as well as its fiscal impact.

"The Joint Commission has finally done what we were either unable or unwilling to do for ourselves: demand a greater and more powerful role in the strategic management of technology for nursing" (Simpson, 1991, p. 26).

In healthcare today, informatics is used as an instrument for efficient decision making, financial planning, and management, yet nursing frequently has not kept up with the advances and has not participated in the design and development of systems that directly impact on clinical decision making. In 1962, Peplau forewarned "that computers would change nurses and nursing" (p. 239). She specifically advised that decisions about relations between nurses and automated health services must be guided by the purpose of nursing (Peplau, 1962). She also exhorted nurses to maintain control of their own practice, including the management of information to support practice.

Thirty years later, the American Nurses Association formally designated Nursing Informatics as a nursing specialty, and The Council on Computer Applications in Nursing reemphasized Peplau's thoughts in a report stating that "nursing must control its own future through its ability to develop and control its own information handling processes. It is important for nursing's control of its own practice that *nurses* (emphasis theirs) control the information systems that support nursing" (Simpson, 1992, p. 26).

It is clear that nursing information systems must be matched to the practice of nursing. Clinical decision making should be supported by informatics, not driven by it. Nursing's failure to adequately capitalize on the power and potential of computer technology is directly related to lack of education and training. Today, only four academic programs prepare registered nurses in nursing informatics at the graduate level (Simpson, 1992) and studies have shown that 20 to 30 percent of nurses either are uncomfortable with computers or have no experience with them (Perry and Mornhhinweg, 1992). Ongoing education, from the entry level practitioner through the nursing administrator, is essential for nurses to grasp what computers can do and the impact that computers, with well-designed information systems, will have on practice, ability to make decisions and on the quality outcomes for patients.

REFERENCES

Benner, P. (1984). *From novice to expert: Excellence and power in clinical nursing.* Menlo Park, CA: Addison-Wesley Publishing Co.

Brennan, P.F. (1988). Modeling for decision support. In M.J. Ball, K.J. Hannah, U. Gerdin Jelger, and H. Pererson (Eds.), *Nursing informatics: Where caring and technology meet* (pp. 267–273). New York: Springer-Verlag.

Carnevali, D.L. (1984). The diagnostic reasoning process. In D.L. Carnevali, P.H. Mitchell, N.F. Woods, & C.A. Tanner (Eds.), *Diagnostic reasoning in nursing.* Philadelphia: J.B. Lippincott Co.

Carnevali, D.L., & Thomas, M.D. (1993). *Diagnostic reasoning and treatment decision making in nursing.* Philadelphia: J.B. Lippincott Co.

Childs, B.W. (1992). "If we build it, will they come?" *Healthcare Informatics, 9*(6), 4.

KPMG Peat Marwick (1988). TDS Healthcare Systems Corporation bedside terminal study, 1–50.

Korpman, R. (1990). On-line health care—Patient care automation: The future is now. Part 4: From philosophy to implementation. *Nursing Economic$, 8*(6), 419–427.

Leske, J.S., & Werley, H.H. (1992). Use of the nursing minimum data set. *Computers in Nursing, 10*(6), 259–263.

Marr, P.B., Duthie, E., Glassman, K.S., Janovas, D.M., Kelly, J.B., Graham, E., Kovner, C.T., Rienzi, A., Roberts, N.K., & Schick, D. (1993). Bedside terminals and quality of nursing documentation. *Computers in Nursing, 11*(4), 176–182.

Nauert, L.B., Lower, M.S., & Cox, K.R. (1993). Bedside computers and quality documentation. *Nursing Management, 24*(7), 106–113.

Ozbolt, J.G. (1987). Developing decision support systems for nursing. *Computers in Nursing, 5*(3), 105–111.

Peplau, H. (1962). Automation: Will it change nurses, nursing, or both? In American Nurses Association *Clinical Papers.* Kansas City, KS: The American Nurses Association.

Perry, W.F., & Mornhhinweg, G.C. (1992). Nursing practice: Promoting computer literacy. *Nursing Management, 23*(7), 49–52.

Schroeder, P. (1992). From the editor. *Journal of Nursing Care Quality, 7*(1), viii.

Simpson, R.L. (1992). Informatics: Nursing's newest specialty. *Nursing Management, 23*(8), 26.

Simpson, R.L. (1991). The joint commission did what you wouldn't do. *Nursing Management, 22* (1), 26–27.

Sinclair, V.G. (1990). Potential effects of decision support systems on the role of the nurse. *Computers in Nursing, 8*(2), 60–65.

Thompson, C.B., Ryan, S.A., & Kitzman, H. (1990). Expertise: The basis for expert system development. *Advances in Nursing Science, 13*(2), 1–10.

Time-Life Books (1987). *Artificial Intelligence.* In Understanding computers series. Alexandria, VA: Time-Life Books.

Werley, H.H., Lang, N.M., & Westlake, S.K. (1986). The nursing minimum data set conference: Executive summary. *Journal of Professional Nursing, 2*(4), 217–224.

Woolery, L. (1990). Expert nurses and expert systems. *Computers in Nursing, 8*(1), 23–28.

PART II

MANAGING NURSING RESOURCES

Christina M. Fitz-Patrick
DeEtta F. Hayes

CHAPTER 9

The Strategic Planning Process

Plan ahead for needed dollar$.
–*Anonymous*

INTRODUCTION

Today's turbulent times in healthcare are forcing decisionmakers to plan as never before in order to remain viable and competitive in an ever-changing environment. To maintain its competitive edge, the for-profit sector has used strategic planning for many years. Confronted with the rapid increase of modern technologies and advanced methods of communication, the business world has responded with careful planning. However, it was only in the mid-1970s, with escalating health costs and increased governmental regulation, that healthcare leaders began to understand the value of strategic planning (Marriner-Tomey, 1992). Indeed, it was about this same time that healthcare leaders began to refer to healthcare as an industry, and realized that survival would require significant changes in business attitudes and operations.

OPERATIONAL VERSUS STRATEGIC PLANNING

Today's nurse managers and administrators are well versed in operational planning. **Operational planning** is done each year and is a short-range plan that is closely tied to goals and objectives. Each manager plans a staffing and expense budget based on historical data, anticipated projects, and changes that will affect staff and care delivery in the coming year. Such planning is "tight," since it is developed within a variety of financial constraints. In addition, an operational plan is more specific to an organization's immediate needs and expectations. For example, the department of nursing must attend to daily operations consistent with certain basic standards, including adequate nurse-patient ratios based on acuity, compliance with regulatory standards, and a commitment to service excellence.

Expense budgets include daily operations plus capital expenditures for equipment replacement as well as expected changes and new projects. An example of a new project might be expansion of an eight-bed telemetry unit to sixteen beds. This would involve a capital expense for additional equipment, as well as a cost analysis for additional staff and educational expenses. Such a project would require collection of historical data to establish need, a marketing survey, physician support, and anticipated reimbursement projections.

During the operational planning process, it is necessary to focus on organizational goals in order to develop achievable unit and departmental goals and objectives. Usually before the budget process begins, nursing goals and objectives are developed with staff input, from cues based on past and current operations. Although goal setting is more specific, good managers understand the need to be flexible, continually evaluating and reassessing established goals and objectives allowing for additions, changes, and even discarding any that appear unrealistic or unachievable. For example, nursing administration in an eighty-bed oncologic hospital has as a long-range goal, implementation of a shared governance model. The nurse managers know that in order to accomplish this goal, it will be necessary to promote autonomy and empower the staff. One of the ways to achieve this would require demonstration of staff expertise in oncologic nursing. Therefore, unit objectives may include staff certification in the speciality. However, expecting 100 percent compliance may be unrealistic and could fail to attract and retain nurses. By building in reasonable timeframes to accomplish this goal, and allowing for other educational options, such as a graduate degree in oncology, management would demonstrate its flexibility and understanding of individual values and needs.

In contrast to this position, Marriner-Tomey (1992) states, "Strategic planning clarifies organizational beliefs and values . . ." (p. 4). Bryson (1988) elaborates that "strategic planning requires broadscale information gathering, an exploration of alternatives, and an emphasis on the future implications of present decisions. It can facilitate communication and participation, accommodate divergent interests and values, and foster orderly decision making and successful implementation" (p. 5). Therefore, strategic planning generates a broad-based global statement that sets the tone in guiding an organization forward.

Strategic planning is often viewed as synonymous with long-range planning since it usually covers a three- to five-year period. Its development integrates the organization's mission statement with its philosophy. After an indepth analysis of the internal and external environments, goals and objectives are developed that are less specific, but assistive in identifying strategic issues. Identification of strategic issues provokes a variety of key questions for each department head in the organization. From these questions, department heads and staff assess, plan, and evaluate for their areas of responsibility.

This chapter discusses the strategic planning process at the corporate level, at the chief nurse executive (CNE) level, and at the nurse manager level. Implications for nursing staff will be described. Decision-making examples in the strategic planning process are also presented.

THE STRATEGIC PLANNING PROCESS

In order to develop, implement, and evaluate effective nursing programs in keeping with an organization's vision, it is essential that the CNE have a firm sense of the organizational culture and history and a clear understanding of the entire strategic planning process. A good starting point is with Bryson's (1988) eight-step strategic planning process that "should lead to actions, results, and evaluations" (p. 48). These steps include:

1. Initiating and agreeing on a strategic planning process
2. Identifying organizational mandates
3. Clarifying organizational mission and values
4. Assessing the external environment (opportunities and threats)
5. Assessing the internal environment (strengths and weaknesses)
6. Identifying the strategic issues facing an organization
7. Formulating strategies to manage the issues
8. Establishing an effective organizational vision for the future

Initiating and Agreeing on a Strategic Planning Process

In most organizations the strategic plan is initiated by the chief executive officer (CEO) and developed with the administrative team, which would include chief executives from nursing and medicine. However, in many larger organizations there is a department for planning and development that would provide guidance and act as a resource during the entire process. Whatever the situation may be, it is essential that strategic planning be perceived by everyone involved as a valuable management tool that is extremely useful in the decision-making process. It is during this initial phase that roles and responsibilities are clearly defined and resources are allocated.

Clarifing Organizational Mandates

Organizational mandates are, according to Bryson (1988), "the musts it confronts" (p. 49). The following mandates would be included in any strategic plan, since they impact on an organization's operation and existence:

- Legal: State and federal laws, city statutes
- Professional: Education, research, professional organizations
- Community: Optimal, cost-effective care, competent staff
- Education: Students and staff
- Staff: Adequate work environment, benefits, ancillary and administrative support

Unless these and other mandates, unique to the situation, are clearly identified and analyzed, an organization may unknowingly restrict its opportunity to grow and prosper. Attention to this key element cannot be overlooked, since it is crucial to the success of the planning process.

Clarifying Organizational Mission and Values

Mission and values clarification is closely tied to identification of stakeholders. Bryson (1988) defines a stakeholder as, "any person, group, or organization that can place a claim on an organization's attention, resources, or output, or is affected by that output . . . the key to success in public and nonprofit organizations is the satisfaction of key stakeholders" (p. 52). **Key stakeholders** may include, but are not limited to, patients, staff, physicians, administration, board of directors, the community, and where applicable, the union.

Once the stakeholders are identified by the strategic planners, the mission statement will become clearer and more easily developed. The mission statement, necessarily broad in scope and usually brief, explains the reason for an organization's existence. It is the focal point that provides direction and guidance for the leadership as goals are pursued and achievements are evaluated. It is, according to Ives (1991), ". . . the ultimate standard for measuring the achievements of the organization" (p. 38).

However, a mission statement is not confined only to the leadership. Indeed, outstanding leaders understand the value of sharing a well-defined mission statement with employees through staff meetings, orientation programs, and brochures such as employee handbooks and annual reports. As Bryson (1988), sees it, ". . . an important and socially justifiable mission is a source of inspiration to key stakeholders, particularly employees. Indeed, it is doubtful that any organization ever achieved greatness or excellence without a basic consensus among its key stakeholders on an inspiring mission" (p. 49). For example, the following mission statements reflect such thinking:

- University Hospital is committed to providing quality patient care to the community, to advancing professional and ethical practice through education, and to promoting technological and research advancement. Key to this mission is the firm belief that each and every individual within the organization shares and participates in fostering this mission.
- Community Hospital's Department of Nursing is committed to providing family centered care by competent professional nurses and support staff within a reasonable financial framework. Fulfilling this mission depends on the valued participation of each person associated with the nursing department.

Assessing the External Environment

One method for assessing the environment is referred to as the SWOT analysis (Strengths, Weaknesses, Opportunities, and Threats). This assessment is a vital component in the strategic planning process. In this step of the strategic planning process, the environment external to the healthcare orgnization is considered in light of potential threats or opportunities. Although the external environment is fraught with unstable socioeconomic factors and constricting governmental regulations over which an organization has little control, there are opportunities that exist in which "lemonade can be made from lemons." This was demonstrated when acute care service reimbursement became regulated by the government in an effort to control escalating healthcare costs. Many facilities shifted their services and procedures to outpatient status which shortened length of stay, reduced costs, and placed reimbursement into a less restricted category. Faced with decreased length of stay and increased outpatient services, organizations realized that inpatient census and the subsequent revenue would significantly drop. Many administrators viewed this as an opportunity to increase volume by being price competitive with other facilities. This was accomplished by hospitals becoming preferred providers for local businesses. Preferred provider status also increased an organization's competitive edge by including occupational health and worker compensated care with a firm's employee healthcare benefits.

Assessing the Internal Environment

This step of the strategic planning process involves surveying the healthcare organization for internal potential strengths and weaknesses. Organizations have a wealth of information at their disposal. In addition to the hard data of assets and expenditures, many overlook the richness of their history, their culture, and their human resource potential. According to Strasen (1987): "The data base created from the situation audit can include the analysis of many different factors and/or parameters in the environment from past, present, and future perspectives" (p. 216). Steiner (1979) proposes that an indepth analysis will provoke a variety of questions for the planning team, especially as they relate to the consumer and to resource availability. Such questions include:

- Who is the consumer we serve and how is our service perceived?
- What resources require maximum attention?
- How will their availability impact on future goals and objectives?

For example, a large university hospital long established as a leader in healthcare, medical and nursing education, and research has begun to feel the effects of increased operating costs and a shift to more medicare, medicaid, and uninsured patients. The facility is a strong presence in the city, possessing a reputation for excellence and a genuine concern for patients and staff. Employee turnover rate is among the lowest in the city, especially low for nursing. The planning team is acutely aware of the opportunities and threats in the external environment, significantly the cuts in medical education funds and the revenue loss for care of the uninsured and indigent (Figure 9-1). Based on this information, their assessment of the internal environment includes strengths:

- Financial status
- Support from physicians and alumni
- Programs and services
- Employee suggestion program
- Equipment and technology
- Administrative team
- Staff expertise
- Location and marketing
- Patient satisfaction

Their assessment of the internal environment includes weaknesses:

- Union demands and relations
- "Lag" time for Management Information Systems (MIS)

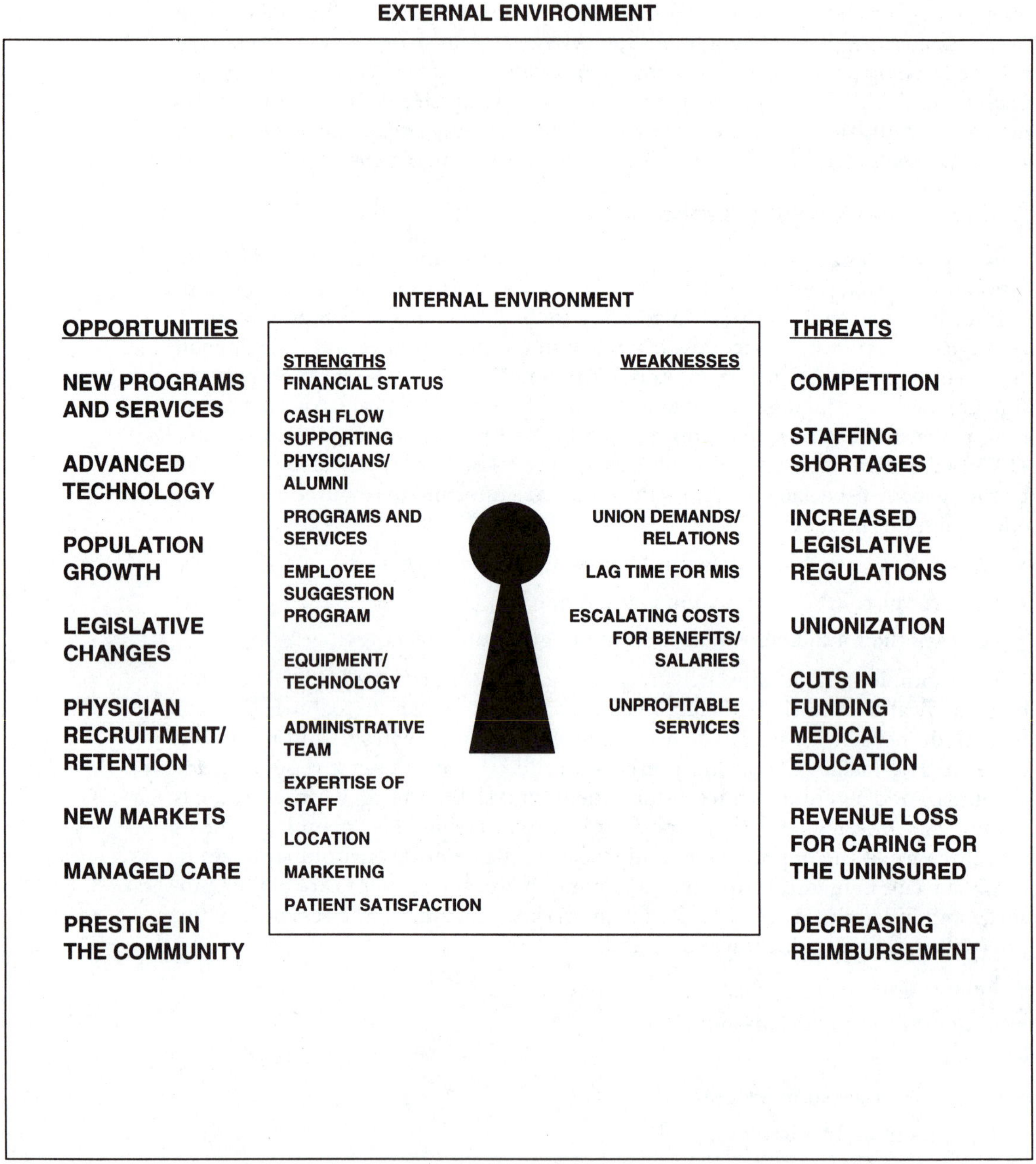

EXTERNAL ENVIRONMENT

INTERNAL ENVIRONMENT

Figure 9-1 Key to Success in Strategic Planning: SWOT Analysis.

- Escalating costs for benefits and salaries
- Demand for improved technology
- Unprofitable services
- Potential for fixed costs from third-party payors

Identifying Strategic Issues

Bryson (1988), recommends that a "statement of a strategic issue should contain three elements . . ." Summarized, they include:

1. A short, concise description of the issue
2. A listing of the factors that make the issue a policy question
3. A definition of the consequences of failing to address the issue

Each of these elements must be present in order to define a strategic issue.

The university hospital mentioned in the previous example has identified and ordered five primary issues based on the SWOT analysis. The first issue is *elimination of or drastic reductions in state funding.* This issue is the most significant to University Hospital because its impact is so far reaching. It will affect healthcare clients, the community, local employers, physicians, students, and hospital staff. Failure to address this primary issue will severely restrict resources, with the potential of placing patients at risk. Employers will suffer the consequences of escalating health benefits cost, since it is likely that the hospital will be unable to provide cost-effective managed care. In addition, decreased resources will limit educational and research provisions. Limited resources will also affect physician practice by restricting technological growth. Also, physicians and staff will feel the effects on their incomes. Indeed, staff cutbacks will most surely occur, greatly diminishing the amount of ancillary and administrative support for both physicians and nurses.

Issue two is *revenue loss as a consequence of treating the uninsured and indigent.* This issue is socially significant, since a vast majority of the public believe that cost-effective, optimal healthcare is a right. Furthermore, the public is demanding a national healthcare policy that they expect will meet their needs and decrease their contributions. In addition, although the public is less concerned with the indigent and uninsured, they do expect the healthcare community to provide for those without health insurance. Failure to address this issue will place decision making in healthcare policy in the hands of politicians whose agendas are most often not in agreement with the medical community. The issue, if unaddressed, will create a profound moral dilemma for physicians, nurses, and families.

Issue three is *decreasing funds for worker's compensation.* University Hospital's mission statement includes provision of a preferred provider, managed care concept for many local businesses. The hospital expects that this concept will control and maintain cost effectiveness for local employers. In the event that worker's compensation benefits are substantially reduced, the hospital will suffer a loss of revenue in addition to their ability to effectively manage employer plans.

Issue four is *escalating costs for salaries and equipment.* This issue is closely linked to issue one. Educational mandates require maintenance of a solid university with the ability to continue providing top quality medical education, including qualified teaching staff, a viable school of medicine, and a stable environment in which to practice. Staff mandates include equitable wages and benefits, a safe working environment, and adequate administrative and ancillary support. The consequences of failure to address these issues are obvious for the survival of the school and hospital.

Issue five is *union demands that the organization might face.* As a stakeholder, the union has its own agenda to increase membership and keep that membership on the payroll. With the threat of a decrease in or elimination of state funding, the hospital will be faced with the possibility of freezing wages and reducing the workforce. The union will obviously see this as a threat to its position and influence. Problems with the union would hamper the hospital's daily operation and could potentially risk patient care delivery. The hospital's solvency and reputation in the community will suffer if there is the slightest question regarding compromised care and services. The significance of these issues must be clearly understood by the CNE. It is his or her responsibility to advise the managers about the impact these issues will have on nursing goals and objectives and on daily operations. Maintaining a balance between conceptualizing the overall picture and attending to daily operations is likely to be a difficult task for some in nursing management. However, it is an excellent opportunity for CNEs to create the kind of environment in which managers can learn and develop their decision-making skills.

Formulating Strategies to Manage the Issues

According to the literature (Strasen, 1987; Garner, Smith, and Piland, 1990; Bryson, 1988), it is during this phase of planning that specifics such as new programs, alternative strategies, organizational goals and objectives, policies, and standards begin to emerge. This is an activity requiring energy and enthusiasm; a time when the leadership must stress the value and importance of establishing innovative and creative methods of goal achievement. It is also the time to encourage managers to reassess and validate compliance with present policies and standards. Historically, decisionmakers have been less attentive to this part of the process, viewing it as "busy work." Indeed, it is important for the nursing management team not to get caught up in detail work at this time, but rather to determine responsibilities with timeframes for accomplishment. University Hospital has developed several strategies in response to key issues over the next two years. The hospital expects to:

1. Develop and implement a system of shared services with satellite facilities
2. Continue to market itself as a regional referral center in an effort to remain competitive with local community hospitals
3. Optimize MIS capabilities by integrating all existing systems, enhance inter- and intradepartmental electronic communication, and further refine systems according to specific departmental needs
4. Expand existing space for outpatient services to increase volume.

Items 1 and 4 will require establishment of two new programs, while items 2 and 3 will expand programs already in place. The implications for nursing are clear, and it is within this framework that the CNE and nursing management will develop departmental and unit goals covering a two-year period. Nursing will:

- Act as a resource in education and management for satellite hospitals
- Assist in the further development of standards of care, quality assessment programs, policies, and procedures across satellite facilities
- Continue to identify patient populations that could utilize services across the multihospital system
- Assist in the development of a centralized recruitment and retention program
- Continue to educate the nursing staff in cost-effective management of patient care delivery
- Vigorously promote and participate in the "Suggestion Program" for employees to identify cost-saving strategies for the institution
- Select a system that will streamline nursing documentation and decrease the time spent on clerical duties while integrating the system hospitalwide
- Explore the feasibility of bedside computers
- Participate in the assessment, planning, organizing, and implementing the expansion of outpatient services
- Evaluate patient care delivery systems that focus on cost effectiveness and support patient care services to maintain positive patient outcomes
- Develop critical pathways to decrease length of stay
- Evaluate the present patient education program for each department
- Identify union demands and provide a supportive, colleagial atmosphere to discourage and eliminate the need for union representation for professional nurses

Establishing an Effective Vision for the Future

Formulation of strategies is closely linked to an organization's vision. Vision statements are brief, challenging, and inspirational (Bryson, 1988). Inspiration is what moves people to stretch beyond the predictable, to exceed an organization's expectations while fostering firm ethical standards. Kouzes and Posner (1987) describe vision as "an ideal and unique image of the future" (p. 85). Inspired visions of the future enhance positive thinking and energy. Without vision an organization restricts the growth and creativity of its staff and may unwittingly promote mediocrity from within.

DECISION-MAKING MODELS

Obviously, the preceding example is a nearly perfect textbook case that is unlikely as such to be encountered in the real world. What happens in a hospital with a much different environment and with a much different culture? The following is a case study that describes the political decision-making process that would take place in a more realistic setting. The discussion contains key elements of the political model described in Chapter 1 (Chaffee, 1983), such as the diversity of values, considered alternatives, change, and implementation, as well as the political skills necessary to make things work. The political model described in the literature (Bryson, 1988; Chaffee, 1983) is most conducive to the initial phases of planning, since it acknowledges the diversity of organizational and personal interests, values, and goals among key players. The model's most basic and significant point is that it is inductive, and defined not by consensus but by conflict (Bryson, 1988). A possible consequence of diversity is conflict (Chaffee, 1983), which is not necessarily undesirable. Indeed, to ignore or attempt to avoid conflict will only lead to frustration and failure (Bryson, 1988). Instead, wise leadership recognizes the inevitable presence of conflict and its positive nature, which encompasses a broad spectrum of talent, experience, and energy among the participants. By redirecting these qualities, the leadership will be able to focus on issue resolution from which policies and programs evolve. It is a dynamic process, one that continually assesses and evaluates stakeholder interests until some semblance of concensus is reached.

Scenario 9-1

The board of directors and administration of a 350-bed city hospital realizes that the blue-collar, ethnic neighborhood they have long served is changing. At one time, the community consisted mainly of large, close-knit families with strong ties to the hospital. Indeed, it was the only place where many agreed that they or their children be hospitalized. In recent years, however, many families are seeing their children marrying and moving to the suburbs, leaving behind in the community an aging population. Consequently, obstetrical and pediatric services have seen a large decrease in patients, with a subsequent increase in the medical-surgical volume, especially in cardiac care. This resulted in a dramatic shift in reimbursement, with over half of the past year's funds coming from medicare and medicaid.

Fortunately, the leadership identified the trend early on, recognizing that in order to remain viable, tough decisions needed to be made. Clearly change was inevitable, and the political decision-making model came into play. Stakeholders in the organization had a wide variety of values and a long history of emotional ties to the organization. There was an atmosphere of mistrust and disagreement about the "how and who" should address the issues at hand. Even though all levels of staff had access to the strategic plan, which included alternative strategies, there was considerable misunderstanding and emotions ran high, clouding the broad picture. There was strong resistance to accepting changes brought about by socioeconomic conditions affecting the local community. Ironically, this resistance came primarily from the organization's major strength, its stable and loyal staff. Faced with significant resistance and a certain amount of distrust, the leadership within the organization had to lobby vigorously among the most powerful to convince them that major changes would be necessary, the most dramatic change being the eventual elimination of obstetrics and pediatrics while focusing on an increase in adult services, chiefly in cardiac care, cardiac rehabilitation, long-term care, and home care.

While Community Hospital stakeholders wanted to remain a full-service organization, it was obviously not realistic in today's marketplace. Administration decided to follow the lead of many other organizations by forming alliances with other area hospitals in order to share services and resources. In the example given, the pediatric department was closed, while plans were made to gradually phase out obstetrics. Pediatric patients seen in the emergency department were referred and transferred to a nearby children's facility. Obstetrics had experienced a significant drop in deliveries to an all-time low of 480 in the past year. Obstetricians were joining medical staffs in suburban hospitals since their patients were moving into those areas.

Based on the population changes, the decision was made to develop and implement a marketing strategy that focused on the cardiac patient. The plan promoted the hospital's image as an expert in the adult cardiac care field, emphasizing prevention, establishing a "chest pain" center, a heart catheterization unit, and a cardiac rehabilitation department. Not surprisingly, the hospital was considering as a long-range goal the possibility of doing open-heart surgery.

The entire process of pursuing alternative strategies was difficult, yet challenging, for all. Specifically, it had profound implications for nursing. Both pediatric and obstetrical nurses felt a real sense of loss, while having to reassess their career plans. With the support and understanding of nursing administration, nurse managers in those departments, who also were experiencing strong feelings, had to skillfully negotiate with their staff in an attempt to retain as many nurses as possible. Most of them had been with the hospital for many years, lived nearby, and were vested in a generous pension plan. Several chose to remain with the hospital to work in other areas, while others decided to leave and look for pediatric and obstetric positions in other facilities. Significant changes such as these are painful yet necessary in order to eliminate the risk of having to close doors!

As seen in the literature (Baldridge, Curtis, Ecker, and Riley, 1977; Chaffee, 1983) and as the name implies, the political decision-making model is based on expert negotiating skills, and decisions may not always be supported by individual goals. Negotiating is not for the novice, but for risk takers who possess an understanding of an organization's vision and how that vision is influenced by the changes taking place in healthcare. Effective negotiators are experienced in lobbying and in winning support in order to build strong alliances and gain power. In this situation, and as Chaffee (1983) indicates, the model works well in loosely connected departments of professionals who share a wide variety of values. Large, complex healthcare facilities may be viewed as this type of structure.

NURSING'S ROLE IN THE STRATEGIC PLANNING PROCESS

A retreat for nursing administrators and managers is an excellent way to meet and plan. At a retreat, the CNE reviews the organization's mission statement, its philosophy, its strategic plan, its internal analysis, and their relationship to the department of nursing. Discussion of the internal analysis will necessarily include an assessment of how the SWOT analysis affects nursing. Each of the threats and weaknesses will have raised issues and provoked many questions at the corporate and administrative levels and will do the same for the nursing retreat participants. In this forum, the CNE serves as facilitator for the brainstorming among the group. The nurse managers actively participate in the decision-making process. They outline the direction with guidelines, formulate action plans, and develop timeframes to accomplish their plans within the resource limitations of the organization.

Responsibility for sharing the process and the plans with staff lies with the nurse managers. Pertinent information, especially models, should be posted and informal discussions with staff are to be encouraged. Such informal discussion and staff meetings are excellent ways to develop valuable feedback and creative problem solving. Furthermore, it is a sure way to promote cohesiveness beneficial to the staff as well as to the organization. Goal accomplishment is enhanced and teamwork thrives when staff members have access to valuable information that indicates where the organization is headed. When staff understand nursing's role in the scheme of things, there is a sense of goodwill with other departments and a reduction in the feeling of isolation.

SUMMARY

Strategic planning is yet another tool for nursing to master in order to meet the ever-increasing demands placed on leadership. It is no easy task to embark on an unfamiliar path; nevertheless, it can be a stimulating and exciting challenge for all levels of nursing staff. Understanding an organization's nature, its culture, and mission enhances the planning process. Good plans serve most organizations well. Outstanding plans are dynamic, even chaotic and will, in a positive environment, bring together employees who share common goals. Solid yet flexible planning is the basis for decisions that will stabilize and move an organization forward.

REFERENCES

Baldridge, J.V., Curtis, D.V., Ecker, G.P., & Riley, G.L.(1977). Alternative models of governance in higher education. In J.V. Baldridge & T.E. Deal (Eds.), *Governing academic organizations.* Berkeley, CA: McCutchan.

Bryson, J.M. (1988). *Strategic planning for public and nonprofit organizations.* San Francisco: Jossey-Bass.

Chaffee, E.E. (1983). *Rational decision making in higher education.* Boulder, CO: National Center for Higher Education Systems.

Garner, J.F., Smith, H.L., & Piland N.F. (1990). *Strategic nursing management.* Rockville, MD: Aspen Publishers.

Ives, J.R. (1991). Articulating values and assumptions for strategic planning. *Nursing Management, 22*(1), 38–39.

Kouzes, J.M., & Posner, B.Z. (1987). *The leadership challenge.* San Francisco: Jossey-Bass.

Marriner-Tomey, A. (1992). *Guide to nursing management.* St. Louis, MO: Mosby-Year Book, Inc.

Steiner, G.A. (1979). *Strategic planning: What every manager should know.* New York: Free Press.

Strasen, L. (1987). *Key business skills for nurse managers.* Philadelphia: J.B. Lippincott, Co.

Elisabeth T. Hallman
Robin B. Allen

CHAPTER 10

Financial Decision Making in Nursing

Proportion your expenses to what you have not what you expect.
—English proberb, cited in Safire and Safir, 1990

INTRODUCTION: THE PAST IN PERSPECTIVE

Almost two centuries ago, Napoleon recognized the importance of making a good decision. Prior to the turn of this century, financial decisions in healthcare appeared simple. Hospitals were supported financially by philanthropy, and the concept of insurance coverage for hospitalization was unheard of. The hospital billed one flat daily rate to every patient. This all-inclusive rate covered any service the patient received. Although this appears to be an oversimplified method, it is important to remember that hospitals at that time had few services and an undifferentiated product line.

As technology advanced, new surgical procedures were introduced, new pharmacologic advances were discovered, and new services were provided. Patients began to pay a separate fee for each service in addition to the flat rate. It became apparent that the cost of these new products and services far outstripped the flat fee patients were being charged. This à la carte approach to payment created havoc among the patients, and hospitals realized they had to change how the patients were charged for their services. By 1930, to help spread the costs, an all-inclusive rate for inpatients, based on their length of stay and accommodations, was again being utilized by many hospitals.

During the 1920s and 1930s, the concept of reimbursable costs for direct patient care to hospitals by the federal government as well as nongovernmental agencies was introduced. In 1966, the United States government became the largest purchaser of medical care with the advent of the Medicare program, which improved access to the healthcare system for those people 65 years and older.

The 1930s through 1970s saw medical care costs escalating at an astonishing rate, due to the rapid expansion of healthcare services. Cost-based reimbursement, increased demand for services, rapid technological advancements, inflationary pressures on the economy, nursing shortages, and the cost of insuring physicians against malpractice claims were just some of the reasons the costs escalated so dramatically. By the end of the 1970s, third-party payers were reimbursing two-thirds of all healthcare costs on a retroactive basis, and it was evident that any efforts towards cost containment, up to that time, had been unsuccessful. Healthcare financial systems were in need of a drastic change.

Between 1983 and 1986, the Medicare program phased in a reimbursement strategy based on a **prospective payment system (PPS).** PPS provided a predetermined specific rate based on the patient's diagnosis. This program was adopted, in some form, by many third-party payers also. **Diagnostic related groups** (DRGs) altered the incentives for payment to hospitals and created a cost consciousness that had heretofore been absent in the healthcare industry. The terms "lean and mean" and "survival of the fittest" became financial buzzwords as resources became more limited and hospitals struggled with these changes.

Today, this cost-conscious, economically constrained, competitive environment creates a major challenge. The goal of any financial decision we make is to produce a high quality nursing product in a cost-effective environment. Yet these goals are frequently at war with each other, and it is our challenge to create a fiscally responsible environment in which to offer a quality nursing product.

As we attempt to create a quality nursing product, we must determine what decision-making models will assist us to make these decisions in the most cost-effective manner. Two models will be woven into this chapter, the **multiattribute utility theory (MAUT)** and **value analysis.** The MAUT is a framework which provides a precise, step-by-step method to assess and quantify multiple variables. The value analysis model allows the prioritization of decision options utilizing a matrix of criteria with assigned value scores. Most managers intuitively make decisions on a daily basis, and while there are no right or wrong decision making models, MAUT and value analysis are just two examples of models that may help quantitatively support the financial decisions to be made.

DEFINITIONS OF VARIOUS BUDGETS

In order to discuss the various types of budgets found in nursing organizations, a preliminary discussion of the theoretical basis for any type of budget will be offered. Goals and objectives are defined for the hospital organization, as well as the nursing organization. The budget can then be described as translating those objectives and goals into numerical terms. Budgets are plans for how you expect to measure the outcomes of the care that is delivered. In other words, budgets are quantitative tools only and are useful in determining if the outcomes as defined are met.

Budgets can be developed for periods of time from one year to several years for the purpose of forecasting for the future. The yearly budgets are usually divided into specified time periods so that outcomes can be measured on a regular basis. The term "budget" denotes dollars; however, at times there are budgets, such as personnel budgets, that may have no dollars attached but use personnel or full time equivalencies (FTEs).

There are various names for the most common budgets: cash budgets, operating budgets, capital budgets, and program budgets. There are also various methods used to develop these budgets: fixed or static budgets, planned program budgets, flexible budgets, and zero-based budgets. In order to define the process of budgeting more accurately, each of the major types of budgets will be defined.

The Cash Budget

The cash budget is not used in the nursing organization, but the nursing organization needs to be aware of the impact of the cash budget on the operating budget. A **cash budget** is just what it says—the cash that flows in and out of the organization. The revenue received from insurance companies is an example of inflow, while salary is an example of outflow. These obviously have to match to some degree so that the hospital does not have shortfalls in the outflow budgets.

The Operating Budget

The **operating budget** is the most germane to the nursing organization, as it reflects day-to-day financial activity. Nursing units are considered cost centers, which may include revenue or income and expenses. However, most nursing cost centers do not include revenue. The operating budget for a nursing unit consists of the salary dollars for the staff as well as any expenses, such as patient care supplies required to provide patient care on the unit—the nonsalary expenses. It is helpful for staff nurses to realize that their unit has specific salary dollars attached, and personnel decisions have to be made with the impact on the operating budget of the unit in mind. Any overtime or extra staff needed on the unit may require extreme scrutiny to validate that the expenses are in the operating budget, and therefore, if incurred, will still keep the cost center in line with its budgeted dollars.

The Capital Budget

The third type of budget is the **capital budget.** Capital budget items can be defined in various ways, such as items costing over a certain dollar amount, or items expected to have a defined lifetime, such as $300 or 3-year lifespan. Usually capital budget items are very costly and are therefore not included in the operating budget. On nursing units these items may include a cardiac or hemodynamic monitor, furniture, computers, or renovation of the unit.

The Program Budget

Program budgets are intertwined with capital budgets and used for new projects or special types of events that are expected to occur. The program budget may have labor or personnel expenses attached, and it may also have equipment requirements attached. Usually the equipment part of a program budget will be incurred in the capital budget, whereas the labor dollars will eventually flow into the operating budget, perhaps in the first year, but oftentimes in future years. An example of a program budget is the opening of a new intermediate care unit. All of the costs attached to the opening of that unit have to be accounted for and budgeted for. There may be renovation costs, equipment costs, and naturally, there will be new salary costs attached to those particular types of beds. All of these costs will flow into the appropriate budgets after they are identified in the new program budget. Program budgets look at costs over long periods of time and try to make long-range projections as to the feasibility of the new programs.

THE PRESENT: THE PROCESS OF BUDGET DEVELOPMENT

The Cash Budget

The cash budget is the foundation for meeting current necessary expenses. In any organization, many expenses, such as the payroll, are paid on a regular basis, while revenue collections frequently lag behind by months. This lag time may be caused by internal mechanisms such as billing procedures, or by external issues such as the timeframe in which third-party payers, such as private insurance, government programs, and health maintenance organizations (HMOs), meet their obligations. Even though revenue projections, the anticipated income, may be positive, the collection delays may result in a cash crisis. Therefore, it is essential to have a solid cash budget to meet regular planned expenses, as well as a cushion to meet unexpected cash needs.

A hospital walks a fine line with a cash budget, because it must maintain enough reserves to meet current expenses, both planned and unplanned, but not have so much in cash reserves that it will affect the institution's ability to reduce its debt, purchase capital, or invest in new programs.

While it is not the institution's primary budget, due to its operational importance, the cash budget must be carefully developed and actively managed. This budget will provide a schedule of cash receipts and cash disbursements. This budget is constructed, first, by gathering information about the primary budgets: the revenue, expense, and capital budgets. The next step is to utilize the information gathered from above to convert the revenue budget to the expected receipts portion (anticipated income) of the cash budget and to convert the expense and capital budgets into the disbursement (anticipated payments to be made) segment of the cash budget. A minimum balance is determined as a buffer and the above information is then consolidated into the cash budget, and the process is completed as outlined in Table 10-1.

The cash budget is useful for more than projecting cash surpluses and shortages. It is a powerful tool in planning investment and borrowing strategies. Although it is the financial manager who is responsible for the cash development preparation, it is essential that nursing be aware of the importance of this budget and its impact on cash management decision making for the capital, operating, and program budgets.

The Operating Budget

"The expense statements are out and we are over budget!" How many times have you heard that comment as a manager or even as a staff nurse? For many of us it is

***Table 10-1* • Cash Budget (in Thousands of Dollars)**

	Month 1	Month 2	Month 3
Cash Balance (Beginning)	$25	$25	$25
Receipts			
Inpatient	$600	$500	$750
Outpatient	350	300	375
Other Operating	25	27	25
Nonoperating	5	10	14
Total Receipts	980	837	1164
Cash Available	$1,005	$862	$1,189
Payments			
Salaries	$500	$550	$540
Supplies	275	290	310
Plant & Equipment	65	200	100
Payment on Loans	2	125	125
Total Payments	$842	$1,165	$1,075
Cash Balance (Tentative)	$163	($303)	$114
Less Minimum Balance	25	25	25
Amount to Be Invested (Borrowed)	$138	($328)	$89
Cash Balance (Ending)	$25	$25	$25

heard on a regular basis. But just what does it mean? The comment refers to the fact that the operating budget, the budget that should reflect the day-to-day, shift-to-shift financial activity of the unit, or the cost center, or the institution is not in line with the original projections made at the start of the current fiscal year. How did this happen? Usually actual expenses exceeded projected or budgeted expenses and/or the actual revenue was less than the budgeted revenue. Why did it happen? To answer that we need to explore the process by which the operating budget is developed.

The goal in developing the operating budget is to convert the corporate strategy into an operating plan and then to express the operating plan as a budget (Berman and Weeks, 1979). The corporate strategy will encompass the hospital's mission statement—to deliver quality, compassionate healthcare to the community in a cost-effective manner regardless of race, color, creed, or financial ability—as well as the institution's financial goals for the coming year—an expense increase of 5.2 percent is anticipated while generating a positive operating margin of 4.7 percent. An operating plan will take into consideration all services (inpatient, outpatient, support), and define the goals for each of these services for the coming year based on healthcare industry assumptions, economic conditions, state and local initiatives, historical data, and financial goals for the institution. Once the goals are defined, they should be prioritized and then broken down for revenue producing (radiology, laboratory) and nonrevenue producing (maintenance, environmental services, nursing unit) areas. These financial units are usually referred to as **cost centers.**

At the cost center, such as the nursing unit level, a projection of the volume of services to be provided is determined, based on the assumptions above and translated into patient days or an appropriate volume indicator, such as patient visits. In cost centers with patient day information, the number of hours of nursing care each patient on that unit requires is determined and a staffing pattern is developed. This staffing pattern determines the number of positions or full-time equivalencies (FTEs) required to deliver direct patient care. The formula for calculating FTEs is: Standard hours of care * Patient days/2080 = Required FTEs.

Standard hours of care include:

- Direct patient care hours
- Indirect hours such as conference time and sick, vacation, and holiday hours

Indirect hours may be considered nonproductive time and may include the amount of time necessary to account for sick time, vacation time, holiday time, education programs, and days off. Indirect care hours may also include those unit-based people not involved in direct patient care, such as medical clerks, nurse managers, clinical nurse specialists, and inservice educators. This terminology may vary from institution to institution but the composite parts are the same. The combination of direct, indirect, and nonproductive hours multiplied by the patient days will yield the FTE complement necessary to staff the unit. The base salary dollars for each FTE are then determined by multiplying the number of annual hours worked by the hourly rate. Added to the base salary dollars will be any differentials, bonuses, and raises projected for the year. These calculations result in the salary budget for the fiscal year. Since salaries and benefits represent 60 percent to 70 percent of the operating budget, it is essential that the nurse manager work with realistic numbers and accurately calculate and project these figures.

The other expenses related to the operating budget are non-personnel costs. These are expenses incurred and supplies consumed by the department as it delivers patient care: medical-surgical supplies, linen, nutrients, office supplies, conferences, leases, dues, books, and tuition. Calculations of these expenses are derived from past usage as well as projected additional consumption. Many of these nonpersonnel expenses are volume driven, and as such the nurse manager has control over the usage and should carefully monitor. The nonvolume driven expenses can be controlled through careful planning during the budget development process.

The development of revenue projections for the operating budget has changed significantly since the advent of the prospective, case-based reimbursement system. Today, hospitals must develop their revenue budgets based on a projection of the DRGs, as well as a projection of the third party payer mix—commercial carriers versus health maintenance organizations (HMOs), state-subsidized insurance programs, Medicare, and nonpayers (Table 10-2).

The actual fiscal performance is measured on a regular basis, usually monthly, cost center by cost center. The variance report or expense statement allows each cost center manager to adjust his or her spending patterns on a regular basis to reflect what is actually occurring, keeping in mind the budgetary constraints as well as the operating plan and goals developed for the fiscal year. Ongoing budget analysis should not be considered punitive, but a mechanism to evaluate the effectiveness of the care delivery system and the appropriateness of the goals.

In looking at the justification process necessary with operating budgets, Finkler (1984) makes two important points. One is that the operating budget is a living document and therefore must be something viewed on a regular basis and not something is prepared once a year and then put into a drawer never to be seen again. The other important point Finkler makes is that responsibility equals control when it comes to the budgeting process. If a manager does not have control over the items in the budget, then he or she cannot be held responsible for the expenses incurred in that budget or any variances. Keeping those two thoughts in mind, the operating budget can be viewed as a daily working document, a monthly document as well as a yearly document. For a manager to control the expenses in an operating budget, there must be daily controls that would include monitoring of census activity on a unit, acuity of the patient, or the length of stay of a particular patient population. Daily monitoring for nursing cost centers also requires looking at staffing patterns, as well as time spent on education and/or hours spent participating in things other than direct patient care.

If daily monitoring is maintained, monthly monitoring of the cost center becomes much easier. Most institutions issue, on a monthly basis, what is normally referred to as a labor analysis or worked hours report, which is very beneficial to the manager. This document gives such information as the number of worked hours administering direct patient care on the unit; the number of sick, vacation, or holiday hours; the number of overtime hours; and also, the number of hours spent by personnel floating (in and out of the unit). All of this information is very valuable in analyzing a monthly expense and/or variance report (Table 10-3).

In the budget preparation process, consideration should be given to fluctuations in spending throughout the year. For example, vacation time or nonproductive time is budgeted more heavily during the summer months. Another example is tuition reimbursement that is paid out as an expense, based on an academic year, at various points and is not equal monthly. If these considerations have been taken into account at preparation time, the monthly variance report should be fairly easy for the manager.

Negative as well as positive variances to the budget must be reviewed. Positive variances or items under budget may be useful information for historical purposes and for future budgeting preparations. Each line item must be reviewed for exact rationale. Professional staff salaries would be separated from technical support salaries; therefore, such things as overtime can be identified for specific categories of workers and perhaps a justification can be given based on the acuity of the patients.

Another important consideration for nursing is the actual cost per patient day on a unit. A monthly budget statement may indicate that the expenses are under budget for the month, however, the number of patient days during which care was provided on that particular unit may also be under. In other words, it may not be good enough to be under budget alone, but to be under budget based on the actual cost per patient day.

Table 10-2 • **FY 94 Budget 4928/5928 OB/GYN Clinic Nonpersonnel Expenses**

Volume	July	Aug	Sept	Oct	Nov	Dec
OP VISITS—OBSTETRICS	295	340	301	332	316	339
OP VISITS—GYNECOLOGY	260	259	188	289	260	236
OP VISITS—FAMILY PLANNING	8	8	8	8	8	8
OP VISITS—ENDOCRINE	12	12	16	12	5	8
OP VISITS—ONCOLOGY	22	21	16	27	23	14
TOTAL OUT PATIENT VISITS	597	640	529	668	612	605

Non-Personnel	July	Aug	Sept	Oct	Nov	Dec
100DENTAL	231	231	231	231	231	231
101FICA	2669	2669	2669	2669	2669	2669
102TUITION	0	0	180	0	0	0
105PENSION	0	0	0	0	0	0
107HOSPITALIZATION	4034	4034	4034	4034	4034	4034
109GROUP LIFE	159	159	159	159	159	159
110DISABILITY	181	181	181	181	181	181
127CONSULTING	8909	8909	8909	8909	8909	8909
129PHYSICIAN	39079	39079	39079	39079	39079	39079
136HONORARIUMS						
137OTHER FEES	250	250	250	250	250	250
165TELEPHONE	35	35	35	35	35	35
184FOOD	291	291	291	291	291	291
201REAGENTS	108	108	108	108	108	108
203PHARMACY	42	42	42	42	42	42
214OTHER SURGICAL	450	450	450	450	450	450
217INSTRUMENTS	17	17	17	17	17	17
218MINOR EQUIPMENT	100					
219OTHER MEDICAL	935	935	935	935	935	935
301REGENTS	252	252	252	252	252	252
302OTHER LAB	33	33	33	33	33	33
303PHARMACY	96	96	96	96	96	96
305IV SETS						
306IV SOLUTION						
307OXYGEN	30					
311SYRINGES	10	10	10	10	10	10
312NEEDLES						
313SURGICAL PACKS						
314OTHER SURGICAL	220	220	220	220	220	220

Jan	Feb	Mar	April	May	June	Total
335	301	335	322	336	322	1951
263	231	249	249	249	249	1490
8	8	8	8	8	8	48
11	8	13	10	11	12	65
29	29	35	29	31	29	182
646	577	640	618	635	620	3736

Jan	Feb	Mar	April	May	June	Total	FY'93 Budget	% Change
231	231	231	231	231	231	2766	2766	0.00%
2669	2669	2669	2669	2669	2669	32022	32022	0.00%
1180	0	0	0	0	2180	3540	573	517.80%
0	0	0	0	0	0	0	0	0.00%
4034	4034	4034	4034	4034	4034	48402	48402	0.00%
159	159	159	159	159	159	1908	1908	0.00%
181	181	181	181	181	181	2175	2175	0.00%
8909	8909	8909	8909	8909	8909	106912	75576	41.46%
39079	39079	39079	39079	39079	39079	468950	472680	–0.79%
						0	0	0.00%
250	250	250	250	250	250	3000	4440	–32.43%
35	35	35	35	35	35	420	0	100.00%
291	291	291	291	291	291	3492	0	100.00%
108	108	108	108	108	108	1296	1149	12.79%
42	42	42	42	42	42	504	807	–37.55%
450	450	450	450	450	450	5400	10407	–48.11%
17	17	17	17	17	17	204	1009	–79.78%
100						200	2296	–91.29%
935	935	935	935	935	935	11220	22667	–50.50%
252	252	252	252	252	252	3024	2781	8.74%
33	33	33	33	33	33	396	1273	–68.89%
96	96	96	96	96	96	1152	1036	11.20%
						0	0	0.00%
						0	0	0.00%
30						60	125	–52.00%
10	10	10	10	10	10	120	0	100.00%
						0	0	0.00%
						0	2	0.00%
220	220	220	220	220	220	2640	1953	35.18%

Table 10-2 • (Continued)

Non-Personnel	July	Aug	Sept	Oct	Nov	Dec
315ANESTHESIA MATERIAL						
317INSTRUMENTS-MEDICAL	15	15	15	15	15	15
318MINOR MEDICAL	7	7	7	7	7	7
319OTHER MEDICAL	353	353	353	353	353	353
322CATHS						
401OFFICE	118	118	118	118	118	118
402OFFICE/OTHER	213	213	213	213	213	213
417INSTRUMENT						
418OTHER NON-MEDICAL	44	44	44	44	44	44
503CLEANING						
507DATA PROCESS						
509PLASTICS	36	36	36	36	36	36
518ISSUES-OTHER						
600TEMPORARY HELP						
602OUTSIDE PRINT	167	167	167	167	167	167
611MAINTENANCE						
614OUTSIDE MAINTENANCE	100	100	100	100	100	100
615OUTSIDE PHOTO						
690OTHER	120	120	120	120	120	120
691PROFESSIONAL BILLING	7662	7662	7662	7662	7662	7662
700MEMBERSHIP	90					
702BOOKS	25	25	25	25	25	25
703TRAVEL-LOCAL	20	20	20	20	20	20
704TRAVEL	125	125	125	125	125	125
705POSTAGE	90	90	90	90	90	90
706MEETING	450		450		450	
750ANNUAL DINNER			6000			
754RECRUIT ADVERTISEMENTS						270
758ADVERTISEMENTS						
818OTHER						

Jan	Feb	Mar	April	May	June	Total	FY'93 Budget	% Change
						0	0	0.00%
15	15	15	15	15	15	180	928	–80.60%
7	7	7	7	7	7	84	0	0.00%
353	353	353	353	353	353	4236	5177	–18.18%
						0	0	0.00%
118	118	118	118	118	118	1416	1200	18.00%
213	213	213	213	213	213	2556	0	100.00%
						0	300	–100.00%
44	44	44	44	44	44	528	650	–18.77%
						0	0	0.00%
						0	0	0.00%
36	36	36	36	36	36	432	396	9.09%
						0	371	–100.00%
						0	0	0.00%
167	167	167	167	167	167	2004	3468	–42.21%
						0	0	0.00%
100	100	100	100	100	100	1200	2232	–46.24%
						0	0	0.00%
120	120	120	120	120	120	1435	4356	–67.06%
7662	7662	7662	7662	7662	7662	91944	91941	0.00%
						90	100	–10.00%
25	25	25	25	25	25	300	700	–57.14%
20	20	20	20	20	20	240	636	–62.26%
125	125	125	125	125	125	1500	1500	0.00%
90	90	90	90	90	90	1080	604	78.81%
450		538				2338	2599	–10.04%
						6000	6000	0.00%
					270	540	600	–10.00%
330				300		630	700	–10.00%
						382229	382229	0.00%

In developing justifications for the variance reports, quality of care and the efficiency of the staff must be reviewed. Any new technology may affect the hours of care to be provided. Policy changes may affect variance report justifications.

In looking at the process of monitoring expenses, decisions must be made on a daily basis. The manager must be comfortable making these decisions based on his or her knowledge of patient care as well as new developments that may be occurring in the hospital or on the unit.

The Capital Budget

In the capital budgeting process, there are many steps that require decisions to be made by the nurse manager. The first step in the process is to review all equipment on the unit and identify whether the equipment is movable versus fixed, non-medical versus medical, replacement versus something that might be required for a new service. The goals and objectives of the organization and the nursing unit must be considered when reviewing equipment needs. The next step is to describe the item as new or replacement. In looking at replacement, it may be necessary to establish a way to replace equipment that is not part of the prioritization in the capital budget. In other words, if medication carts need to be replaced every five years, there would be a plan spanning multiple years, and this expense would not have to be restated in every capital budgeting process. The estimated cost for any item and how soon it would be needed also needs to be identified.

The nurse manager then may be asked to prioritize his or her requests. In looking at prioritization, various decisions may flow into that process, such as who will benefit from the new equipment and how would that benefit be measured. How will that new piece of equipment affect the overall quality of patient care, who has used this particular type of equipment, and what is its benefit (Kropf, 1992)? One acceptable method of prioritization, which could be used in the following scenario, is the process called value analysis (see Chapter 9). This is a decision matrix that rates each capital item numerically and thus establishes the prioritization (Goldman, 1990). Table 10-4 is an example of a value analysis matrix, which can be used to assist a decisionmaker in capital purchase decisions. (See Scenario 10-1, p. 161).

These criteria are transformed into a value analysis matrix with a valuation scale in Table 10-4. In the case of the obstetrical department, physicians would provide over 75 percent support, employee morale would be enhanced, as staff would feel they had state-of-the-art equipment to accompany their technical skills, and the ultrasound machine would definitely be used by patients, for a **total relationship score** of 60. Safety would be enhanced for patients, as physicians could more closely monitor the stages of fetal development, availablilty would be improved by adding a new machine so patients would not have to drive across town to another lab, and physican diagnostic turnaround time would decrease, yielding a **quality of service score** of 60. Purchase of the ultrasound equipment would represent a growth position in the industry lifecycle, a return on the investment could be expected in less than two years, with a life expectancy for the new machine of twenty years, yielding a **financial viability score** of 55. The grand total for this value analysis matrix would be 175, 5 points less than the the highest possible score of 180, and much higher than the lowest possible score of 45.

Table 10-3 • **Department of Obstetrics & Gynecology Expense Variance Analysis**

MONTH MARCH 1993

COST CENTER '5928	**UNIT:**	**OB/GYN CLINICS**
I. VOLUME ANALYSIS	**OB/GYN VISIT**	**(INCLUDES COLPO, GEN GYN, OB, ONCO)**
	MTD	**YTD**
BUDGET	643.00	5689.00
ACTUAL	690.00	5390.00
VARIANCE	–47.00	299.00
DAYS/MONTH	23.00	158.00
ADC	30.00	34.11
% OF BUDGET	107.31%	94.74%
***TOT PTS PER CLINIC STAT**	1304	9152

II. PERSONNEL EXPENSE ANALYSIS

	MONTH ACTUAL	**MONTH BUDGET**	**VARIANCE**	**ACTUAL COST/PT**	**BUDGET COST/PT**
RN	21536.00	21731.00	195.00	31.21	33.80
(006 + 010)				16.52*	
OTHER	17214.00	18541.00	1327.00	24.95	28.84
(001 + 004 + 008 + 014)				13.20*	
TOTAL SALARY EXPENSES	38750.00	40272.00	1522.00	56.16	62.63 WO/ACCRUAL
				44.41*	
	YTD ACTUAL	**YTD BUDGET**	**VARIANCE**	**ACTUAL COST/PD**	**BUDGET COST/PD**
RN	197380.00	192074.00	–5306.00	36.62	33.76
(006 + 010)				21.57*	
OTHER	169302.00	163284.00	–6018.00	31.41	28.70
(001 + 004 + 008 + 014)				18.50*	
TOTAL SALARY EXPENSES	366682.00	355358.00	–11324.00	68.03	62.46
				40.07*	
FRINGE BENEFITS	**MONTH ACTUAL**	**MONTH BUDGET**	**VARIANCE**		
	8092.00	9083.00	991.00		

JUSTIFICATION/COMENTS REGARDING THE VARIANCE

001 WILL BE > BUDGET BY $6337 FOR FY. ADM. POSITION DELETED IN 6/92 BUT NOT VACATED TIL 9//92.

004 TIMING VARIANCE WITH A. SCHNEIDER. WILL BE ON LINE BY END OF FY'93.

008 DECREASING OVERTIME FOR BILLERS AS PART OF ACTION PLAN.

014 OVERAGE DUE TO SALARY COST TRANSFER FROM 2643 FOR S. HORNE WHO WAS LATERAL TRANSFER.

014 ANTICIPATE OVERAGE IN FEB DUE TO SALARY COST ENTRY FOR 12 PP FOR J. WILLIAMS FROM EPOC TO CLINIC.

014 INCREASED VOLUME HAS RESULTED IN INCIDENTAL OVERTIME.

Table 10-3 • *(Continued)*

III. NON-PERSONNEL EXPENSE ANALYSIS (EXPENSES > 10% OR $100 OVER BUDGET)

EXPENSES LINE	MTD ACTUAL	MTD BUDGET	MTD VARIANCE	VARIANCE
127CONSULTING FEES	12472.00	6298.00	–6174.00	–15535.00
129PHYSICIAN FEE OTHER	35468.00	39390.00	3922.00	15533.00
136HONORARIUMS	0.00	0.00	0.00	–500.00
137OTHER FEES	300.00	370.00	70.00	–3590.00
165TELEPHONE	0.00	0.00	0.00	–331.00
184FOOD	0.00	0.00	0.00	–2265.00
201REAGENTS	0.00	96.00	96.00	–537.00
203PHARM SUPPLIES	0.00	153.00	153.00	365.00
214OTHER SURGICAL SUPPLY	0.00	970.00	970.00	6239.00
218MINOR MEDICAL EQUIPMENT	48.00	460.00	412.00	1715.00
219OTHER MEDICAL SUPPLY	0.00	1889.00	1889.00	–12304.00
301REAGENTS	235.00	232.00	–3.00	501.00
302OTHER LAB SUPPLY	30.00	106.00	76.00	427.00
303PHARM SUPPLY	0.00	87.00	87.00	102.00
306IV SOLUTION	11.00	0.00	–11.00	22.00
307OXYGEN	0.00	0.00	0.00	83.00
311SYRINGES	2.00	0.00	–2.00	–20.00
312NEEDLES	0.00	0.00	0.00	–10.00
313SURG PACKS	0.00	0.00	0.00	–64.00
314OTHER SURG SUPPLY	174.00	163.00	–11.00	–405.00
315ANESTHESIA	0.00	0.00	0.00	–63.00
317INSTRUMENTS, MED	43.00	0.00	–43.00	684.00
318EQUIPT, MED	0.00	0.00	0.00	–254.00
319OTHER MED SUPPLY	260.00	490.00	230.00	1546.00
401POMERANTZ	142.00	125.00	–17.00	–139.00
402OFFICE SUPPLY	49.00	0.00	–49.00	–990.00
417INST&MINOR EQUIPT	0.00	25.00	25.00	–1405.00
418NON MED SUPPLY	0.00	21.00	21.00	–104.00
509PLASTICS	80.00	33.00	–47.00	–338.00
518ISSUES	0.00	31.00	31.00	236.00
600TEMP HELP	0.00	167.00	167.00	–2663.00
602OUTSIDE PRINT	348.00	289.00	–59.00	1397.00
614OUTSIDE MAINTENANCE	0.00	186.00	186.00	1217.00
690OTHER	196.00	363.00	167.00	391.00
691BILLING	11399.00	7821.00	–3578.00	–13622.00
702BOOKS	75.00	25.00	–50.00	–206.00
703TRAVEL	385.00	53.00	–332.00	79.00
704TRAVEL	0.00	25.00	25.00	515.00
705POSTAGE	0.00	–8.00	–8.00	–225.00
706MEETING EXPENSE	0.00	0.00	0.00	1161.00
750ANNUAL DINNER	0.00	0.00	0.00	392.00
754RECRUITMENT—ADVERTISING	0.00	0.00	0.00	600.00
‘758GEN ADVERTISING	0.00	0.00	0.00	700.00
818OTHER EXPENSE (INSURANCE)	0.00	26975.00	26975.00	250985.00

JUSTIFICATION
HD10 SALARIES
ON-CALL EXPENSES
ROSENSWEIG HONORARIUM PAID IN OCT
PLAYROOM SERVICES
NO PHONES INSTALLED
SNACKS FOR PATIENTS PER CITY CONTRACTS
PREGNANCY TESTS

NORPLANT BLANKET ORDER, WAS DC'D
WILL BE $7604 OVER BUDGET FOR FY '93
INCREASE USE OB PATIENT BILI LAB STIX
USE APPROPRIATE FOR PATIENT VISITS
NOTHING NEEDED
USE APPROPRIATE FOR PATIENT VISITS
NO OXYGEN ORDERED
DEPO INJECT & TINE TESTS FOR TB
SAME AS ABOVE
NO PACKS ORDERED
INCLUDED GLOVE USAGE DUE TO INCREASED VOL

STAPLE REMOVERS
SCOPETTES FOR COLPOS
USE APPROPRIATE FOR PATIENT VISITS
STATIONARY SUPPLIES FOR CLINIC & HD10
SUPPLIES FOR CARE COORDINATORS
YTD OVERAGE DUE TO COLPOSCOPY EQPT

CUPS USED FOR URINE TESTS
NOTHING ORDERED
BILLER ON LOA REPLACED BY TEMP THRU 11
EDUCATIONAL MATERIAL FOR PATIENTS
MAINTANENCE CONTRACT

INCREASE IS VOLUME DRIVEN
PDRS
WOMEN'S MARKETING CONFERENCE
CHILDBIRTH CONFERENCE
LETTERS TO PATIENTS WHO MISS APPTS

SIVITZ SYMPOSIUM
NOTHING SPENT
NOTHING SPENT
TIMING VARIANCE

Table 10-4 • Value Analysis Matrix

RELATIONSHIP MANAGEMENT

Criteria Valuation Scale

Physician	Over 75% Support	(20)	50% to 70% Support	15	25% to 50% Support	10	Less than 25% Support	5
Employee	Morale Enhancement	(20)	Productivity Enhancement	15	No Effect	10	Some Negative Effect	5
Patient	Utilized by Patient	(20)	Care Related	15	Not Care Oriented	10	Not Related	5

Relationship Management Total **60**

QUALITY OF SERVICE

Criteria Valuation Scale

Safety	Enhance Safety of All	(20)	Enhance Patient	15	Meets Requirements	10	No Significant Issues	5
Access	Add Technology	(20)	Improve/ Equal Current Technology	15	Enhance Technology Access	10	No Effect Seen	5
Prod-uctivity	Decrease Resources Needed	(20)	Resource Reallocation	15	Resource Allocation	10	Increase Resources Needed	5

Quality of Service Total **60**

FINANCIAL VIABILITY

Criteria Valuation Scale

Industry Life Cycle Issues Position	Innovation	(20)	Growth	(15)	Consolidation & Stabilization	10	Decline	5
Return on Investment	Under 2 Years	(20)	2–4 Years	15	4–5 Years	10	No return	5
Life Expectancy	2 Years	(20)	15 Years	15	10 Years	10	5 Years or Less	5

Financial Viability Total **55**
GRAND TOTAL **175**

Whether or not a value analysis system is used, an explanation needs to be given for the capital request. This might include how the equipment would change patient care, any patient volume that may be driving the request, or the obsolescence of an item that needs to be replaced. The lifetime revenue generation is also a vital piece of information. In looking at any piece of equipment or capital item,

Scenario 10-1

The Obstetrical Department Labor and Delivery needs to decide if an ultrasound machine should be purchased. An ultrasound machine would generate the ability to do more procedures and therefore to generate more revenue for the hospital. The following information in the categories of relationship to management, quality of service, and financial viability in Table 10-4 must be analyzed in order to make a capital budgeting decision:

- Physician support
- Effect on employees
- Effect on patients
- Ability to enhance patient safety
- Patient accessibility
- Productivity based on resource need and allocation
- Position in the industry lifecycle
- Return on investment
- Life expectancy

the quality of care issue and how the equipment will benefit the patient care of the organization must always be kept in mind. Once the analysis is completed, the decision will ultimately be made based on the organizational objectives and outcomes of the value analysis.

The Program Budget

As identified earlier, program budgeting looks at the future of an organization. A program budget will take a specific idea and generate the information necessary to determine if the program is a feasible one. The first component in preparing a program budget is to identify all aspects of the program; after identification, a cost-benefit analysis decision-making strategy can be applied. Benefits may be in nonfinancial terms, such as quality issues, or as a tradeoff with another type of program. These details must not only look at the nursing costs associated but must cut across departmental barriers.

Scenario 10-2

A teaching institution is considering the possibility of expanding its recovery room hours to include nights and weekends. This need was identified because of ongoing operative procedure scheduling constraints as well as surgeon availability. The multiattribute utility theory (MAUT) provides a methodology to evaluate this decision. The following steps may be used to walk through the process of MAUT.

Step 1 involves *determining the appropriate viewpoint for the decision.* In this instance, the viewpoints of management as well as physicians should be considered; therefore, a committee composed of representatives from anesthesia, nursing, finance, surgery, and support departments should be formed.

The second step is *identifying decision alternatives.* In this case the alternatives could include:

- Expand hours to include weekends and nights
- Modify current hours
- Make no changes in the hours

Step 3 is *identifying attributes for evaluation.* The following operational issues should be considered before determining the attributes to be evaluated:

- Current operating room schedule
- Current delays in operative procedures due to scheduling
- Current hours of physician practice patterns, including weekends
- Potential for change in physician practice patterns
- Current recovery room hours
- Impact on interfacing departments

Several financial items should also be considered. These are addressed in Table 10-5 under the headings of revenue, cost, and turnover. **Revenue attributes** include associated revenue with an increased number of cases. The **cost attributes** include associated salary costs for nursing, anesthesia, and ancillary personnel, capital expenditures—stretchers, equipment, and operating expenditures for supplies. The **turnover attributes** assess physician, nurse, and patient turnover based on the individual's satisfaction with ability to practice or services offered.

In step 4 *factors are identified to evaluate the attributes.* In this instance, revenue associated in Table 10-5 with an increase in cases, costs associated with an increase in staff, an increase in capital needs, an increase in operating supplies, and physician, patient and staff satisfaction can be measured. While satisfaction may appear unquantifiable, satisfaction may be measured in terms of turnover of physicians, patients, and nurses and the cost to recruit and train physicians and nurses and attract new patients.

Step 5 is *establishing a utility scale.* On a scale of 1 to 10 (least to most) each committee member would rank the factors of each attribute (revenue, cost, turnover) in terms of contribution to his or her decision. In Table 10-5, under the utility scale columns, one member ranked the attributes.

Step 6 involves *transforming each factor value to a utility scale* by tabulating the average scores for each attribute. For example, under revenue the utility value for revenue greater than $400,000 is 10, or most desirable.

Step 7 is *determining relative weights for each attribute and factor.* In this case, the committee could rank the attributes of revenue, cost, and turnover in terms of the importance in the decision. For example, if they ranked the attributes 1, 2, 3 (1 being least important and 3 being most important) the contribution value to the decision would be 50, 33, and 17 percent. The values assigned are based on the perspective of this particular committee, and could be assigned any relative number. For example, by

Table 10-5 • Multiattribute Utility Theory

Attributes					
Revenue		**Cost**		**Turnover**	
($000's) Factors	Utility Scale (1–10)	**($000's) Attributes**	Utility Scale (1–10)	**#PTS, RNS, DRS) Attributes**	Utility Scale (1–10)
>200	10	>100	1	30	1
150–199	8	80–99	2	20–29	3
100–149	6	60–79	4	10–19	5
50–99	3	40–59	6	1–9	7
0–49	1	20–39	8	0	10
Less than	0	Less than	10		
	1=LEAST DESIRABLE 10=MOST DESIRABLE		1=LEAST DESIRABLE 10=MOST DESIRABLE		1=LEAST DESIRABLE 10=MOST DESIRABLE
Relative Weights	50%		33%		17%

changing the values to 2, 2.5, and 3, the assigned contribution value for the factors in Table 10-5 would be 40, 33, and 27 percent.

Step 8 involves *calculating the total utility for each of the decision alternatives* (Table 10-6). The calculation involves selecting a factor from each attribute that would be the outcome of the alternative and multiplying the utility score of each factor times the ratio weight for that attribute.

Step 9 is *determining which decision alternative has the greatest utility score.* For example, using Table 10-6, for the expand alternative, the revenue attribute that received a utility score of 10 would be multiplied by the relative weight of the revenue attribute of 50 percent—10 times 50 percent equals 5. This process would be completed for all alternatives for each attribute, revenue, cost, and turnover and the accompanying utility scale. Thus the recommended action would be to expand services, as this alternative received the highest score, 7.36.

Step 10 is *performing a sensitivity analysis* to see if a change in weights or differential scaling would alter the decision.

Table 10-6 • Alternatives, Attributes, and Corresponding Utilities

Alternative	**Attributes Revenue**	+	**Cost**	+	**Turnover**	=	
Expand	(10*Rel Wt) 5	+	(2*Rel Wt) 0.66	+	(10*Rel Wt) 1.7	=	7.36
Modify	(7*Rel Wt) 3.5	+	(8*Rel Wt) 2.64	+	(7*Rel Wt) 1.19	=	7.33
No Change	(1*Rel Wt) 0.5	+	(10*Rel Wt) 3.3	+	(10*Rel Wt) 1.7	=	5.5

The costs and benefits of undertaking such a project should now be clearly identified. This would not be a unilateral decision to implement this program, and MAUT would ensure input and consensus from multiple disciplines. If this program were approved, the salary dollars would be transferred to the appropriate operating budgets, and any equipment costs would flow into the capital budget. As you can see, identifying all the potential impact areas of a new program, and insuring that all costs and benefits are identified is a large undertaking.

THE FUTURE

How will we make financial decisions in the twenty-first century? How will we analyze the effectiveness of decisions? It's hard to say, but one thing is for certain—with the economic conditions and healthcare reform as the cornerstones, solid, fact-based financial decisions will create a fiscally sound healthcare system. Nursing's impact will be dramatic as practice is streamlined, and new and exciting ways are created to deliver quality healthcare in a cost-conscious world.

SUMMARY

In the 1920s and 1930s, calculating charges for healthcare was simple due to the small number of technologies and services available. As time progressed, both services and costs escalated. Finally, in the 1980s, prospective payment systems based on DRGs were implemented by government and private third-party payers in an attempt to control costs. Healthcare organizations turned attention to the process of budgeting.

In this chapter, a review of the various types of budgets was given. The process of budget development was discussed, with examples of budget variance analysis as a decision-making tool provided. Case scenarios demonstrating value analysis and the multiattibute theory of decision making were reviewed.

The future will demand even more applications of fact-based decison-making theories and strategies to maintain tight control of the use of healthcare dollars with the move to models of community-based healthcare delivery and more participative management. All nurses, whether functioning in clinical or administrative roles, will need to maintain financial savvy in making decisions concerning healthcare finances.

REFERENCES

Berman, H., & Weeks, L. (1979). *The financial management of hospitals*, 4th ed. Ann Arbor: Health Administration Press.

Finkler, S. (1984). *Budgeting concepts for nurse managers.* Orlando: Grune & Stratton.

Goldman, E. (1990). Making the best decisions. *Healthcare Forum Journal, 33*(1), 30–35.

Kropf, R. (1992). Managing for technology to improve service. *Healthcare Executive,* 7(1), 25–26.

Safire, W., & Safir, L. (1990). *Leadership.* New York: Simon & Schuster, Inc.

Robin B. Allen
Linda A. Sinesi

CHAPTER 11

Human Resource Management

Think wrongly if you please, but in all cases think for yourself.
—*Doris Lessing, b. 1919, British writer (cited in* Quotable Women, *1989).*

INTRODUCTION

Many decisions are made by nurse managers that influence human resource issues in acute care, ambulatory care, and community settings. Nurse managers must interview, hire, and evaluate all employees. Each one of these situations involves making decisions, all of which may have far-reaching effects. Nurse managers may also need to discipline employees. These situations usually involve complex decisions and ones in which the manager must be comfortable with every aspect of the process. This chapter will offer some insight into the manager's decision making in all of these situations, as well as in the more complex areas of retention incentives and substance abuse.

THE SELECTION PROCESS: HIRING

One of the most important responsibilities of nurse managers is the selection of new employees. The challenge is to hire the best applicant for each job opening. Careful selection is important because of the many costs associated with employee turnover. According to the National Association of Health Care Recruiters, the minimum average cost for each new hire in 1988 was $20,000. This cost reflects expenses for recruitment materials, salaries, hiring expenses, and lost staff productivity during orientation (Glover, 1989). In addition to the financial expense, turnover may cost the hospital dearly in terms of employee morale and satisfaction, and in the ability to effectively provide nursing services. Careful decision making will lead to better employees who will stay longer and will reduce the costly cycle of continual hiring and turnover.

The Interview Process

The key to effective decision making is mastering the skill of job interviewing. The interview provides the opportunity to obtain data useful for making sound employment decisions. Employee selection is a complex decision-making process that draws upon the manager's perception, communication skills, insight, and logic.

What characteristics should the nurse manager look for in prospective employees? What characteristics form the basis for making a hiring decision? Does the prospective employee have

- A positive attitude?
- The willingness to work?
- Flexibility?
- Reliability?
- The ability to do the job?
- The temperament for the job?

The nurse manager must be able to visualize the candidate as part of her working staff. The manager should ask, "Can the candidate do the job? Will the candidate do the job? and, Will the candidate's professional needs and goals be met in this position?" (LaRocca, 1982). During the interview process, an attempt should be made to determine if the applicant has the skills to do the job, if the applicant has the motivation to do the job, and if the job is the right fit for the applicant at this time. The manager should also offer factual information about the position and about the organization to provide the applicant with a basis for accepting or rejecting a job offer, if made. Both the interviewer and the applicant must attempt to determine the extent to which the position will be enjoyable and challenging to the applicant.

Never hire a borderline candidate just for the sake of filling the position. It is far better to be selective and wait for the right employee than to hire in desperation. A bad hire means a bad termination sooner or later. It is important to be selective and patient, and not to fall victim to pressure and short-range hiring.

Obstacles and Pitfalls in Hiring

What are the obstacles to effective hiring decisions? The nurse manager should be aware of the following obstacles, as defined by Metzger (1982), and try to minimize these obstacles in the hiring process.

- ***Personal Biases***—Examine personal biases that would affect your hiring decisions. If you had to choose between two equally qualified candidates, would you hire the black or the white, the female or the male, the older or the younger?
- ***Lack of Defined Expectations***—Be sure you have clear expectations based on objective, performance-based criteria for the position. Candidates should be evaluated against the expectations, not against each other.

- ***Making Early Decisions***—Hiring decisions should be made once all the information is obtained, rather than on the basis of first impressions. Studies have shown that once managers have formed an impression, they tend to pay attention only to information that reinforces it (Del Bueno, 1982).
- ***Halo or Horn Effect***—Applicants should not be rated on the basis of one positive or one negative characteristic.
- ***Central Tendency or Leniency Effect***—Beware of the tendency to rate all candidates in the average range (central tendency), or to rate all candidates highly (leniency effect).
- ***Cloning Effect***—Avoid the urge to hire people in your own image. Managers may make the mistake of trying to hire employees who have similar characteristics to their own or those who will not appreciably change the work group.

Under federal law, job discrimination based on sex, race, color, religion, national origin, or age is prohibited. State law governing employment varies, so it is important to become familiar with the laws in your state. Any inquiry designed to elicit information as to national origin, race, color, ancestry, age, religion, or handicap is unacceptable unless based upon a bona fide occupational qualification (BFOQ).

A **BFOQ** is a qualification that is absolutely necessary to perform a job. For example, if the job requires the ability to speak Spanish, you may ask "Do you speak Spanish," but you are prohibited from asking "Is Spanish your native tongue?" To avoid problems, do not pursue a conversation that is legally out of bounds. If the applicant tells you she speaks Spanish because she was born in Puerto Rico, it is up to you to close the subject (Martin, 1989).

Del Bueno (1982) advises concentrating on the qualities important for the performance of the job to avoid falling prey to these obstacles. Careful preparation for the interview is essential. First, it is important to review the job description of the position to be filled. The interviewer must be familiar with the job requirements and must be able to clearly articulate expectations for job performance.

The Interview

Once the manager has reviewed the job description and defined the expectations for the job, the interviewing process can begin.

Study the application prior to the interview with special attention to the following: number of previous positions and length of stay at each, breaks in employment, and reasons for leaving. Note any inconsistencies or concerns and prepare questions to further explore these areas during the interview.

The interview should be divided into the following segments: introduction, structured questions, and closing remarks. During the introduction segment, the interviewer should attempt to put the applicant at ease. The interviewer should clarify the position the applicant is applying for, ask the applicant to talk about previous work experience, and determine why the applicant is looking for a job change at this time.

The structured question segment is the area where the most important information is obtained. In this segment, the interviewer should ask questions and seek to clarify and verify the applicant's answers. Statements like "Tell me more about that," questions such as "Can you give me an example?" or "How did you go about handling that problem?" will assist the interviewer in clarifying. A statement, "If I understood you correctly . . ." and a question "Are you saying . . . ?" will assist the interviewer in verifying. Be an artful listener. Make use of the pregnant pause. A moment of silence can bring out additional information. A long pause after the applicant answers your question will indicate you feel more needs to be said. For example, the manager might ask "Why did you leave your last job?" The applicant might answer, "Because there was not room for advancement." Instead of going on to the next question, pause and wait for the applicant to add to his or her answer. At this point, the interviewer should attempt to resolve any concerns about the applicant. Ask questions related to your concerns to elicit additional information.

The use of a structured interview or standardized format may be very helpful in forming comparative judgments between two or more applicants for the same position (Kaiser, 1978). It may also be useful as a historical database for evaluating hiring patterns and when making decisions about retention strategies. Interview questions should be based on the job requirements and typically include four types of questions (Purcell, 1980).

- ***Situational Questions***—The manager will describe a typical job-related situation and ask the applicant to discuss how he or she would handle the situation. To test the applicant's ability to prioritize, the manager may ask, "What would you do first?"
- ***Job Knowledge Questions***—The manager will ask questions that will assess knowledge essential to job performance. The manager may ask the applicant to describe the symptoms of hypoglycemia.
- ***Job Sample/Simulation Questions***—The manager will ask questions related to job content. For example, the applicant may be asked to calculate an IV drip rate. These questions are generally task related and may require the applicant to actually perform the task.
- ***Work Requirement Questions***—The manager will ask questions designed to assess the applicants "willingness" to meet the job requirements. Areas such as willingness to rotate shifts or work weekends will be explored here. While it is permissible to ask questions related to required work schedules, it is illegal to ask those related to willingness to work religious holidays.

It is important for effective decision making to ask key questions and to keep questions open-ended. Examples of open-ended questions include those that begin with why, who, what, when, where, how:

- "Why are you interested in this position?"
- "Who is your role model?"
- "What are some of the things you particularly liked about your last job?"
- "What questions do you have about the position?"
- "Where would you rank this job with other jobs you have had?"
- "How do you feel your supervisor rated your job performance?"

Questions should always require a fuller explanation. Avoid questions such as:

- "You are looking for a position as a Registered Nurse?"
- "Are you willing to work weekends?"
- "Did your supervisor rate your job performance fairly?"
- "Do you have any questions about the position?"

All of these questions lead to yes or no answers.

Finally, the manager must prepare for questions the applicant may ask you. Applicants may ask questions on the following topics:

- ***Nursing Care***—"What is the method of patient care delivery?" "What is the nurse/patient ratio?"
- ***Nursing Service***—"What is the philosophy of nursing?" "Is there a regular meeting of a joint committee of doctors, staff nurses, and hospital administrators concerning patient care issues?"
- ***Orientation***—"What is included in orientation?" "How long is the probationary period?"
- ***Performance Evaluation***—"How will I receive feedback regarding my performance?" "Will my salary increases be based on performance?"
- ***Professional Advancement***—"Are inservices offered at a variety of times to facilitate attendance?" "What is the policy on attendance at outside workshops/conferences?" "What are the requirements for promotion?"
- ***Salary***—"What will my starting salary be?" "When will I be eligible for an increase?" "Are there differentials for evenings, nights, weekends, holidays, call time?"
- ***Hours***—"What are the shift start times?" "Is the schedule posted at least two weeks in advance?" "Will I be required to rotate shifts?" "How often?"
- ***Vacation/Holidays***—"How many paid holidays will I receive?" "Which ones?" "Will I be paid for vacation days not taken?"
- ***Health Insurance/Benefits***—"If I don't use all my sick days, can I add them to my vacation time?" "Is there an employee discount for prescriptions?" "Do you have a retirement plan?" "Does the health care organization pay full premiums for healthcare?"

In the closing segment, the interviewer should ask the applicant if there is anything that has not been covered. If interested in the applicant, a tour of the healthcare delivery setting should be offered. It is often helpful to introduce the applicant to several staff members. Remember, not only is the applicant trying to obtain the position, you are also trying to hire the applicant. It is often helpful for the applicant to meet the staff in order for both of you to evaluate the fit of the applicant to the position. The manager will be attempting to evaluate not only what is being looked for in a prospective employee, but also what the applicant is looking for in a prospective employer.

Ask the applicant if he or she is interested in the position. Discuss the course of action to be taken (i.e., your timeframe for making the decision, when the applicant can expect to hear from you). Be clear as to how follow-up will occur.

Regardless of the outcome, the interview process is an opportunity for the nurse manager to create good feelings toward the organization. The applicant will base his or her judgment of the healthcare organization on how the interview process is handled.

Reference Check

The next step in the process is the **reference check**. The reference check is used to validate impressions gained from the interview and to verify basic information such as position title, job responsibilities, and dates of employment (Kieffer, 1991).

In these litigious times, many companies have adopted the policy of releasing dates of employment only. It is often helpful for the manager to do the reference check, because it is possible to gain clues about an applicant's past performance by listening not only to what the previous employer says, but how it is said. Listen for silences, tone of voice, and hesitation.

There is an interviewing technique that may decrease an interviewer's dependence on the reference check. Simply ask the applicant what he or she believes the previous supervisor will say when you make your formal reference check. The question implies you will be checking, and when asked the right way evokes very honest responses. Other questions you may ask are: "Do you think your previous supervisor would describe your strengths and weaknesses accurately?" If so, "What do you think he would tell me?" The answers to these questions may uncover some areas that will need further clarification or investigation.

The last step is to contact the applicant and either make a job offer or tell the applicant he or she has not been selected.

PERFORMANCE APPRAISALS/EVALUATION

According to Jones and Hauser (1991), "performance appraisals should measure job specific performance criteria" (p. 40). There is an implication in this that a clear and concise job description is necessary in order for the nurse manager to complete a performance evaluation. Any prospective employee should request a copy of the job description prior to employment. Sheridan (1987) states that a job description will offer the fastest clues as to the employer's expectations. Job descriptions need to include a description of the job, the qualifications for the job, to whom the individual reports, and the functions and responsibilities of the particular position. Performance standards can be derived directly from the job description if the job description is written in behavioral terms. This particular chapter will not deal with development of job descriptions, but will define the various performance appraisal techniques and types. One important point to be made prior to any further discussion on performance appraisal is the need for managers to focus on managing performance and not just evaluating performance (Kanin-Lovers and Bevan, 1992).

Instrument Types

There are various instrument types available to use for the performance appraisal. All can be acceptable if coupled with the appropriate job description and the establishment of standards. The job description and the standards must be shared with the employee upon hire and annually thereafter. There may also be times when it is necessary to develop particular standards or goals with an employee who is having difficulty in a specific area. Some of the instrument types are:

- ***Essay Technique***—The employee's strengths and weaknesses are identified in relationship to the job description. This is done in a narrative form.
- ***Graphic Rating Scale***—This is a scale in which a range is given, such as satisfactory to unsatisfactory.
- ***Forced Choice Rating***—The evaluator reviews groups of statements and determines which best fit or least fit the individual being rated.
- ***Critical Incident Technique***—This is known by nurse managers as anecdotal notes—incidents that are considered critical to performance of the job.
- ***Rank Order Method***—This method has a number of variations, one of which would be to list all employees on the floor from most valued to least valued. Rank ordering appears to lend itself to general perceptions by the evaluator rather than concrete facts.
- ***Paired Comparison Ranking***—Another method of ranking in which selected criteria are used to evaluate employees against each other.
- ***Management by Objectives***—Predetermined goals and objectives are established and then the performance appraisal evaluates whether they are met. In this method, the employee is considered to be an integral part of the process (Schweiger, 1986).

Evaluation

There are various reasons given in the literature to support the use of performance appraisals. Probably the most important is to give feedback to the employee about how he or she is doing on the job. This can be extremely important when dealing with disciplinary issues or with other types of actions necessary to review the standard of care being given on a nursing unit. It can also be a time for mutual goal setting (McGee, 1992). Another reason for performance appraisal is to help with decisions regarding compensation. It is very important during the budgetary process to have all the information available on merit increases, if such a system exists. If the performance appraisal system gives raises based on years of service rather than merit, then this may not be as important in the budgetary process. There are human resource personnel who strongly believe that the performance appraisal should not be linked with any wage increases given to an individual. This requires employees who are motivated by knowing they do a good job rather than motivated by material consequence. As stated briefly before, personnel decisions—promotion, layoffs, discharges, or any other decisions about how personnel are used on a particular unit—should be based on performance appraisals. Performance appraisals are only a continuation of the communication process and are not formal meetings to discuss issues that the employee was not aware of before the performance appraisal meeting (Pennock, 1992).

In the next section, disciplinary action will be discussed in greater detail, and the important part that performance appraisals play in that system will be reviewed.

As stated earlier, job descriptions and performance appraisals must be shared with an employee at the time of hire and must be reviewed on an ongoing basis. If this is done during the interview process, it assures that all employees on a unit have heard the same expectations. It may be helpful to review the expectations in a staff meeting as well as at the time of individual appraisals.

The Process of Evaluation

The processes of performance appraisals are varied, but in most organizations they are conducted from the "top down." Most of us are familiar with the superior-subordinate relationship whereby the superior evaluates the subordinate. Self-evaluations have become fairly common in the nursing industry. This can be enlightening not only for the employee but also for the manager. When an employee evaluates him- or herself, he or she is required to give some thought to areas where he or she may not be performing to the level of others in the health-care delivery setting. Sometimes a point of comparison with peers is provided in the process. The process helps the supervisor to see where the expectations may have been misdirected. As an example, if an employee does not see that she is having a problem with nursing documentation, but the supervisor feels that documentation is a major problem in this individual's performance, the supervisor may question whether the employee understands the expectations. If this is so, once again, the expectations should be reiterated with the individual. The self-evaluation also will give the supervisor a better understanding of the individual, especially if the individual is a relatively new employee and the nurse manager has not had adequate time to observe this employee's performance.

Another suggestion is the subordinate-superior evaluation whereby the subordinate evaluates the supervisor. As one might surmise, this can be a difficult process, and must be viewed as nonthreatening, and one in which the supervisor can gain information to help his or her growth. A simple tool may be used, such as one in which the manager is rated on various components: leadership ability, concern for others, responsibility, and cooperation. The employee should always be given anonymity when completing this, because many employees feel inhibited and fear retribution. If done in a positive manner, this type of tool can supply a lot of information to the supervisor to enhance growth and to realize his or her full potential.

One concept that has become more widely used in recent years, especially with regard to shared governance and professional practice literature, is the use of the peer review. This process can be extremely threatening to the staff nurse, in fact more so than a superior evaluation. The process must be clearly defined, so that all individuals understand and are able to work through their anxieties regarding the process. The process, which has been used in some organizations, includes a compilation method using the self-evaluation and perhaps a peer evaluation of choice, a random peer, or several peers. This may allay some fears if the staff nurse can choose one of his or her peers to do the evaluation in conjunction with someone he or she has not chosen, and also if his or her own self-evaluation plays a part in the overall performance appraisal. Another component of peer review may be a peer review committee, which can be extremely threatening, because the peer review committee would be privy to the overall rating of the individual. Confidentiality must be maintained in order for the process to work appropriately. One word of caution in using peer review is that a "**halo effect**" has been documented in the literature (Farh, Cannella, and Bedeian, 1991). When used only for developmental purposes, the halo effect is gone; however, evaluative situations cause raters to be more lenient, less differentiating, and less reliable. Some of these effects may be alleviated with formal training in peer review.

A decision-making process must occur in every performance appraisal. Whether that be the supervisor determining where the employee fits on the performance scale, or whether that be a peer trying to complete an evaluation form. In either case, all of the facts and perceptions must be looked at, and a valid determination must be made as to the actual performance of the individual. In establishing a peer review system, the people on the unit must first decide if they want to have such a system, and then decide what the process will be after a decision is made to implement. There is no clear definition of how the decision-making process works in this situation because so many emotional factors enter the process. As said earlier, a peer review system can be extremely threatening to an individual and to organizational cohesiveness when used.

Scenario 11-1

You have a peer review system in place and an employee has received his performance appraisal and reacted negatively. The employee would like to see each evaluation and speak with the peer who completed it to determine what he did wrong. How would you handle such a situation? What decisions would you make on behalf of the staff and on behalf of the disgruntled employee?

In this situation, it might be best if the Peer Review Committee sits down with the employee and discusses the employee's concerns. The Committee may be able to shed light on the reviewer's comments while maintaining anonymity. If anonymity has been guaranteed as part of the process, then that needs to be respected. There also may be other grievance procedures in place in your organization that can be of benefit to an unhappy employee.

COUNSELING AND DISCIPLINE

"Creativity is an element of the decision-making process" (Das, 1987, p. 72). This may seem an odd thing to say when describing the discipline or counseling process for employees. Another axiom within the human resource literature is the one of avoiding discipline. Discipline is only one method of changing behavior; other strategies should be employed before the formal discipline process. Some believe self-discipline is the only form that has a long-term impact (Kiechel, 1990). There definitely is a negative connotation to the word counseling; however, counseling can be a creative strategy used by the nurse manager or at the request of the employee. Nurse managers should find that a large percentage of their time is spent counseling employees, but not in the formal sense within the disciplinary process. The needs of an individual employee can be viewed in the same context as nurses look at patients. Using the nursing process, a nurse assesses needs, plans a strategy, implements a strategy, and then evaluates the outcomes. In many ways, this is the same process that the nurse manager must undertake in order to be objective and fair in dealing with his or her employees.

Steps of the Disciplinary Process

Another axiom used in the discipline process is never to counsel an employee in a public place. A private setting should always be used, and confidentiality maintained. There are identified steps to the formal disciplinary process, and the most elementary is a verbal counseling. The nurse manager may use an anecdotal note to document the conversation. There are varying thoughts about the use of anecdotal notes and many human resource administrators feel that any contact with an employee regarding a disciplinary issue should be documented and placed in that person's permanent employee record. If a verbal counseling is done and not documented, then the counseling is not viewed as the first step in the disciplinary process.

When a situation warrants a written counseling, this is considered the first step in a progressive disciplinary process. In the written counseling process, the documentation should include what the error or infraction was, and what action is being taken on the part of the employee to remedy the situation. If the situation continues, the next step in the process is a written document, carrying more weight than a written counseling. This may be called a warning notice, or some other name that implies a progressive pattern. Once again, the facts are recorded and also what needs to be done to remedy the situation. The third step in progressive discipline is usually the suspension of the employee. This allows an employee to consider his or her options and also what it would be like to be unemployed. Sometimes the loss of pay will change behavior that was not changed based on the counseling or warning notice. The last step in the progressive discipline is the termination of the employee, and once again, this should be used as a last resort when all other attempts at behavior change have been exhausted.

Individual organizational policies may differ, but in most, a progressive discipline policy implies the same actions for the same infraction. In other words, absenteeism is viewed differently in a progressive disciplinary process than is a work performance issue. An employee may be to the point of suspension for absenteeism, but may be only on a written counseling for work performance. There also may be specific guidelines within an organization as to who can give the disciplinary document to the employee, as well as who must approve the process prior to implementation. In many organizations, termination of an employee can only be done after discussion with the human resource department or expert.

Documentation of problems is extremely important, and good records must be kept regarding occurrences warranting discipline. Good records, according to Shideler (1989), reflect six elements:

- Accuracy
- Objectivity
- Relevance
- Clarity
- Timeliness
- Consistency

Verification that the employee has been made aware of the incident should also be included.

Scenario 11-2

You have a female employee who has a tardiness problem because of childcare responsibilities. According to your hospital disciplinary policy, the individual had previously been given a written counseling document and a warning document. The problem has continued, and it is now time to suspend the individual. What could be your creative strategies to avoid such an action? Try to include in your thought process the individual's home schedule, the work schedule and work flow on your unit, and the childcare responsibilities of the individual. Perhaps a remedial solution can be found for someone who probably cannot afford to have the pay loss, and for whom the suspension will not change the behavior. Is the employee a good worker and one you wish to retain? Is the workflow such on the unit such that you could stagger the employee's start time? Could the employee start later and thereby be on time? Would this change disrupt the unit or could adjustments be made in the assignments to accommodate the worker?

Grievance Process

Employees have a right to grieve disciplinary actions if they do not agree that the actions are valid. In most organizations, this grievance procedure is defined in the employee handbook and is very similar to those found in a union environment. The employee must notify a supervisor of the manager or the human resource department or expert of his or her intent to grieve the action of the manager. Usually five to ten working days are provided for the person to do so. At that time, the supervisor will hear the grievance by speaking with the employee as well as the manager. A decision to uphold the decision of the manager or to negate the disciplinary actions is then made by the supervisor.

If the employee does not agree with the action of the supervisor, an appeal can be made to the human resource department or expert, once again within a specified period of time. A person in the human resource department hears the grievance and either upholds the action or once again can negate the disciplinary action. This process continues up through the supervisory levels; in most instances there are three to four steps in the process. A final decision is usually made by one of the executives of the organization. At any level in the grievance process, the hearing person may change the discipline if he or she feels that a more appropriate action should have been taken.

Cautions

Nurse managers, in handling disciplinary issues, should be cautious in the use of discipline and attempt to avoid the formal disciplinary process if at all possible. The manager should be assured that all facts have been investigated, that all people involved have been talked to, and that the action being taken is similar to previous actions for similar problems. One of the very difficult things in large nursing organizations is for nurse managers to know precedents for disciplinary issues. Sometimes inequities can be avoided by speaking with a supervisor who may have more of an understanding of the total organization. Employee handbooks with disciplinary actions defined specifically help the manager to make appropriate decisions. Explicitly stated policies also help employees to know where they stand and what can possibly happen to them for infractions of established rules.

According to Rutkowski (1987), there are a few steps that a manager can take when determining disciplinary actions to insure that a wrongful discharge action will not be sought against the employer. In deciding whether to take action, the following points should be assessed:

- Is there legitimate reason for discharge which may be defined by the institutional policy?
- Is there evidence that stated policies were not followed?
- Is there consistency and objectivity in documentation in all steps taken?
- Has there been reasonable handling of the situation, which means the investigation of all facts and discussion with any other personnel who have a need to know?
- Is there assurance that the action is consistent with hospital policies and stated or implied promises?

Rutkowski (1987) goes on to encourage managers to ask themselves the question, "Would I feel comfortable stating my reason for discharge in an open hearing, before a jury and/or a judge?"

An employee has the right to go to the EEOC (Equal Employment Opportunity Commission) if he or she feels that his or her rights have been violated. The employee also has the right to a hearing before the unemployment board if unemployment insurance is denied based on a disciplinary action. Both of these types of hearings may require a manager to testify before a hearing board. Prior to the hearing, human resource department/experts will coach the manager in the hearing process and appropriate verbal statements. These are very difficult hearings, especially for new nurse managers. The guidelines given previously in this chapter can in many cases avoid the need for such hearings. If the disciplinary action is appropriate to the situation, hopefully the employee will realize that his or her actions were inappropriate and will also realize that attempting further appeals would be unnecessary and not in his or her best interest.

Discipline and Substance Abuse

One issue explored in the current nursing literature is one of appropriate disciplinary action for narcotic or alcohol abuse. There are various State Board regulations; however, most employee advocates believe that rehabilitation needs to be offered to the employee, rather than termination from employment. In the not-too-distant past, termination was the only option when an employee showed signs of alcohol abuse or diverted narcotics for self-use. Now there is more knowledge of the problem and more realization that the problem is fairly common in the nursing community. Rehabilitation is necessary to keep nurses in the workplace. Many institutions will approach the employee, allow the employee to acknowledge the problem, and then offer some type of rehabilitative services. Institutional policy may vary depending on State Board regulations. In the state of Pennsylvania, the State Board of Nursing is notified if there is an abusing employee; however, that employee can enter one of the rehabilitation programs approved by the State Board and will not forfeit his or her license for the first infraction. The one exception to this is evidence of selling or obtaining drugs for someone else, or being convicted of a crime. This type of program enables nurse managers to work with the employee and to offer help rather than a punitive action. A suggestion for all nurse managers is to know State Board regulations, and to encourage the institution to have a written policy of discipline for the impaired professional.

The nurse manager may have difficulty working through the decisions that need to be made. It is not a process that is done frequently, and therefore, the nurse manager does not always feel comfortable that he or she is making the appropriate decisions. Once again, gather all of the facts while maintaining the confidentiality of the employee. Sometimes the process is difficult, especially when the manager must initially acknowledge the problem. This may also happen when a physician instead of a nurse is suspected. The neophyte nurse manager will need assistance working through the process. These are probably some of the most dramatic disciplinary situations, because patients are affected, as is the employee's life and possibly an entire career.

RECRUITMENT AND RETENTION

Recent statistics indicate that the national hospital vacancy rate for nurses has decreased; however, changes in healthcare delivery settings will accelerate the future need for nurses in excess of availability (Shearer, 1993). In the mid-1980s, the healthcare industry began a cultural transition from the traditional labor-intensive high-tech mentality to a service-oriented customer-focus mentality (Eisenberg, 1986). In today's environment, the employee recruitment process must not only be concerned with the technical skills, but also the interpersonal skills of prospective employees.

Family issues affect workers more than at any time in the past, due to the changing demographics of the workforce of the 1990's. Today, more women and dual income or single-parent wage earners make up the workforce. The changes in the workforce are creating a demand for organizations to remove family-related barriers to productivity by designing work-family benefits programs. This is happening at a time when economic constraints are forcing many organizations to reduce benefits (McDermott, 1993).

Traditionally, nurses' concerns about the workplace have fallen into four categories:

- Working conditions
- Nursing administration support
- Salary and benefits
- Scheduling

One must shift the search for solutions to the problems of nurse recruitment and retention from the outside environment to the workplace itself. Nurses have some power to control the hospital environment, and nurse managers have the responsibility to look critically at traditional thinking, systems, and methodologies. The nursing management team must ask: "Is the system meeting the needs of today's workforce, or is the workforce asked to tailor lifestyles and needs to the system?"

Regardless of the hospital's patient mix or geographic location, certain characteristics are common to those facilities that successfully recruit and retain nurses. This conclusion was supported in the study, "Magnet Hospitals: Attraction and Retention of Professional Nurses," conducted by the American Academy of Nursing's Task Force on Nursing Practice in Hospitals in 1982 (McClure, 1982). In this study, hospitals that were successful at recruitment and retention created a practice environment valuing quality care, nurse autonomy, open lines of communication, innovation, bringing out the best in the individual, and striving for excellence. The study credits the nursing leadership of the organizations with promulgating these values.

Retention Incentives

Nurse managers should not underestimate the importance of the influence staff nurses have on the recruitment and retention process. Some of the best retention incentives are free. Treating staff with courtesy, respect, and complimenting staff are strategies nurse managers can use with great success. The least expensive and most effective recruitment is done by satisfied staff. Conversely, staff members who are unhappy in their jobs have a negative impact on the recruitment and retention process.

Maraldo (1991) states that proper utilization of nurses once they enter the workforce is the key to ending the nursing shortage. Many sources agree that today's managers must develop strategies that would restructure the workplace to offer nurses greater work schedule flexibility and increased autonomy and control over nursing practices.

Incentives to attract and retain nurses have grown in popularity. Organizations are offering incentives such as tuition reimbursement, permanent shifts, shift bonuses, weekend bonuses, weekend plans (full-time pay for working two twelve-hour shifts on weekends), recognition programs, clinical ladders, collaborative practice models, and shared governance, to name a few. Recruitment and retention strategies must go beyond offering basic incentives. They should encompass the nursing organization's values and demonstrate the organization's caring for the individual.

Nursing organizations must recognize that healthcare is in a constant state of change and therefore continuously update strategies to keep pace with that change. Successful organizations will be aware of the needs of the workforce, will respond to those needs, and will effectively communicate how employee needs are met for both existing and potential employees (Finkler, 1993).

Plan for Recruitment and Retention

With these factors in mind, what questions should the nursing management team consider when developing a recruitment and retention plan? The following will lend some direction to a plan.

- What is the target population for recruitment? What are the recruitment needs? What clinical specialties have vacancies (ICU, Medical-Surgical, Psych)? Does one wish to recruit new graduates or experienced RNs, full- or part-time staff?
- What are the recruitment goals? How many positions are currently vacant? Will anticipated turnover be considered? How many positions does one wish to fill? Will this decision be based on the average daily census of the unit or number of patient visits? What are the budget constraints?
- Does one need incentive programs for recruitment and retention? What is currently being done to retain nurses? Does one anticipate adding any nurses? Which specialties? What is the cost and the benefit of the incentive?

The multiattribute utility theory (MAUT) may be a helpful decision-making approach for the manager faced with developing a recruitment and retention plan. Multiple considerations will influence how the nursing organization will choose strategies. The MAUT can be used to identify and analyze multiple variables to provide a common basis for arriving at a decision. This technique is well suited for those decisions in which group input is critical. This method has both an intuitive and an empirical element, and encourages decisionmakers to identify and agree on alternative options and the attributes that best compare the performance of each option (Garre, 1992).

SUMMARY

Decision making is always complex, but in the arena of human resources, it becomes even more so because of the direct impact of the decision on the individual. All human resource decisions must be well thought out to protect the individual as well as the organization. New managers must rely on more experienced individuals for their insight and direction into many of these situations. Only with time do managers become comfortable making these decisions by relying on their own experience.

REFERENCES

Das, Y. (1987) Decision making. In K.W. Vestal (Ed.), *Management concepts for the new nurse manager* (pp. 71–86). Philadelphia: Lippincott.

Del Bueno, D.J. (1982). Picking winners: A primer for hiring staff. *RN, 82*(2), 96–100.

Eisenberg, B.(1986). Strategic human resource plans help providers survive changing conditions. *Modern Healthcare, 16*(7), 154–156.

Farh, J., Cannella, A., & Bedeian, A. (1991). Peer ratings: The impact of purpose in rating quality and user acceptance. *Group and Organizational Studies, 16*(4), 367–386.

Finkler, S. (1993). *Financial management for nurse managers and executives.* Philadelphia: W.B. Saunders.

Garre, P. (1992). Multi-attribute utility theory in decision making. *Nursing Management, 23*(5), 33–35.

Glover, S.M. (1989). *Recruitment and retention.* Baltimore: Williams & Williams.

Jones, D., & Hauser, M. (1991). Putting teeth into pay-for-performance programs. *Healthcare Financial Management, 45*(9), 32–44.

Kaiser, P. (1978). Ten steps to interviewing job applicants. *American Journal of Nursing, 78*(4), 627–630.

Kanin-Lovers, J., & Bevan, R. (1992). Don't evaluate performance—manage it. *Journal of Compensation and Benefits,* 7(5), 51–53.

Kiechel, W. (1990). How to discipline in the modern age. *Fortune, 12* (10), 179–180.

Kieffer, M. (1991). The reference check: What you need to know. *Healthcare Executive, 91* (11/12), 18–19.

LaRocca, S.L. (1982). Interviewing and selecting staff. *Nursing Management, 13*(9), 22–24.

Maraldo, P. (1991). Empowerment, not numbers will end the nursing shortage. *Health Care Financial Management, 45*(9), 20–30.

Martin, P. (1989). Hire right, hire smart: The artful interview. *Working Woman, 87* (3), 71–76.

McClure, M. (1982). *Magnet hospitals: Attraction and retention of professional nurses.* Kansas City, MO: American Nurses Association.

McDermott, M. (1993). Finding the fit. *Profiles*, 6(4), 54–58.

McGee, K. (1992). Making performance appraisals a positive experience. *Nursing Management, 23*(8), 36–37.

Metzger, N. (1982). Interviewing skills: Selecting the right candidate. *The Health Care Supervisor, 82*(10), 41–49.

Pennock, D. (1992). Effective performance appraisals (really!). *Supervision, 53*(8), 14–16.

Purcel, E.D. (1980). Structured interviewing: Avoiding selection problems. *Personnel Journal, 80*(11), 907–912.

Quotable women: A collection of shared thoughts. (1989). Philadelphia: Running Press.

Rutkowski, B. (1987). *Managing for productivity in nursing.* Rockwell, MD: Aspen.

Schweiger, J. (Ed.) (1986). *Handbook for first line managers.* New York: Wiley.

Shearer, J.L. (1993). Health care reform: Nursing's vision of change. *Hospitals, 67*(8), 20–26.

Sheridan, D. (1987) Becoming a successful employee. In K.W. Vestal (Ed.), *Management concepts for the new nurse manager* (pp. 187–199). Philadelphia: Lippincott.

Shideler, D. (1989). Documenting disciplinary situations. *Supervisory Management, 34*(7), 15–20.

Robin W. Wells

CHAPTER 12

Leadership

> . . . the very speed of change introduces a new element into management . . . already nervous in an unfamiliar environment, to make more and more decisions at a faster and faster pace.
>
> —*Toffler, 1980*

INTRODUCTION

Where does leadership reside in the organization? It resides within each member of the organization. The scope of each leader's influence will vary widely and be subjected to various constraints. The importance of the dissemination of leadership potential cannot be underestimated for organizational health and personal growth.

It is important to recognize that within each organizational level, there are leadership abilities and desires. According to Bennis (1989), ". . . learning to lead is a lot easier than most of us think it is, because each of us contains the capacity for leadership" (p. 3). In fact, almost everyone can point to some leadership experience. This may be played out through formal or informal leadership roles. These roles may be formally granted (positional), given (elected or selected), borrowed (an ineffective formal leader lends his power to another), or conferred (group consensus that another person should take leadership).

The breadth and depth of leadership depends upon the equilibrium of the organization, availability of resources, scope of power granted, timeframes, relation to others, and recognition potential. Stable organizations have clearly defined leadership roles and team expectations as well as adequate resources. Transitional organizations often experience the rise of informal leaders and power struggles as they compete for limited resources. Organizations in start up or in crisis often turn to charismatic or autocratic leaders who do not share power because of severe time and resource constraints.

Organizational and/or situational stability demands different leadership styles for various types of decision making. An effective leader must:

- Know the steps of the decision-making process
- Understand the three types of decisions most commonly made
- Determine whether the decision should be made by an individual or a group
- Decide an approach or decision strategy
- Choose devices and/or techniques to assist the decision making
- Determine a method to successfully implement the decisions

According to Lancaster and Lancaster (1982), "the factor that weighs most heavily in the success or failure of . . . (leaders) is the quality of the decisions they make . . . especially . . . in an era fraught with rapid changes that necessitate a rational, systematic approach to making decisions" (p. 23).

LEADERSHIP THEORY

What is leadership? **Leadership** is the "process of influencing the actions of a person or group to attain desired objectives" (Koontz, O'Donnell, and Weihrich, 1986, p. 397). Leadership cannot occur in a vacuum, it involves a leader and at least one follower.

Who becomes a leader? For more than forty years (1904-1948), trait theorists believed that leaders were born, not made. They studied a variety of personality traits, physical characteristics, and specific abilities. No physical characteristics were consistently found in successful leaders (Yukl, 1981), but a group of traits and skills were found that appeared to be characteristics of successful leaders (Table 12-1).

Yukl (1989) and Stogdill (1974) both recognized that certain abilities and personality traits could increase the probability of leader effectiveness, but not guarantee it, and that the key to effectiveness depended on the leadership situation. In other words, Stogdill found that results varied from situation to situation, and he concluded that it took more than innate ability for a person to become a leader. ". . . The pattern of personal characteristics of the leader must bear some relevant relationship to the characteristics, activities and goals of the followers" (Stogdill, 1974, p. 64). Situation theory emphasizes environmental factors that enable the leader to get the work done effectively. However, opponents of the situation theory (proponents of the Great Man theory) noted that many crisis situations require a leader, and yet many situations do not produce a leader to resolve the problem (Schriesheim and Kerr, 1977).

The next natural step in leadership theory development was to take a wider view of situation theory by looking beyond the situation into the workings of the organization at large. The organizational view became known as **systems theory,** which means, ". . . viewing the organization in terms of its larger environment and treating the organization both as a whole and as a set of intricately related parts" (Burack and Torda, 1979, p. 42). Systems theory recognizes that the organization impacts on the relationship between a leader and subordinates in terms of prescribed work roles and centralization of decision making.

Table 12-1 • **Traits and Skills Most Frequently Characteristic of Successful Leaders**

Traits	Skills
Above average intelligence	Good communication
Self-starting	Creative
Adaptable to situations	Knowledge about tasks at hand
Perceptive	Alert to social environment
Possess emotional maturity and integrity	Organized
Goal oriented	Conceptually skilled
Assertive	
Self-confident	Technical (knowledgeable about methods & processes)
Decisionmaker	Human relations
Reliable	
Influential	
Energetic	
Tolerant of stress	
Responsible	
Originality	

(Adapted from Yukl, G.A., Leadership in Organizations, *2nd ed. Englewood Cliffs, NJ: Prentice-Hall, 1989); Hein, E.C., and Nicholson, M.J.,* Contemporary Leadership Behavior: Selected Readings *(Boston: Little Brown, 1986); Bass, B.M.,* Stogdill's Handbook of Leadership: A survey of Theory and Research *(New York: Free Press, 1981).*

Leadership Behaviors

Leadership behavior explains the overt actions of leaders engaged in the functions of planning, organizing, directing, and controlling. Leadership style is a variety of traits and behaviors used to influence others, which taken as a whole, corresponds to a style of leadership. It can be either **autocratic** (boss-centered/task oriented) or **democratic** (subordinate-created/ people oriented). All leadership style descriptions can be placed on a continuum. No approach is inherently inappropriate; the approach taken by the leader depends upon the situation, and the system in which the decision making occurs. It is perfectly reasonable for a leader to behave one way in situation and/or organization A, and another way in situation and/or organization B. For example, during a cardiac/respiratory arrest, an autocratic style of leadership is necessary to complete the task of advanced cardiac life support. The focus is on the patient, not the feelings of the team members or consensus of the treatment protocols. On the other hand, a more democratic approach is expected from the chair of the advanced life support committee when protocols are chosen and decisions made for treatment implementation and cessation.

Autocratic behaviors include an authoritarian approach (no questions asked!) and one-way communication (top down). This leader structures the task to be completed, minimizes obstructions to enable efficient task achievement, and then rewards the workers. The process is task oriented, with a technical focus on production and close subordinate supervision. The autocratic leader initiates and controls the process through centralized decision making. This style is effective in crises, because it permits rapid decision making and demands work efficiency.

However, according to Gillies (1989),

> . . . even in situations of high stress and high need for task information (as in a critical care unit), authoritarian leadership may provoke aggression in employees with low self-esteem. Furthermore, authoritarian leadership encourages dependence in subordinates by engendering fear of criticism, fear of disfavor, fear of financial loss, and concerns that the leader can accentuate or relieve at will through manipulation of praise and blame (p. 374).

Staff who are achievement-oriented often prefer an autocratic leader. Staff who are affiliation/relationship-oriented probably will not. In general, autocratic leaders enable workers to produce a greater quantity of work while democratic leaders enable workers to produce higher quality work.

Democratic behaviors include an egalitarian approach (questions elicited) and two-way communication (up and down). The leader provides the vision that outlines the task to be achieved and elicits ideas and plans from the workers. The worker is valued over production. The process is worker-oriented with a focus on interaction, supportive group methods, and consideration of the worker in the decision-making process. The democratic leader controls the process through the use of positional and personal power to motivate the workers, while retaining responsibility for the final decision. One way for the leader to retain power over the decision-making process is by using a veto. Often when using the democratic approach, both leaders and followers misconstrue this to mean, "whatever the group decides, the group does." By retaining veto power, the leader ensures that an appropriate decision is made that considers the workers as well as the organization's vision and resources. According to Gillies (1989), "Although democratic leadership facilitates coordination of diverse viewpoints, exploration of those viewpoints leads to over-long discussion of peripheral and often trivial issues resulting in critical time loss. Therefore, democratic leadership often improves employee morale at the price of decreased productivity" (p. 375).

An effective leader should develop a full range of leadership behaviors. It is important to become comfortable in assessing each situation before determining the appropriate behaviors to use. A "continuum of leadership" was introduced by Tannenbaum and Schmidt, (1973) depicting a range of leadership behaviors from autocratic (boss-centered style) to democratic (subordinate style). He described a continuum of seven types of leadership behavior, beginning with maximum use of authority and ending with a large area of subordinate freedom. Examples of these leadership behaviors can be seen in Table 12-2.

As depicted in Table 12-2, as one progresses from autocratic to democratic behaviors, a third style of leadership style merges. This is known as **participative**

Table 12-2 • **Continuum of Leadership Behaviors**

Style Continuum	Behavior
1. Leader makes and announces decision.	AUTOCRATIC
2. Leader sells decision to subordinates.	AUTOCRATIC
3. Leader presents task or goal and action ideas and invites questions.	PARTICIPATIVE
4. Leader makes decision, which is subject to change if subordinates object or present a better idea.	PARTICIPATIVE
5. Leader presents task or goal, elicits action ideas, then makes the decision.	PARTICIPATIVE
6. Leader defines task or goal and limits, asks . subordinates to recommend a decision.	DEMOCRATIC
7. Leader defines task or goal and limits and through delegation, asks subordinates to make decision subject to veto.	DEMOCRATIC
8. Leader abandons group without defining task or goal or setting limits. Expects subordinates to function independently.	LAISSEZ-FAIRE

Adapted from Tannenbaum, R. and Schmidt, W.H., How to Choose a Leadership Pattern, Harvard Business Review, *51, 164–170 (1993).*

leadership. The leader analyzes the situation, proposes action, elicits comments from the workers, and then makes the decision. At the opposite end of the continuum from autocratic behavior is a laissez-faire ("let alone") leadership. This style is truly an absence of leadership caused by abandonment of the group by the leader. The laissez-faire leader presents no limits in terms of vision, direction, organizational resources, and supervision. The workers are forced to function on their own without clear accountability.

Tannenbaum and Schmidt's (1973) model expanded the focus from leader-only behavior to the inclusion of subordinates in the decision-making process. Then Hersey and Blanchard (1982) added a third dimension: the maturity of the followers. Their three-dimensional model included:

- Task versus relationship behavior of the leader (autocratic versus democratic)
- The environment in which the leader is functioning (situation/system)
- The maturity of the group members

According to Marriner-Tomey (1992),

> this model is consistent with Argyris' immaturity-maturity continuum, which indicates that as a person matures, she progresses from a passive to an active state and from dependence to independence. With maturity, she passes from a need for structure and little relationship through a decreasing need for structure and increasing need for relationship to little need for either (p. 267).

In terms of selecting an effective leadership style, the leader needs to assess the maturity of the individuals who make up the group and determine whether they have low, moderate, or high maturity. Low maturity groups have a high task and a low relationship orientation that respond best to autocratic leadership styles (telling). Moderate maturity groups are either high task/high relationship or high relationship/low task, which respond best to participative leadership style (telling or participating). High maturity groups have low relationship/low task needs which respond best to a democratic style (delegating).

Until 1989, literature on leadership contained four variables that affect the leader. These include characteristics of:

- The leader
- The subordinate
- The situation
- The environment

In 1989, Yukl proposed an integrated conceptual framework that demonstrated that "leader behavior is influenced by a variety of factors, including leader attributes, situational demands and constraints, and information about intervening variables and end results" (p. 268). He believed that ongoing research was necessary to develop this framework into a comprehensive leadership theory.

The emergence of **Total Quality Management (TQM),** with its revolutionary restructuring of the workplace and organizational culture, has lead to the relabeling of leadership styles as either **transactional** or **transformational.** Transactional leadership is necessary to implement role changes in subordinates and can occur through three levels of interactions: telling, selling, or participating. Survival transactions involve telling the subordinate what to do and how to do it with little consideration for leader-subordinate relationship needs. The next two levels of selling and/or participating are called interpersonal transactions, because they consider the leader and subordinate needs. Each of these three transactions is based upon information exchanges rather than through intense interpersonal relationships. Transformational leadership is used to motivate subordinates to commit to revolutionary ideas (such as a new organizational structure or culture) through articulation of a clear vision of the future and use of intense interpersonal relationships. The leadership goal is to transform the subordinates' individual values to equal those of the leader. Subordinates are empowered to work to their potential and encouraged to be responsible and accountable through delegation. Transformational leaders are viewed as organizational teachers, because they encourage experimentation and risk-taking and view mistakes as learning opportunities.

Another trend is to shift the focus from the attributes of the leader to attributes of the follower. According to Kelley (1988), "Organizations stand or fall partly on the basis of how well their leaders lead, but partly also on the basis of how well their followers follow . . . Bosses are not necessarily good leaders, subordinates are not necessarily effective followers" (pp. 142, 143). Kelley (1988) has identified five followship patterns, as shown in Table 12-3, based on the degree of independent, critical thinking and a passive/active scale.

Table 12-3 • **Five Categories of Followers' Roles and Behaviors**

Roles	Behavior	Leader Characteristics
Sheep	Passive, uncritical, dependent	Low self-confidence, poor judgment, uses telling
Yes People	More active, uncritical, dependent	
Alienated, Followers, "Turned Off"	Critical, independent in thinking, passive, rarely disagree with leader	Controlling through telling and selling
Survivors	Adept at all four behaviors, active/passive; independent/critical thinking; dependent/uncritical thinking; demonstrates what leader wants!	Varies
Effective Followers	Independent/critical thinking, active	Delegates clear vision, high self-confidence

Adapted from Kelley, R.E., In Praise of Followers, *Harvard Business Review, 88 (6), 142–148 (1988).*

The essential qualities of effective followers are described by Kelley (1988) as:

- They manage themselves well
- They are committed to the organization and to a purpose, principle, or person outside themselves
- They build their competence and focus their efforts for maximum impact
- They are courageous, honest, and credible (p. 144)

An emerging leadership role is the cultivation and appreciation of effective followers.

Today's leaders must assess each situation in terms of the following:

- The task (difficulty, complexity, time availability)
- The group (size, communication, background, and maturity)
- The group's need for task versus relationship behavior
- The leader's repertoire of behaviors and skills
- The effectiveness of the followers
- The environment in which the task/goal resides

Based on this information, the leader must choose the appropriate leadership style and initiate those behaviors. Leaders who are able to adapt their style are most likely to reach the best decisions.

THE BOSS'S LEADERSHIP STYLE

What type of leadership style is needed to facilitate decision making? That depends on where the leader falls in the organizational hierarchy. The most frequently used leadership style is related to:

- The boss
- Positional, personal, and professional power
- Scope of responsibility
- Departmental maturity
- Organizational size and culture

Of these, the most frequently overlooked factor is the leadership style of the boss.

The leadership repertoire of the boss must be assessed to gain insight into the types of situations that trigger specific leadership behaviors. This is important, because the leader's behavior in a specific situation puts limits on the managers reporting to him or her. For example, if a manager is told a final decision, the only leadership option is to tell his or her subordinates. If the boss tells managers in a department meeting that sick time can be accrued to 240 hours as of January 1, there is little to do except to provide subordinates with that same information. The subordinates may not understand that neither they nor the manager can impact this decision. On the other hand, if managers are asked to participate in the decision making, they may have the opportunity to gather information from their subordinates. The manager's leadership behavior may be selling and/or participating. In the accrual example, subordinates might have the opportunity to put forth concerns such as:

- An incentive program to convert sick days to vacation time or cash
- Ways of handling long-term illnesses
- The possibility of increased use of sick days on a regular basis so the time would not be lost

On the other hand, if delegating decision making is highly valued by the boss, managers are likely to look for these opportunities unless they can justify why this behavior is inappropriate for their subordinates.

STRENGTHS OF SUBORDINATES

In addition to knowing the boss's repertoire of leadership behaviors, managers must also assess the subordinates' maturity levels and acceptance of specific leadership actions. It is important to assess how an individual responds in a given situation, as well as how a group of individuals responds to the manager as a leader. Each subordinate will fall at some point on the maturity continuum—from a need for high structure/low relationship to less structure/high relationship and then to little need for either. This transition is not related to age, is not necessarily stable across situations, and may reverse during high-stress situations. Consider the maturity level of a newly graduated nurse (GN): Her needs are for structure so that she can successfully complete her patient care tasks with little regard for a personal relationship with the leader. In six to twelve months, as task-related behavior becomes more routine, energy can be used to form relationships. However, the first time the GN is unexpectedly reassigned to another unit (pulled), the need for high task structure will reemerge and the new leader must anticipate this and plan to spend time helping the GN structure the workload for success. Paying attention to individual needs will help make managers successful decision makers.

GROUP BEHAVIOR

Managers should identify the informal leader, observe what behaviors the informal leader uses to influence the group, and compare this with the leadership style the manager must assume in a given situation. In the capped sick time hour situation, the formal leadership style had to be either tell or sell. If the manager chose to sell the decision, the informal leader might be helpful in the process. The advantage to the informal leader is that he or she gets the high relationship with the manager (formal leader). The advantage to the formal leader is that the staff gets to process the decision through the informal leader. The risk to the formal leader is that the informal leader can sabotage either the formal leader or the decision.

In addition to determining leadership behavior, deciding whether to convene a group is a critical leadership decision. Groups are resource intensive, may discourage opposing views through pressure to conform, and require a skilled formal leader to reach an organizationally acceptable decision. Groups are convened when the decision needs to be understood and accepted, and the implementation requires cooperation. "Since groups possess greater knowledge and information than any of their members individually and are less limited in the approaches used to solve a problem, they can deal with more complex problems than individuals can" (Sullivan and Decker, 1992, p. 25). However, there must be time available, with a deadline set, and the process should not lead to unacceptable levels of conflict. During groupthink, decision making may become frivolous, high risk, or subverted, because no one individual can be held responsible or accountable. Thus the leader may wish to retain veto power.

OTHER SITUATIONAL CONSIDERATIONS

Decisions are made under conditions of certainty, risk, or uncertainty. In making a decision where the problem can be clearly defined, where all possible alternatives are known, and where all scenarios can be played out for risk analysis, the condition of certainty exists. In today's healthcare environment, this is extremely unusual.

In a risk situation, alternatives, associated costs, and the potential for success must be estimated. Each of these must be given a probability percentage ranging from 1.00 (certain to happen) to 0 (certain not to happen). For instance, in making a decision concerning a plan to recruit GNs, one indication of success is purported to be the hiring of five GNs in the next sixty days. The probability of this happening in any given marketplace in July and August is a 0.10. It is known that only extremely dissatisfied GNs will leave their current place of employment within their first two months of hire. And, GNs who plan to start work in the fall have already committed themselves to positions prior to graduation and are not seeking employment during these months. Under conditions of risk, the probability of each alternative must be assessed by the leader as accurately as possible. If a group is assigning probability and there is a great disparity, the leader should not immediately settle for the middle ground. The group members at the extreme must explain to the leader and to the group's satisfaction their rationales. As the rationales are explored, one of the probabilities which at first seemed extreme may be accepted by the group as reasonable. This would never have occurred if the leader had permitted the group to quickly accept a compromise probability.

The most common decision-making condition the leader will encounter is that of uncertainty. All alternatives, risks, and consequences of the decision are not known. There are three approaches for the leader to use:

- Maximax (optimistic)
- Maximin (pessimistic)
- Risk-averting (middle of the road)

To be successful, the leader must take a logical/rational perspective to gather as much information as possible before using past experience and intuitive skills to make the final decision. The following tools including several discussed in Chapter 3 are available to assist in this process:

- Decision trees
- Best/worst case scenarios
- Expert information systems
- Consultants

Decisions made under conditions of risk and/or uncertainty are influenced by the culture of risk taking within the organization and are related to the availability of expendable resources. In times of scarcity, organizational risk taking falls. Leaders need to assess the organization's most likely response to decisions requiring a high level of risk and match their recommendations to it.

DECISION-MAKING OBSTACLES

All decision making occurs within the framework of the organization's culture. The first factor for the leader to assess is *the milieu surrounding each situation.* There are several potential organizational/cultural conditions that the leader needs to understand. They include:

- The degree of organizational rigidity/inflexibility surrounding key issues such as resource allocation, the role of nursing, male response to female decisions, and tolerance of specific leadership styles.

- The knowledge of organization icons and sacred cows and the strength of the organization's past history in current issues.
- The range of risk taking and the circumstances surrounding the choice. For example, does the organization careen from taking no risks to taking extreme risks, or are moderately safe decisions the norm?
- An assessment of the events that precipitate decision making: Are decisions only made during crises? Does the leader have to be a "squeaky wheel" to get decision approval? Are corporate games played out during the decision-making process? How are leader power struggles resolved?

The single most important decision the leader makes is deciding which organization to join. During the hiring process, it is imperative to make sure that personal and professional values match those of the organization and that the leader's dominant leadership style will be facilitated by the organization's culture.

The second milieu obstacle in decision making is caused by a *lack of motivation* among leaders, subordinates, and groups as well as within organizations as a whole. Lack of motivation is often caused by mismatches between employees and the organization's culture, or during times of extreme uncertainty and organizational change. Assess the values of potential employees during the hiring process in order to prevent value clashes. In some situations, the leader can relieve tension caused by value conflicts that emerge during the decision-making process. This can be achieved through the use of humor or the creation of satisfying independent activities.

The third milieu obstacle is the *scarcity of key resources* that impact the leader's ability to make decisions. These include:

- Time
- Access to experts
- Meeting facilities
- Assembling a group
- Computer support
- Secretarial assistance
- Materials

These often require bargaining and/or bartering skills to obtain. Make sure that the minimum amount of resources is available before proceeding to make a major decision. At budget time, remember to build in funding to support decision-making activities. This may include funding for the purchase of microcomputers, specific software programs, flip-charts, report holders, and consultants.

The fourth obstacle in decision making is *lack of skill* in the leader, the subordinates, the group, or the organization. Important skills include problem recognition and definition, information seeking/gathering, in-depth analysis, accurately developing alternatives, and assessing risks. Additionally, the leader needs to have well-honed verbal, networking, and writing skills. It is important to identify the skills that are missing or require further development. Obstacles are a fact of life! By learning how to minimize them, the leader improves his or her chances for a successful decision outcome.

Creativity

Sullivan and Decker (1992) define creativity as, "The ability to develop and implement new and better solutions . . . creativity is an essential part of the critical thinking process" (p. 243). Creativity draws upon the activities of the right brain rather than the rational/logical left brain. It is the leader's responsibility to encourage creativity during decision making and to be skilled in specific techniques. A common group of creativity-enhancing techniques explained in detail in Chapter 3 are:

- Brainstorming
- Best/worst scenarios
- Nominal group technique
- Delphi technique

Use of these techniques requires suspension of value judgments, eliciting an abundance of imaginative ideas, and connecting imaginative ideas together.

A second group of techniques for stimulating creativity, called **synectics** (Gordon, 1968), is based on the use of four different types of analogies:

- Personal analogy (individuals identify with the problem)
- Direct analogy (make comparisons with parallel concepts)
- Symbolic analogy (use impersonal images to describe a problem)
- Fantasy analogy (suspend judgment and reality)

The leader must decide whether it is important to generate a large number of ideas or to identify one different idea.

If a problem is identified that has not been worked and reworked in the organization, the first set of methods might be the most useful in generating a large variety of ideas. These ideas might be new to the organization, but well-known to others. In situations where well-known solutions are not sufficient, the second set of techniques should be tried to elicit a new and different idea. For example, after all known techniques were used to improve staffing, an organization still had a staff retention problem. The Baylor Plan was conceived to address the three interrelated issues of adequate staffing, weekend coverage, and staff retention. A leader must recognize the importance of using both sides of the subordinate's brain and to create opportunities for creative problem solving.

SUMMARY

Leadership styles and skills are critical to facilitate decision making in today's healthcare organization. In times of risk and uncertainty, the leader must assess the task, the situation, the maturity of the subordinates, the usefulness of a group, and common obstacles in selecting a leadership style. Developing a wide range of leadership skills and maintaining a flexible approach will ensure decision-making success. Decision making does not occur in a vacuum. An effective leader must work with and through others instead of always making decisions alone.

REFERENCES

Bass, B.M. (1981). *Stogdill's handbook of leadership: A survey of theory and research.* New York: Free Press.

Bennis, W. (1989). *On becoming a leader.* New York: Addison-Wesley.

Burack, E.H., & Torda, F. (1979). *A manager's guide to change.* Belmont, CA: Lifetime Learning Publications.

Gillies, D.A. (1989). *Nursing management: A systems approach.* Philadelphia: W.B. Saunders.

Gordon, W.J. (1968). *Synectics.* New York: McGraw-Hill.

Hein, E.C., & Nicholson, M.J. (1986). *Contemporary leadership behavior: Selected readings.* Boston: Little Brown.

Hersey, P., & Blanchard, K.H. (1982). *Management of organizational behavior: Utilizing human resources.* Englewood Cliffs, NJ: Prentice Hall.

Kelley, R.E. (1988). In praise of followers. *Harvard Business Review, 88*(6), 142–148.

Koontz, H., O'Donnell, C., & Weihrich, H. (1986). *Essentials of management.* St. Louis: McGraw-Hill.

Lancaster, W., & Lancaster, J. (1982). Rational decision making, managing uncertainty. *Journal of Nursing Administration, 12*(9), 23–28.

Marriner-Tomey, A. (1992). *Guide to nursing management.* St. Louis: Mosby-Year Book.

Schriesheim, C.A., & Kerr, S. (1977). Theories and measures of leadership: In J.G. Hunt & L.L. Larson (Eds.), *Leadership: The cutting edge.* Carbondale, IL: Southern Illinois University Press.

Stogdill, R.M. (1974). *Handbook of leadership.* New York: Free Press.

Sullivan, E.J., & Decker, P.J. (1992). *Effective management in nursing.* New York: Addison-Wesley.

Tannenbaum, R., & Schmidt, W.H. (1973). How to choose a leadership pattern. *Harvard Business Review, 51,* 164–170.

Toffler, A. (1980). *The third wave.* New York: Bantam Publishing House.

Yukl, G.A. (1981). *Leadership in organizations.* Englewood Cliffs, NJ: Prentice-Hall.

Yukl, G.A. (1989) *Leadership in organizations,* 2nd ed. Englewood Cliffs, NJ: Prentice-Hall.

Yvonne Troiani Sweeney
Sharon M. McLane

CHAPTER 13

Empowerment

To encourage others is to strengthen the team.
—*Anonymous*

EMPOWERMENT AND AUTONOMY

It's difficult to pick up a book or article on management or leadership in recent years without encountering references to empowerment. Since **empowerment** is the cornerstone of this chapter, we want to begin by establishing a definition.

Mason, Costello-Nickitas, Scanlan, and Magnuson (1991) define empowerment as enabling others to recognize and feel their strengths, abilities, and personal power. Block (1987) articulated the concept of empowerment as a fundamental respect for people, their abilities, their freedom as individuals, and their dignity. Chandler (1992) explains empowerment as enabling others to act. "People are empowered when responsibility, authority and accountability are meted out in equal measure" (Manthey, 1989, p. 17).

Synthesizing these definitions, we can define empowerment as recognition of the fundamental ability of staff to make effective decisions regarding the work they do, and providing them with the necessary resources and support to make those decisions. However, empowerment of staff just doesn't happen by itself; it is a carefully nurtured partnership between leaders and staff. Empowerment requires leaders who are truly committed to coaching, mentoring, and leading staff as they utilize their skills, abilities and knowledge in making decisions. "Management must believe that the people who perform the work know more about the work than anyone else; therefore, they are the right people to make decisions about how that work should be done" (Manthey, 1989, p. 17). Empowerment also requires staff who are willing to accept the responsibility, authority, and accountability to affect their practice and work environment. If management fails to provide and promote an environment that supports empowerment, or if staff fail to accept the responsibility, authority, and accountability requisite to empowerment, the outcome is nonetheless the same—staff become embroiled in a victim mindset and a sense of powerlessness over change.

Empowerment, as described by Mason et al. (1991), is ultimately a commitment to yourself and others, a confirmation of yourself, your values and dreams. It requires an awareness and respect for your abilities and strengths and willingness to employ them in collaboration with the abilities of those with whom you associate and work. Mason et al. (1991) continue to describe empowerment as having three integral components: positive self-esteem, developing self-efficacy with the skills necessary to achieve personal and group goals, and an increasing awareness of the complex social and political realities that influence your life and situation.

Employing these definitions, we can see that empowerment is a concept with both personal and external connotations; empowerment embodies a management philosophy that allows and supports staff to make decisions regarding their professional practice and work environment, and personal self-awareness and purpose as individuals and professionals.

Inherent to the concept of empowerment is an absence of desire by the staff for "parental" caretaking by the organization or leader, replaced by a sense of accountability and ownership in the future of the organization on the part of its employees. Consistent with empowerment is the belief that we can make a difference and that we each have a real stake, personally and professionally, in the outcomes of the healthcare organization in which we practice. It is an acceptance that we each have a responsibility to make things happen, rather than waiting for somebody to fix the problems. Empowerment is also an attitude, and as individuals we have a choice regarding whether we wish to embrace the principles of empowerment, as individuals or as leaders. The result of that choice directly impacts our "fit" in the organization in which we are employed or the organization in which we may wish to be employed.

As we can see, empowerment begins within each of us: It is an acceptance of responsibility and accountability for ourselves and our lives, a recognition that we have power and influence over our future and day-to-day experiences. The seeds of empowerment lie within each of us, and therein rests much of the responsibility for empowerment.

Inescapably intertwined with empowerment is the concept of autonomy. **Autonomy** is the knowledge that you have choices and options, that you are not other-directed but rather self-directed. To be empowered, a person must first believe in and accept his or her personal autonomy. Unfortunately, many people believe they are not autonomous individuals, but rather victims of the "system." The reality is just the opposite. Within each of us is the ability to be autonomous. Block (1987) defined autonomy as the decisions we make to act on our own choice. We each have choices—a choice to act on our own behalf and on behalf of what we believe in, or the choice to do nothing and react to the choices and decisions of others. Recognition of our personal autonomy is the first step toward empowerment and the first step in risk taking also. Autonomy is acceptance that we are responsible and accountable for the outcomes of our actions and can no longer blame others when those outcomes are not what we originally desired. Autonomy, particularly in the workplace, does not mean working in isolation, but rather functioning as a unique professional, sharing professional expertise, knowledge, skills, and abilities in equal collaboration with physicians, clients, administration, and other members of the healthcare team (Mundinger, 1980).

The choices indicated by autonomy imply a direction or vision of what we want for our personal future or for the future of the organization in which we spend a major portion of our lives. Therefore, the initial step toward autonomy is to put into words the future we wish for our personal lives or for our nursing unit and organization (Block, 1987). Block goes on to describe **vision** as something for which we are willing to take risks, something that keeps us focused on our customers and describes how we contribute to the mission and business of the organization, and something that captures our imagination and engages our spirit. A vision is a provocative statement of what we want, and helps to create a focused and connected team with a purpose—a purpose each member understands and recognizes, and which guides individual and group decisions.

To this point, we have focused to a significant degree on empowerment as an internal value, one of self-awareness. Within the structure of an organization, empowerment carries a somewhat different connotation. Empowerment involves the creation of an environment in which staff collaborate as peers with other members of the healthcare team—the leader, administration, physicians, other departments—contributing their professional expertise to decisions that affect the welfare of patients and the quality of patient care. It is the role of the leader to lead and coach staff in creating a vision of a true professional practice environment. Porter-O'Grady (1992a) describes the leader's role as that of facilitator, mentor, and coach, someone whom staff can trust and rely upon, and someone who recognizes his or her skills, uses them effectively, and admits mistakes when he or she makes them.

Staff in an empowered environment accept their own accountability for the direction and future of the organization. They recognize that identification of a problem or need is the first step in problem resolution. In an empowered environment, it is no longer acceptable to sit back and wait for ethereal "others" to solve a problem, but rather to become an active collaborator in defining alternatives and solutions. To blame others for shortcomings is to truly blame ourselves for our own lack of initiative to solve the problem.

Last, empowerment involves risk taking, or a willingness to carefully evaluate the alternatives, keeping in mind the vision that has been created, and setting off in new directions to achieve that vision. Keep in mind that risk taking does not mean foolhardy actions, but rather the courage to forge new paths and the recognition that not all effectively designed plans will necessarily result in the desired outcome. Risk takers are supported to take those risks and are willing to evaluate unplanned outcomes in order to develop new ideas to achieve the desired goal.

TEAM BUILDING

Team building is an essential element in creating an environment for empowerment and facilitating the decision-making process. Covey (1989) describes teamwork as interdependence, that is, the paradigm of *we*—*we* can do it; *we* can cooperate; and *we* can create something great together by combining our talents and abilities. Dependent people get what they want through other people; independent people get what they want through their own efforts. Interdependent people achieve their greatest success by combining their own efforts with the efforts of others. Interdependence is a more personally and intellectually mature approach to problem solving and decision making. We are empowered through true independent character as we are enabled to act rather than be acted upon. Independent people who have the maturity to think and act interdependently are good team players (Covey, 1989).

Building effective teams takes time, effort, and cooperation. Creating an environment within the team where team members feel empowered to make decisions is even more difficult, as it requires a great deal of trust. Trust must exist among the team members and with the individuals who have empowered the team to make decisions on their behalf. The team members must agree to work interdependently toward the accomplishment of a common goal. Therefore, interdependence, the need for each member's experience, ability, and commitment, and mutually agreed upon goals are important characteristics of effective decision-making teams. The members must be committed to the idea that working together as a team leads to more effective decisions than working in isolation.

Another important characteristic is **accountability.** The team must be accountable as a functioning unit. Members hold each other accountable for the decisions that are made as a team and accept responsibility for outcomes based on those decisions. Role clarification, well-defined processes and procedures, effective leadership, trust, and open communication are also characteristics that facilitate teamwork and create an environment for empowerment and decision making.

Developing effective decision-making teams, thereby creating an environment for empowerment, is a process that requires hard work and a great sense of commitment by the members. The process of team development was described in Chapter 5 and include four stages: forming, storming, norming, and performing.

The amount of time a team spends in each phase, as well as the intensity of the phase, may vary depending on the maturity and experience of the members in establishing effective teams. The issue of personal maturity is an important one in truly understanding the concept of and achieving interdependence. Creating an effective team requires trust and interdependence. Covey (1989) suggests that true independence of character empowers us to act rather than be acted upon. Interdependence is the ability of people to combine talents and ideas and create something great together. This is *empowerment.*

Several elements (characteristics) are essential in building and maintaining an effective team. They include fostering group member roles, managing meetings, and facilitative leadership (Krumberger, 1992). How well a team functions, including how well it is able to establish and accomplish goals, depends to a large extent on how the team members relate to each other. Understanding both positive and negative behaviors helps the team to be more effective in accomplishing tasks. Contributing directly to the accomplishment of the group's work, for example, are group-building roles, including the initiator, the opinion giver, the clarifier, and the tester. The *initiator* is the individual who assumes a leadership role in presenting ideas and getting things started. We often refer to this person as the informal leader. He or she has the ability to look at issues from different perspectives and often presents different ideas for discussion.

The *opinion giver* presents facts and opinions for him- or herself and on behalf of others. He or she is an information source for the group and has the ability to analyze data. Depending on past experiences, the opinion giver may be a valuable asset to the team, drawing upon those experiences for the benefit of the entire team.

The *clarifier* is helpful in pulling together issues and ideas and restates suggestions and draws conclusions. This person also seeks clarification of the group's values and is counted on by the members for consensus building. The clarifier often acts as a process person for the group and can provide valuable feedback as to the effectiveness of the group process. He or she helps to keep the members focused and on track.

The *tester* is relied upon to test the team's ideas against reality to see if they will work. He or she is very familiar with organizational culture and climate, and is therefore able to determine the practicality or feasibility of ideas.

Group maintenance roles serve to build or maintain the health of the group, both morally and emotionally. These roles may include the harmonizer, the gatekeeper, the consensus tester, the compromiser, the encourager, and the tension reliever (Krumberger, 1992). The *harmonizer* challenges members to explore differences, thereby attempting to reconcile disagreements. The *gatekeeper* focuses on encouraging group members to participate in order to keep lines of communication open. The *consensus tester* monitors the extent of the group's agreement on certain issues. The *compromiser* is interested in ensuring the progress of the group and will therefore sacrifice some part of his or her own position in order to insure that progress. The *encourager* is the nurturer of the group and welcomes any and all contributions the members may have. The *tension reliever* offers a bit of humor at the appropriate times to help counterbalance negative feelings.

Effective relationships are developed and nurtured by the harmonious work of the team leader and the members of the team. Each member must consciously make an effort to work on the process of team development. Eight attributes and nine characteristics of teams that function at a high level are summarized in Table 13-1 (Mossop, 1988).

Table 13-1 • Attributes of High Functioning Teams

Attributes	Characteristics
Participative leadership	Empowerment
Shared responsibility	All members responsible for performance of team
Aligned on purpose	Sense of common purpose
High communication	Open, honest communication Climate of trust
Future focused	Change as opportunity for growth
Task focused	Meeting focused on results
Creative talents	Individual talents and creativity maximally used
Rapid response	Identifies and acts on opportunity

Adapted from Mossop, M.W., Total Teamwork: How to Be a Leader, How to Be a Member. *Management Solutions, 35, 3–9 (1988).*

CREATING A MISSION AND A VISION OF LEADERSHIP

Participative or facilitative leadership is "creating an interdependency by empowering, freeing up, and serving others" (Buckholz and Roth, 1987). One of the very important practices of leadership that facilitates teamwork, decision making, and empowerment is having and sharing a vision. That vision must first start with one's self. As Covey (1989) states, "Begin with the end in mind." Have a clear understanding of your destination. Know where you're going so that you better understand where you are now and so that the steps you take are in the right direction (Covey, 1989). Sharing an inspiring vision involves creating and communicating to other team members an inspiring image of the ideal future state or an image of the mission accomplished and inviting their participation in the pursuit (Krumberger, 1992). Seeking input from the entire team, understanding their values, and listening to their ideas also helps to promote buy-in and a sense of ownership by the team members. Creating a vision of greatness is the first step toward empowerment (Block, 1987). Having a vision gives leadership to the team and channels members' values into the workplace. It becomes a picture of how we want our values to be lived out in the organization (Block, 1987). It is important that there is a personal vision within each of us as well as a vision of the group or team as it expresses a statement of optimism and a dream of how we would like our organization to be.

It is equally important to have a mission statement. While a *vision statement* is an expression of hope (Block, 1987), a *mission statement* is a statement of the business we are in. For example, the mission of a healthcare organization may be to provide high-quality, cost-effective care to a specific geographical population. Within that same organization, the vision may include statements such as, We will strive to create an environment for empowerment and an atmosphere where accountability and risk taking are supported and encouraged.

As we look at the history and growth of nursing organizations throughout the country, we can see that many of these organizations have developed a vision that has created an environment for empowerment by investing the staff nurse with the accountability and authority to make decisions at the bedside relative to clinical practice. Many nursing organizations have implemented, or are in the process of implementing, professional governance structures that promote and support decision making at the clinical level, and that develop nursing professionals as leaders. Such organizations have a vision of greatness, a picture of how they want their organization to look, and a philosophy that provides the direction to get there.

Leadership versus Management

Management is often distinguished from leadership in the cliche "management is doing things right; leadership is doing the right things" (Covey, 1989). Management is efficiency in climbing the ladder of success; leadership determines whether the ladder is leaning against the right wall. The leader is the one who successfully leaps on the fastest train, evaluates the situation and yells, "We're going the wrong way!" But busy, efficient producers and managers might respond, "So what? At least we're going somewhere!" Leadership is an influencing process whereby the leader works with and through others toward the goals of the organization (Ketchum,

1991). When leadership is successful, it results in a change in attitude, and a high level of achievement on the part of the employee. Leadership styles can be extremely liberating, and can create an environment for empowerment and decision making.

Blanchard and Johnson (1982), authors of *The One Minute Manager,* have even asserted that what is important is not what happens while you are there, but what happens when you're not there. Employees of an effective manager and progressive leader will maintain the same level of performance regardless of whether the manager is there to oversee operations. Leaders create visions, set directions, define desirable outcomes, continually monitor the environment for change, and build the commitment and enthusiasm of others to collectively work together toward those ends. Managers organize and facilitate the efforts of groups and individuals and monitor the progress along the way to be sure everyone is on track. Leaders are architects, while managers are general contractors of the building process. We believe in the distinctions between the terms manager and leader, and therefore have used leader throughout our discussions, except when the currently recognized term nurse manager is necessary.

TRADITIONAL LEADERSHIP

Hospital and nursing organizational charts identify lines of direct control and management within the traditional confines described by the bureaucratic model (Porter-O'Grady and Finnegan, 1982). Traditionally, nursing organizational charts have defined a top-down management style, with the nurse executive at the top and the staff nurse at the bottom. Administration and management have traditionally maintained tight control over decisions related to all aspects of nursing. These decisions are usually handed down to the direct caregivers in the form of policies and procedures with the expectation that they will be followed. This leaves little, if any room, for autonomy and accountability on the part of the staff nurse. Consequently, there is often limited buy-in to decisions made, and much confusion as to how these decisions were derived. Nursing organizations that continue to function under the bureaucratic model run the risk of stifling professional growth and development.

For years managers have been searching for the "best" management style. The traditional debate existed between task-oriented (autocratic) management and participation/relationship oriented (democratic) management. Theory development and research in the field of leadership today has described effective leaders as those who use more than one dominant style of leadership and involve their followers (Bass, 1981; Marriner-Tomey, 1992). A more in-depth review of leadership styles was provided in Chapter 12. These newer more participative methods of leadership are more likely to foster the concept of empowerment among staff members.

PARTICIPATIVE MANAGEMENT

In a participative structure, the leader consults with staff, either on an individual or group basis, prior to making the decision; he or she allows the staff to influence the decision. Staff ideas and suggestions are considered by the leader before the final decision is made.

During the past several decades, participative decision making has been strongly supported in many management circles and texts, recognizing the value that staff expertise and knowledge contribute to the ultimate decision. The key difference between the participative model and the empowered decision-making model is that the final decision is made by the leader in the participative model, usually after considering the input of staff. In the empowered decision-making model, the leader facilitates or supports decision making by the staff. Growth of the staff decision-making skills is limited and occurs often by chance in a participative environment.

Scenario 13-1

To clarify the participative decision-making process, let's consider an example. A nursing unit has been provisionally allocated a budget of $15,000 for capital equipment (defined as durable equipment costing more than $500) for the next fiscal year. During the budgeting process, the nurse manager discusses capital equipment needs with staff, and, considering their input, submits prospective requests for two intravenous infusion pumps (approximately $3,000 each), two dopplers (approximately $500 each), and a replacement monitor for patient transport (approximately $8,000).

During the time period between preparation of the capital budget requests and administrative approval of the unit capital budget, staff identify the need for two transport stretchers (approximately $3,500 each). This need is based upon noted delays in patient transport for diagnostic evaluations and a resulting increase in length of stay of approximately 0.5 days. Upon receipt of approval for capital budget funds of $15,000 for the unit, the nurse manager is requested to prepare capital request forms, including justification, for the desired capital equipment. The nurse manager chooses to consult with staff regarding the priority of the original capital budget requests. The staff discuss the unanticipated need for the transport stretchers. Clearly, the only way the unit can meet this new need and remain within the allocated capital budget is to substitute the stretcher for the infusion pumps and the dopplers, or the transport monitor. In a participative management structure, the nurse manager may request staff to indicate why they feel the stretchers are needed and, based upon that input, make the decision regarding the capital equipment to be purchased by the unit.

In contrast, in an empowered environment the leader would support the staff through the decision-making process. At the time the capital budget is approved for the unit, the leader shares with staff (or a designated committee) the approved capital budget dollars and facilitates a discussion of the previously submitted equipment and any changes in patient care unit needs that may have occurred since the original submission. After discussion and consideration by the staff/committee of the trade-offs between the previously submitted and new equipment needs, group consensus regarding the equipment most critical to quality patient care would be determined and submitted for purchase. Further, the leader coaches the staff/committee as it deliberates their choices and the cost-benefit analysis of their alternatives, guiding the staff/committee to consider trade-offs such as the impact on quality of care, the effect of efficiency and cost effectiveness of care delivery, the impact on patient satisfaction and physician satisfaction, the ability to increase revenues, the impact on patient length of stay, equipment maintenance costs, the age of equipment to be replaced (if applicable), the compatibility of the new equipment with present equipment, the training needed for effective use of the equipment, and the ability to establish a patient charge for use of the equipment.

The primary difference between the empowered and the participative decision-making models in this example is the manner in which the ultimate decision regarding capital equipment purchase is made. In the empowered model, the staff are not just consulted, but actually make the decision. The leader facilitates the process by insuring that the group considers and evaluates alternatives and consequences of the final decision, and that the principles of group decision making are carefully observed. The leader facilitates the process, but the staff make and own the decision.

PROFESSIONAL PRACTICE MODELS

Critical elements of a professional practice model have been described as individual professional accountability by the practitioner, coupled with professional responsibility and accountability for all issues relating to the practice—that is, standards of practice and care, assurance of the quality of care provided, responsibility for the professional development of the practitioners, and professional review responsibility (Campbell, 1992). Creating a structure that allows all of these elements to function simultaneously presents a challenge. Porter-O'Grady and Finnegan (1984) are recognized for initiating the first such structure for nursing in the early 1980s, called **shared governance.** Professional practice models have continued to emerge over the past ten years that have as their basis individual professional accountability by the practitioner.

SHARED GOVERNANCE

Shared governance is an organizational structure in which accountability and responsibility for the outcomes of practice reside with the clinical practitioner. The shared governance structure is an accountability-based system founded on individual accountability rather than individual participation in management (Campbell, 1992). Shared governance is not participative management, but a philosophy that supports professional nursing practice.

> The nursing administrator who makes this decision must also realize that once the door has been opened and the people begin to experience shared governance, the door can never be closed again. Therefore, the

> commitment is not just for the short term. It is not periodic or temporary, or just a trial. It is one that makes a statement that will have a lasting impact on the nursing organization (Porter-O'Grady and Finnegan, 1984, p. 123).

The more traditional bureaucratic structure of management very common in nursing organizations has been previously discussed. Bureacracy is a top-down structure that does not support or promote professional accountability. Furthermore, when a bureaucratic structure takes precedence over professional practice issues, care will be compromised, resulting in staff frustration when they are unable to fully participate in the activities associated with their practice (Campbell, 1992). Many organizations have adopted a participative management style in an attempt to decrease conflict that can exist between the nursing profession and the institution in a bureaucratic system. Participative management, however, maintains the traditional bureaucratic hierarchy, as accountability for decision making remains with management. This structure does not transfer accountability to the clinical practitioner and therefore does not promote professional accountability.

The goal of shared governance was to get more nurses invested in their work and profession and to strengthen nursing in the workplace in ways that would empower nursing as a profession and retain the interest of individual members (Porter-O'Grady, 1992a, 1992b). In a shared governance structure, accountability is transferred to the individual professional practitioner. There are several shared governance models that have been described and utilized throughout the country. There is no one right way to structure the model. However, all forms of shared governance should address the following five accountabilities: practice, quality, education, management, and governance (coordination).

In order for a shared governance structure to work in a nursing organization, it must be embraced by the chief nursing officer and expressed as the vision for the future of nursing as a profession and for the organization as a whole. Although the concept of shared governance may not be totally understood by the chief executive officer of the organization, the CEO must agree to generally support the necessary process required to implement it (Campbell, 1992).

Porter-O'Grady (1992a, 1992b) describes shared governance as a vehicle for change, growth, and empowerment for the profession and the professional. It serves as a vehicle for creating and managing change and preparing a desired future. Porter-O'Grady (1992a, 1992b) further explains that shared governance has become a vehicle for building collaborative interdisciplinary relationships that will be models for the future of healthcare delivery.

The Councilor Model

The councilor model of shared governance is the single most frequently implemented model for shared governance. Porter-O'Grady (1992a, 1992b) describes this model as based on the delineation of accountability and an appropriate locus of control. It can be implemented at the departmental and unit levels. In this model, professional accountability is decentralized; locus of control will shift for specified accountabilities and may exist outside the traditional management role.

The councilor model includes five areas of accountability: practice, quality improvement, education, research, and management. For each area of accountability, a council, which is a decision-making body, is formed within the department of nursing and has authority over its defined accountabilities. Typically, four of the councils are clinical in nature, and one is a management council. The majority of the members of the clinical councils are practicing staff nurses, with management representation often acting in an advisory role. A staff nurse will also fill the leadership role (chairperson) on the clinical councils. The management council typically includes the chief nursing officer, nursing service directors, and nurse managers, and staff nurses may also be represented on the council. The management council is chaired by a nurse manager. On all councils, clinical and management, the leadership role is filled by an individual in a position closest to the patient.

A very important step in preparing for the implementation of shared governance is to assess the perceptions and readiness of management and staff. As shared governance is implemented, all individuals must be sensitive to the impact of change on themselves and their relationships with others, particularly between management and staff. Roles will change as shared governance becomes a reality. For example, there will be a transition in the management role from focus on self to focus on group relationships and functions. The manager's style moves from motivation to empowerment. The role of the nurse executive also changes as this individual becomes the link between the professional nursing staff and the executive staff, the board, medical staff leadership, and the community. All individuals in management positions must consider a change in style as they move from a directing to a facilitating relationship with staff. Staff will have greater control over issues related to practice, quality of care, competence, and evaluation, as managers provide support and guidance. In a traditional bureaucratic organization, committees existed to give advice and guidance to management, who then made all final decisions. Within this shared governance model, the councils are invested with the power and accountability for decision making (Porter-O'Grady and Finnegan, 1984).

MANAGEMENT COUNCIL

Under shared governance, management responsibilities become centralized and directed specifically to assure appropriate support of the nursing staff (Porter-O'Grady and Finnegan, 1984). The management council's areas of accountability include human resources, fiscal resources, material resources, support to staff, and organizational systems. The council's work is primarily associated with the allocation of resources to staff and the implementation of decisions made by the clinical councils.

CLINICAL PRACTICE COUNCIL

Along with the management council, the clinical practice council (CPC) provides the foundation for the shared governance structure. It is the primary clinical decision-making group. All other councils will eventually come to depend on the CPC as it defines the parameters of the practice on which the work of the profession builds (Porter-O'Grady, 1992a, 1992b). The CPC is responsible for the development of standards of practice, performance standards, and position descriptions for clinical nurses. The council also develops the conceptual framework for professional practice, and defines and controls the care delivery system, the clinical documentation system, and career advancement programs.

QUALITY IMPROVEMENT COUNCIL

Quality of nursing practice is the second major delineated function for which nurses have accountability. The quality improvement council (QIC) will often depend on CPC activities for planning work. The QIC is responsible for developing the quality improvement plan, assuring the development of unit-based QI plans and activities, setting priorities for continuous improvement, and developing the performance evaluation system. The QIC assesses standards on a regular basis to ensure they are current and being met. They evaluate deficiencies and recommend corrective action. A new area of responsibility for the quality improvement council is establishing mechanisms for peer review and for credentialing and privileging of the professional nursing staff.

EDUCATION COUNCIL

The education council's primary responsibility is for issues related to professional competency. Maintaining ongoing competency and continuing education are also focuses of this council. The education council will develop the vision for education in the nursing organization, including unit-based education plans. It is responsible for developing and maintaining a system to ensure effective communication among the councils and with the entire nursing staff. Other responsibilities include staff orientation, identifying education needs of the staff, determining the appropriateness of programs, and developing a consistent evaluation process for educational programs.

RESEARCH COUNCIL

Most nursing and other professional organizations do not have a formalized or highly developed research function (Porter-O'Grady, 1992a, 1992b). However, several organizations are beginning preliminary work to define the professional accountability for research. Some shared governance structures incorporate nursing research into quality improvement activities. In any case, the research council's responsibilities should include setting research priorities, developing research plans, approval of research activities, publication, and application of research findings.

EXECUTIVE OR COORDINATING COUNCIL

Communication is essential to the success and facilitation of the implementation of shared governance (Porter-O'Grady, 1992a). The coordinating council(CC) can initially play that role. The CC helps to coordinate and moderate all activities among the councils during the implementation phase and for the ongoing development of council activities. This council incorporates the mission of the organization in setting goals and objectives for the department of nursing. It is from this work that all unit-based goals will flow. The CC resolves intercouncil conflict. For example, if there is uncertainty as to which council an issue should go, the coordinating council will make that determination. Maintaining the bylaws and all governance functions are further activities of the CC.

Whatever model is used for the implementation of shared governance, the emphasis must be on the transfer of legitimate authority for decision making to the nursing staff. The implementation of a shared governance structure can take as long as three to five years and requires a great deal of patience, understanding, and commitment. However, the rewards and benefits far exceed the difficulties that may be experienced along the way.

Professional Practice at the Unit Level

Staff in a professional practice model at the unit level are salaried members of a shared governance structure, incorporating peer evaluation as a fundamental part of their practice. This model is so named because it embodies the essential elements of professionalism—practicing self-governance and self-determination, controling the credentialing process of unit members, influencing professional behavior, and expanding knowledge of the profession (Porter-O'Grady, 1992a, 1992b). Clearly, many of these attributes are incorporated in the shared governance structure; the unit-based professional practice model provides the added elements of credentialing and influencing professional behavior through the component of peer review.

In a professional practice structure, decisions affecting patient care are made by the members of the *model*, either directly or through members they have elected to decision-making committees or councils. Administrative decisions that indirectly influence clinical practice are collaboratively made by administrative staff and representatives of the clinical staff.

Using the capital budget example in this type of model, the staff, collectively or through a staff-elected council, develop the capital budget within the guidelines established by the hospital fiscal department. Within the designated capital budget of the unit, staff define and prioritize capital equipment needs as they pertain to patient care. Often, council members consult with the rest of the staff regarding capital budget priorities prior to finalizing capital equipment requests. Upon approval of the capital budget requests, the council once again reviews and prioritizes the equipment initially defined, weighing the cost and benefits to patient care of any newly identified equipment prior to submitting the final capital requisitions.

The role of the leader is that of facilitator, mentor, and advisor throughout the development of the capital budget, supporting the council and staff as they consider alternatives in an environment of limited resources. The professional practice model supports staff growth and involvement in designing their practice and work environment and embodies the essence of empowerment.

SUMMARY

The concept of empowerment as a partnership between leadership and staff was reviewed in this chapter. Empowerment was defined as recognizing the ability of the individual within a healthcare organization to make decisions, and providing that individual with the appropriate resources for decision making. The importance of team building in creating an environment that fosters empowered decision making was discussed. The need for a leader with a view of the future, rather than a manager, for empowerment to take place was highlighted. A scenario involving a nurse manager/leader and staff members in a participative versus empowered decision-making process was presented. Last, views of how decision making occurs in truly empowered nursing organizations with professional practice and shared governance structures were reviewed. On a continuum, empowerment, professional practice, and shared governance are currently on the extreme left. Future insights into management and leadership may shift these concepts to the extreme right.

REFERENCES

Bass, B.M. (1981). *Stogdill's handbook of leadership: A survey of theory and research.* New York: Free Press.

Blanchard, K., & Johnson, S. (1982). *The one minute manager.* New York: William Morrow and Company.

Block, P. (1987). *The empowered manager: Positive political skills at work.* San Francisco: Jossey-Bass.

Buckholz, S., & Roth, T. (1987). *Creating the high performance team.* New York: John Wiley and Sons.

Campbell, C. (1992). Redesigning the nursing organization. In T. Porter-O'Grady (Ed.), *Implementing shared governance.* St. Louis, MO: Mosby-Year Book.

Chandler, G.E. (1992). The source and process of empowerment. *Nursing Administration Quarterly, 16*(3), 65–71.

Covey, S.R. (1989). *The 7 habits of highly effective people.* New York: Simon & Schuster.

Ketchum, S.M. (1991). *Overcoming the four toughest management challenges.* Malvern, PA: Clinical Laboratory Management Review.

Krumberger, J.M. (1992). Group facilitation: Building that winning team. *Nursing Dynamics, 1*(3), 9–15.

Manthey, M. (1989). Empowerment: Change = Change: Empowerment. *Nursing Management, 20*(6), 17.

Marriner-Tomey, A. (1992). *Guide to nursing management.* St. Louis, MO: Mosby-Year Book.

Mason, D.J., Costello-Nickitas, D.M., Scanlan, J.M., & Magnuson, B.A. (1991). Empowering nurses for politically astute change in the workplace. *The Journal of Continuing Education, 22*(1), 5–10.

Mossop, M.W. (1988). Total teamwork: How to be a leader, how to be a member. *Management Solutions, 35,* 3–9.

Mundinger, M.O. (1980). *Autonomy in nursing.* Germantown, MD: Aspen Systems.

Porter-O'Grady, T. (1992a). *Implementing shared governance.* St. Louis, MO: Mosby-Year Book.

Porter-O'Grady, T. (1992b). *Shared governance implementation manual.* St. Louis, MO: Mosby-Year Book.

Porter-O'Grady, T., & Finnegan, S. (1984). *Shared governance for nursing: A creative approach to professional accountability.* Rockville, MD: Aspen.

Patricia M. Haynor

CHAPTER 14

Computer-Supported Decision Making for the Nurse Manager

Information is not, of course, an end in itself, it is the basic input to decision-making.
—*(Mintzberg, 1989)*

INTRODUCTION

Nurse managers are expected to make timely, prudent, outcome- and customer-oriented decisions with reasonable risks for their organizations. To do this, a manager needs to maintain an open systems view of the organization and its environment. The **open systems view** must be both on a macro and a micro level which encompasses day-to-day operational responsibilities as well as the entire organization's direction. Whenever possible, this view should be expanded beyond the organization into the external environment.

One important component of decision making is the congruence of the nurse manager's view with the organization's and leader's vision. The decision-making process should take its lead from the organization's vision statements. Since many different decision scenarios are possible for any given situation, the final decision choice should be the one with the "best fit" with the vision statement. This assures movement toward the organization's goals and objectives to insure long-term viability. Decision alignment with the vision statement also permits the manager to actively demonstrate credible commitment to the direction of the organization.

Another important component of decision making is getting the needed information so that a decision can be made with data that supports it. Data-free decision making is not acceptable in today's world. Data review should be creative in its approach. Different data sets should be compared and contrasted, linkage of diverse data should be attempted, the obvious should be overlooked for the moment, and the unusual sought. Finding data to support a bias does not necessarily lead to a valid decision. A wide range of data gathered and viewed with an open mind leads to various decision scenarios that provide a richer set of alternatives for the manager.

Although data can be either qualitative or quantitative, today's nurse manager receives mostly quantitative data from the organization's computerized information systems. These systems can be hospitalwide or departmentally based. Almost all will be computer based. These are the nurse manager's decision support system. Turban's (1982) definition of a decision support system (DSS) is, "an on-line real-time computerized system especially designed to support managerial decision making. Its major characteristics are ease of use by people with no education or background in computers and its flexibility and adaptability to managerial needs" (p. 35–36). Angehern and Luthi (1990) noted that "Ideally DSSs should behave like human consultants supporting decision making in expressing, structuring, and better understanding of their problems" (p. 17). By 1993, Simpson described the executive information system (EIS), which is based on the idea that "there are key indicators to organizational success and performance. EIS technology represents a shift from data analysis to information analysis. With an EIS . . . information is readily available, screened, compiled and manipulated . . . and presented in color charts, color codes and exception flagging" (p. 32). Accessing and using the data available through DSSs are the keys to being a successful manager in today's healthcare environment.

NEED DEFINITION

The role of the nurse manager is to define the data requirements. Begin by reviewing past decisions and ask the following questions: Was the data

1. accessible, available, and helpful?
2. in a useful form?
3. residing in a computer database?

If the answer to any of these questions is no, then better decision support is needed. First, determine what is needed on a routine basis. Break this down into information that should be received annually, quarterly, monthly, weekly, and daily. Collect all the reports currently received and categorize them by report type and timeframe (Table 14-1).

Table 14-1 contains various types of reports currently used by nurse managers. Depending on an institution's computer system evolution, the number and type of reports will vary widely. However, the trend is to make the reports accessible to the frontline manager who can quickly respond to the data. It's important to define the departmental "must-have" reports and work together to obtain them. Visit other departments and look at their reports, determine who has the information needed, in the form closest to what is needed, and use the information system support (ISS) staff for assistance. Consider whether manual reports can or should be converted. Follow a data paper trail from initial data collection through to final report in order to build a departmental database. Query colleagues in other organizations about their use of decision support systems.

Table 14-1 • **Examples of Report Timing**

Frequency	Report Type
Annual	Operating budget
Quarterly	Turnover, sick time usage, mandatory CE attendance
Monthly	Full time equivalents, vacancy rate, TQM team status, capital expenses, quality assurance monitors
Weekly	Overtime use and cost, absentee rate, unit staffing, compliance to budget
Daily	Staffing, acuity, census
Shift	Actual vs. budget vs. acuity staffing

Once these reports are available, use them. Don't just collect them and put them in a file cabinet. Managers will be held accountable for the information they contain. Today's organizations recognize that the person who plays an important role in goal attainment is the one most able to change a situation. In most healthcare organizations, this is the nurse manager.

DECISION DATA

Characteristics

To help managers make good decisions, data must be accurate, error free, clearly defined, factual, and reliable. How do managers know that the computer generated data set in their report meets these fundamental requirements? The data set must have face and content validity. **Face validity** means that "on the face of it" what is known to be true is reflected in the data. For example, if a room rate is known to be $1,044/day, then the data set reporting the rate should also say $1,044/day. If it says $144/day, the data has no face validity and needs to be corrected. Another example is budgeted hours per patient day (HPPD). If the annual budgeted number was 6 HPPD and the monthly finance reports show 5.2 HPPD, the data is inaccurate on the "face of it". When this occurs, managers must check for other intervening circumstances. In this case, the annual budget may have been adjusted downward without the manager's knowledge, or it could just be an input error. **Content validity** describes the appropriateness of what is in the data set itself. If a room rate dataset contains cost information about repaving the parking lot or daycare costs, the data set becomes suspect. If the HPPD data set contains hours and salary costs for maintenance personnel, questions about the data must be asked. Data sets must reflect reality as managers know it or as others agree upon it, and the data within a data set must have acceptable and agreed-upon relationships to each other.

Factual data clearly defines the parameters and sources of the data. In the HPPD example, the hours and costs contained in the HPPD data set are known to all. The HPPD should include salaries and productive hours of direct care providers. The definition of "direct care providers" does vary by institutions: The most controversial salaries and hours are those of the nurse manager and the unit clerical support. Without knowing the definition of HPPD, it would be impossible for a nurse manager to calculate accurate budget numbers that agreed with those who had the complete definition.

Data bias and premises must also be known. Data can be biased by the way it is defined, by how it is manipulated, and by which pieces of the data are reported or deleted. A classic data bias occurs when overtime is calculated into full-time equivalents (FTEs). This may be done in several ways. One method is to calculate all hours worked (both regular and overtime) into a FTE figure. Another method is to calculate regular hours worked separately from overtime hours. The first method may prevent hiring into vacant positions, because on the FTE report it appears that all positions are filled. The second method clearly defines vacant positions and the cost of not hiring into them is clearly demonstrated as well.

A manager is expected to know the facts, premises, and bias upon which the data set is built and to check the data set for face and content validity. If the definitions and bias are arbitrary and/or counterproductive, efforts should be directed towards correcting them. This is where organizational games are played out, and it is important for nurse managers to understand what is at stake. Data bias is not necessarily intentional; it may have been left over from previous administrations or computer systems, or was a standard operating procedure as defined by an individual department head or an outside regulatory agency. Nurse managers must uncover the bias and premises, use that information during data interpretation, and attempt to get them changed if necessary. However, if the bias and premises are changed, there is the loss of compatibility to previous data sets as well as a period when predictability is lost and the future cannot be anticipated. In other words, this situation can be described as "being in limbo" or "a dark hole." This doesn't mean that bias and premises shouldn't be changed, but rather allowances must be made for them. And last, data must be reliable. The inputs must be the same and the report format should not vary. This insures comparability across time, and permits ease in interpretation and trend recognition.

Sources

Data can come from a single source microcomputer system or from multiple computer systems. There are advantages and disadvantages to both types. A single-source system is a completely integrated or linked database. It is usually easy to access, maintained by experts, and comprehensive in scope. Multiple-source (stand-alone) systems frequently reside in several locations, are maintained departmentally, and are often not linked or integrated into a common database. Access to multi-source computer system information is often determined by the "owner." Data set creation may be independent of other systems.

As a nurse manager, it is important to know in which type of system the data resides and how to access it. Multiple-source systems require the nurse manager to elicit multiple definitions, biases, and premises for data output. The nurse manager also needs an understanding that data compatibility may be limited or influenced by personal relationships with the "owner" and may or may not be received in a timely manner. Multisystem data often leads to data controversy: Who has the "real" or "accurate" data for what?

Data may be internal or external to the organization. In-house data is generated from the daily operation of the organization and may be kept manually or on a computer system. External data may come from regulatory agencies, contracted services, or expert information systems. Knowing where each data set is coming from is imperative, because it may not be comparable or based on the organization's reality.

Formats

In the best of all worlds, computer-generated data should be reported in English, not condensed with uncommon acronyms, abbreviations, or interpretive descriptions. The data should be organized with numbered pages, data fields occurring at the same place from report to report, easily readable print, standard size reports for ease of storage, and report length proportionate to data elements needed. Data totals should appear at regular intervals vertically and horizontally on the reports for ease of use. Columns of summary data should be available to make historical, current, and/or future data comparisons. For example, historical comparisons are valuable for budget preparation, current summaries or today's operating status and future comparisons are used to plan or adjust expenditures for budget compliance.

Computer-generated reports should be structured so that they contain all the information needed in as few reports as possible. Multiple separate reports which require the user to assimilate and integrate data leave room for error and increase the workload. Managers often complain that they are bombarded with information yet have no time to read it. Thus, systems that report exceptions are highly desired.

Exception reports can be extremely helpful timesavers when large amounts of data require ongoing review. These reports highlight only the unusual. However, the danger of exception reporting is that if the nurse manager doesn't know what to request, the data will never be reported. An example of an effective exception report is for staffing compliance. Instead of having to review twenty-one shifts per week for staffing compliance to budget and acuity, an exception report might only list the three shifts that were not in compliance, thus saving the manager the time of reviewing the other eighteen shifts. Additionally, by comparing only the exceptions, trends are easier to recognize and correct. If three exception reports in a row list that the Saturday 3 to 11 shift is not meeting standards, the nurse manager knows exactly where to devote time and energy.

Timeliness

Data becomes useful when it's in the manager's hands. There is usually a time lag between when an event occurs and when the data relating to it is available. Organizations must determine the speed with which data is available. In periods of high stability and adequate resources, longer lag times are acceptable. However, in time of rapid change and resource scarcity, minimal time lags are imperative to the survival of the organization. Today many organizations are allocating significant resources to implement on-line and/or realtime computer systems to minimize lag time. Stand-alone microcomputer systems have been the answer in some organizations for rapid data retrieval. Staffing and scheduling software systems are examples of this. For instance, although staffing and scheduling decisions are made four to six weeks in advance, the daily use of the system provides realtime budget compliance data and fewer monthly finance report surprises. Realtime admission, discharge, and transfer (ADT) computer software can maximize the use of bed utilization and minimize patient waiting. At the same time, a linked ADT and patient acuity system can assist in actualizing accurate care requirements in individual patient care areas. Each of these systems provides the nurse manager with valuable data for timely decision making.

DATA MANIPULATION

Data Trail

When working with data, it's important to ask three questions:

1. Is this raw data?
2. Has this data been refined/manipulated?
3. How is the data reported?

Raw data is just that. It has not been processed in any way. Examples of raw data are: billing invoices, attendance sheets, acuity scores, telephone logs, patient comment letters, and overtime hours. These represent all the data for a given context. Because the data is global in nature, it is difficult to compare, to derive meaning, or to make analytical decisions.

Refined data has been broken into subsets, placed in a context, and given parameters. For example, billing invoices are placed into expense categories and compared with previous monthly expenses and the annual budget. Four weeks of raw attendance sheet data may be refined to highlight employee absence rates per unit, target possible abusers, and show patterns of call-outs. Refined data is used for decision making, because it attempts to elicit meaning from large masses of raw data.

Reports may contain either raw or refined data. If a report contains raw data, one needs to ask the question, Why? Some reasons are:

- There are no tools available to refine the data.
- There are very small quantities of data best reported in a qualitative format since statistical inferences can't be drawn from a small sample.
- The data was collected for the first time and decisions regarding refinement have yet to be made.
- Previously refined data was converted back into its original raw form so that a different refinement approach can be determined.

When a report contains refined data, one cannot assume that it is error-free just because it is in columns, and has headers, mathematical calculations, and comparisons. There are three common types of errors: input, calculation, and classification. **Input errors** can occur as raw data is entered into a computer program, or as refined data is moved from place to place. Computerized calculations are based on formulas. If the formulas are entered incorrectly or out of sequence, all future data manipulations will be **miscalculated.** As raw data is entered into its refinement context, it must be categorized based on underlying assumptions. Human error can lead to the **misclassification** of raw data. If a refined data report contains a classification or data point that on the face of it seems unusual, a misclassification or input error should be suspected and the raw data checked for verification. To check for suspected formula or calculation errors, randomly select a column of figures, do the appropriate calculations, and compare the results.

Methods of Data Refinement

It is important for nurse managers to know how data is refined, even though they may not be doing the actual refinement task. There are three things to learn:

> 1. A conceptual understanding of the software's function for the purpose of controlling needed information . . .
> 2. The assumptions upon which all data and software applications are based . . .
> 3. And to correctly interpret results produced by software packages (Mills, Blaesing, and Carter, 1991, p. 179).

For example, a computerized spreadsheet is constructed from a series of columns and rows used to organize the various pieces of information required to define the report through the use of column or row headings. At the intersection of rows and columns are data cells where raw data is entered or mathematical formulas constructed to refine the raw data contained in other rows or columns. Determining which number to put in which cell is based on the spreadsheet's organization. The refined data is then left to the interpretation of the report reader.

WORD PROCESSING

The most widely used category of business software is word processing programs. Two of the most popular are Word Perfect (Word Perfect Corporation, Orem, UT) and Microsoft Word (Microsoft Corporation, Redmond, WA). Word processing programs have greatly simplified the task of producing business letters and reports. Tasks such as editing pages of text, checking spelling and punctuation, rewriting sentences, and moving whole paragraphs have been made much easier. Certain programs will allow the letter or report to be customized through the use of underlining, bold or italic type, and multiple font sizes and styles. More recent programs have incorporated the ability to merge data from other sources, such as spreadsheets or graphs and charts. The end result is a letter or report, professionally prepared, which is easier to read and understand for the user and easier to produce, store, and retrieve for the producer.

SPREADSHEETS

Spreadsheets are the financial analyst's favorite tool because of their ability to "crunch numbers." A good spreadsheet, in combination with a skilled user, can take large quantities of raw data and reduce it to a meaningful one page report. Spreadsheets are used for categorizing data, performing formula-based calculations, and budgeting "what if" scenarios (modeling). Most spreadsheet programs, with minimal word processing capabilities, have the ability to create graphics and charts for non-numerical data display and alphanumeric charts. Another use of spreadsheet software is forecasting to project the future based on past and present data. Examples of application spreadsheet programs are:

- ANSOS Budget Module (Atwork Corporation, Chapel Hill, NC)
- Smart Forecast II (Smart Software, Belmont, MA)

Examples of general use spreadsheets are:

- LOTUS 1-2-3 (Lotus Development Corporation, Cambridge, MA)
- Quattro-Pro (Borland International, Scotts Valley, CA)

DATABASES

A database program is like a file cabinet of information with a great memory for what it contains. Databases contain discrete bits of information that can be linked or free-standing. The data can be easily retrieved in a variety of combinations for multiple uses. The software is designed to contain (store), count, and categorize large amounts of information. A healthcare example of a database is the ANSOS Staffing and Scheduling System (Atwork Corporation, Chapel Hill, NC). This application requires the inputting of specific information: staff names, titles, credentials, preferred shifts, days off, skills, certifications, licenses, emergency contact numbers, and demographics. Depending on the query to the system, different data sets are compiled: for example, a list of nurses whose licenses expire this year, the number of Licensed Practical Nurses who work the 3-11 shift, the names of staff who live within five miles of the institution, or the names of staff with Advanced Cardiac Life Support Certification (ACLS). A well-known database system for general use is dBASE IV (Borland International, Scotts Valley, CA). For literature searches, CD-ROM disks, or a newer, more powerful mainframe system such as MEDLINE, are available.

PROJECT MANAGEMENT

Managing a major project involves tracking the tasks, resources, and timeframes. This can be very cumbersome in a pen-and-pencil world, because those three aspects are constantly changing. In addition, a change in any one aspect requires a reconfiguration of the other two. Visual representations compress large quantities of data into easy-to-assimilate graphics. Computer software is ideal for this use. Programs such as Microsoft Project (Microsoft Corporation, Redmond, WA) assist the project manager to clearly identify the tasks, resources needed, and timeliness for task completion. Because resources have associated costs, the software assists in developing the budget. The software also permits modeling of various scenarios and produces PERT (Program Evaluation Review Technique) and Gantt charts, which are visual representations of tasks, resources, and timeframes as shown in Figure 14-1.

STATISTICAL PACKAGES

The nurse manager is frequently asked to provide information that is then analyzed statistically. Such research requires analysis of quantitative data using a variety of statistical approaches; for examples, finding the average of a given patient population,

Task Name	Quarter 1	Quarter 2	Quarter 3	Quarter 4
Budget Implementation	July Aug Sept	Oct Nov Dec	Jan Feb Mar	Apr May Jun
Implement New Budget				
A. Salary Budget	—			
1. Preprogram staffing configuration/unit	—			
2. Redefine key indicators	—			
3. Run schedules based on new budget	—			
4. Monitor compliance	—	—	—	—
B. Program Budget				
1. Hire director	—			
2. Write policies & procedures	—			
3. Purchase equipment	—	—		
4. Alter physical plant	—	—	—	
5. Hire staff			—	
6. Begin marketing			—	—
7. Admit patients				—
8. Monitor MD & patient satisfaction				—

Figure 14-1 Gantt Chart: Budget Implementation.

how many patients fell out of bed in a given time period and the most frequent cause, the median bed utilization per unit, or the average length of stay per diagnosis, and the determination of the factors that contributed to it. Software packages such as SPSS-PC (SPSS, Inc. Cary, NC), SAS (SAS Institute, Inc.), and Microstat (Microsoft Corporation, Redmond, WA) permit questions like these to be answered through the use of a microcomputer.

ADDITIONAL SOFTWARE APPLICATIONS

Simulations

Interactive software programs offer excellent opportunities for nurse managers to improve negotiating and critical thinking skills. Negotiating is a skill that can be learned and refined with practice. However, it's difficult to practice the techniques in "realtime," because another person is involved and much could be at stake. Negotiating software, such as The Art of Negotiating (Experience in Software, Inc., Berkeley, CA), guides the user "through several layers of the negotiating process, feeding ideas to be contemplated and possible phrases for use. The software offers negotiators the clarity to gain awareness into their own assumptions as well as opponents assumption." (Mills, Blaesing, and Carter, 1991, p. 182). By sharpening skills on-line, less is at stake.

Decision Support

DSS software is the most exciting type of program, because it tries to help managers perform their most difficult task. Early decision support systems were based on the idea that decisions were logical and rational. Some approaches "introduced rationality by teaching managers to overlay or substitute a step-by-step orderly process on their most natural inclinations" (Zemke, 1988, p. 65). However, Simon stated that "the decisions are not always made logically for a very good reason: What's logical isn't always sensible . . . decisions based on hunches and experiences are often equal in quality to those forced into a logical, rational decision structure" (cited in Zemke, 1988, p. 65).

And so was born the next generation of DSS. An alternative strategy that uses the right brain instead of left-brain techniques emerged. Other software combines both techniques by breaking the process into two phases: an idea phase where an individual can be impulsive or irrational, followed by a rational objective phase to select the solution. This software can be used by individuals or groups. Since this field is changing so rapidly, it is difficult to provide the names of the most widely used programs.

An example of DSS use by a nurse manager might be to identify causes of OR case delays and to determine appropriate interventions. The nurse manager is guided through a series of exercises to identify probable causes and to rank them in terms of "likeliness" using logical/rational techniques. Then the manager is asked challenging questions to help frame logical solutions (left-brain techniques), and finally to imagine more creative solutions (right-brain techniques.)

INFORMATION SHARING SYSTEMS

Another trend in data refinement is through the use of information sharing systems (ISS). These include electronic bulletin boards, computer conferencing, many-to-many communications, and expert networking. Like a telephone, these systems instantly connect managers with others outside their own institutions. The differences lie in the ability to send and receive large volumes of data in a very short time period, send information simultaneously from one to several thousand others, elicit opinions/expert advice from worldwide sources, send data to several others for data refinement, and convene a panel to review and analyze the data while creating a historical log of the interaction. This could be used by nurse managers to post staff positions, to seek educational programs, to poll other nurse managers about specific techniques, or to gather information from others on how to solve a specific problem.

Information sharing systems are user friendly. They have been available in the general market for several years. Two examples are PRODIGY (Prodigy Services Company, White Plains, NY) and CompuServe (CompuServe Inc., Columbus, OH). Now the trend is to create special interest groups (SIGS) that further subdivide into unique areas of interest. These systems and their names/acronyms change frequently, making it difficult to provide a comprehensive list.

A priority in many work sites is the creation of a microcomputer based local area network (LAN) which connects managers and/or workers within the same organization to a common system. Through it they may send memos, E-mail, reports, and data in a paperless manner. This reduces workflow interruptions, the amount of time spent in meetings, excuses for not informing others, and telephone tag. All are designed to help the manager to work smarter, not harder.

Once a manager has used these various techniques for decision making, the next step is to support the decision and sell it to others. Today, being an expert is no longer enough.

USING TECHNOLOGY TO SUPPORT DECISIONS

Issue Definition

The most important part of decision making is defining the issues clearly, succinctly, and in a nonprovocative manner. The problem should be described using refined data in a meaningful format. Graphs and charts should be used to provide clear representation of complex information. Use objective background information and historical data to provide a long-term perspective and to demonstrate the depth of analysis.

Carefully consider which pieces of data should be verbally described and which pieces of data should be visually described—it's true that one picture is worth a thousand words. The impact is much less dramatic if a report states "January and February are the busiest months" rather than "refer to Figure 14-2."

This approach could be strengthened by adding another year or two of historical data as in Figure 14-3.

Don't stun the audience into submission through information overload! Rather, carefully select data that are key indicators of the issue. Exclude irrelevant data and nice-to-know (but not necessary to have) data. Check the selection of key indicators with others for their assessment of the effectiveness of the data to support the issue.

Concerns and Counterarguments

After the issue has been clearly defined and supported with key indicators (refined data), it is important to recognize areas that may be controversial. If a manager is

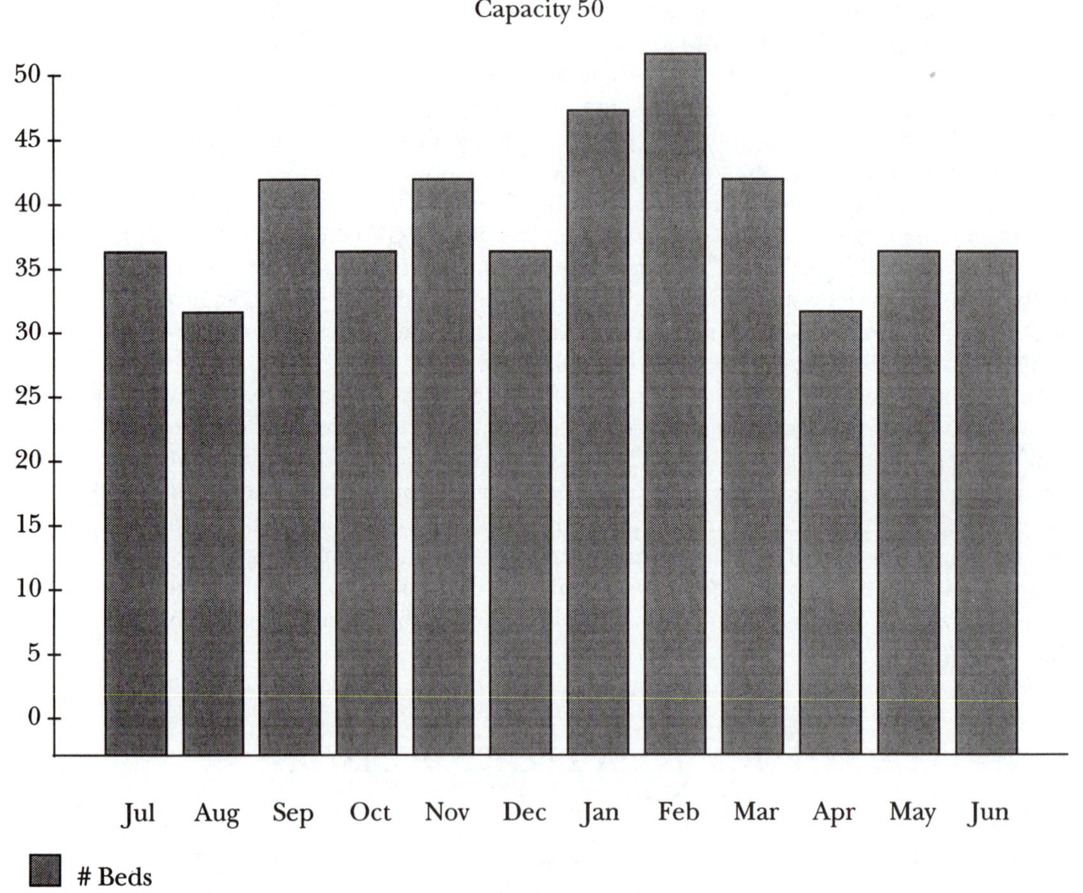

Figure 14-2 Medical Unit A—Monthly Bed Utilization 1993.

trying to justify additional staff to cope with the January and February demands, there are several ways to approach the resolution. In the bed utilization examples in Figure 14-2 and 14-3, staffing could be met by:

1. Hiring 6 FTEs
2. Expecting the staff to work overtime for two months
3. Obtaining temporary staff with additional budget dollars for January and February
4. Not changing budgeted dollars and thus expecting noncompliance in January and February, with end of year budget compliance (regression toward the mean)
5. Obtaining additional budgeted dollars for January and February that can be used to increased part-time hours, pay for X% of overtime hours, and/or hire temporary staff

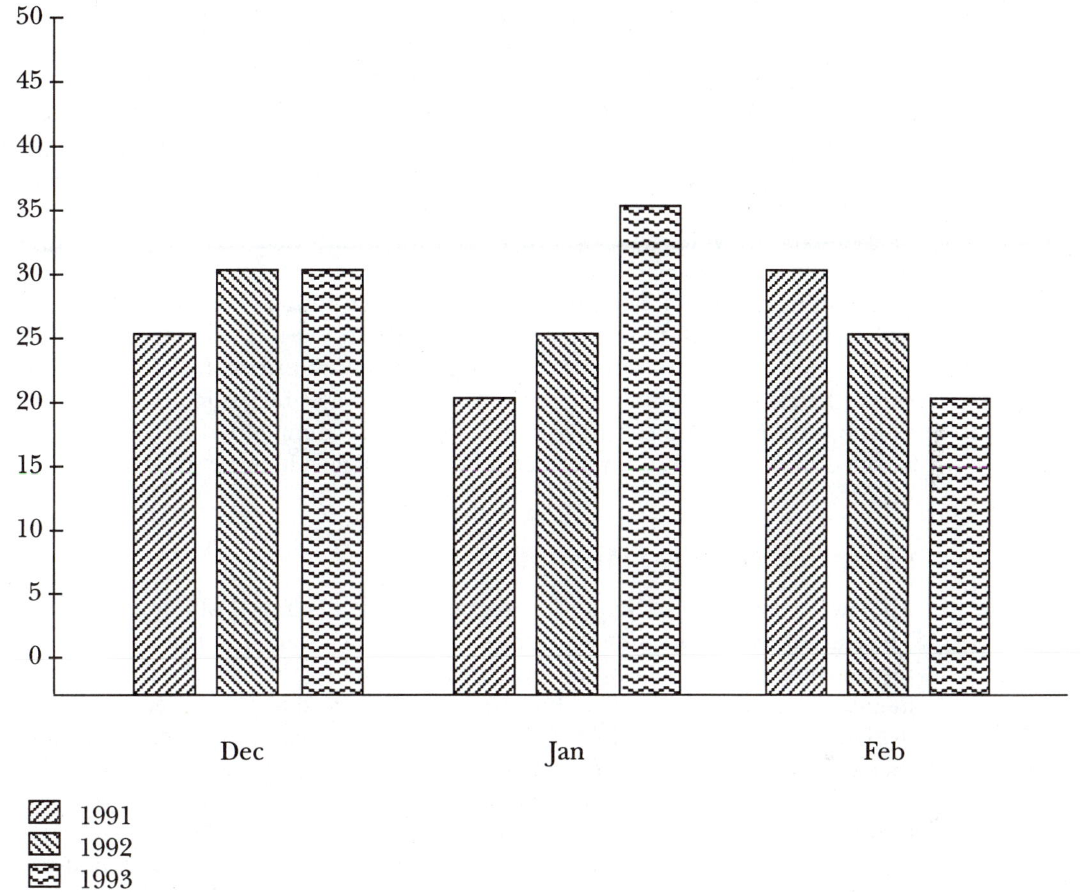

Figure 14-3 Medical Unit A—Bed Utilization December - February 1991—1993 (Bed Capacity 50).

Each approach should be explored with the pros and cons clearly stated and data used to evaluate each option. This can be achieved through the use of "what if" scenarios created on spreadsheets or budget modules.

It is important to include as many alternative ways to solve the problem as possible before systematically creating budget models for each one. After the data is available, it needs to become the basis for accept or reject statements. Anticipate the concern of others about how the data was created and analyzed and ask if the pro and con statements are reasonable.

Rank all options from the highest level of organizational risk to the lowest based upon the data analysis. In the staffing example, option 1, although it may be attractive, carries the highest organizational risk because it represents a permanent cost and commitment. In times of low bed utilization, it may lead to frequent staff reassignments (pulling), and if the census falls significantly, layoffs may be necessary. Option 2 also carries high risk, because it may lead to staff burnout, and attrition with the high cost of subsequent outlay of recruitment and orientation expenses, as well as temporary staffing dollars. The lowest risk option is probably option 5, because the dollars would not be spent if the bed utilization did not increase. The risk analysis section is the one most likely to elicit a conflict in values. When reassessing risk analysis, carefully consider the values of those involved in making the final decision. Be prepared to accept a less than perfect outcome that balances opposing values. The alternative is to cling to one recommendation and perhaps end up with nothing.

Out of this objective process of analyzing options and risks will come the recommendations, which may be different from an intuitive recommendation. The next step is to consider if the objective data led to the recommendation of option 5 (obtaining additional budgeted dollars for January and February), but if the institution in budget month five (December) readjusts the unit staffing budget based on the previous five months usage, this option will not work. In January and February, the extra dollars budgeted in July will no longer be available. In this institution, option 6 may make more sense. Once a recommended strategy has been selected, it is important to plan how to operationalize it and evaluate its effectiveness.

Operation and Evaluation Plan

The first question asked about the recommendation is how it will be implemented. The answer needs to include who will do what, when, where, how, and at what cost. If the recommendation is very time and resource intense, the likelihood of the recommendation being accepted falls dramatically. To be successful, the operation must use the fewest number of people possible for the shortest time, and use currently available system resources. These three approaches will keep the costs reasonable and make a recommendation viable. The timeframe for each activity should be represented on a Gantt or PERT chart.

The plan for evaluating the effectiveness of the decision is as important as the operations plan, because it builds the likelihood of success for future decision making. Consider which data should be identified as key indicators, how frequently they should be reviewed, land by whom. In the bed utilization example, key indicators will be found in the computer-generated monthly budget reports and the staffing reports. The nurse manager should assume responsibility for their monitoring and make the necessary adjustments. The plan should call for these monthly evaluations being shared with the area director or chief nurse executive. Once the data analysis and critical thinking have been completed, it is time to consider how the formal report should be structured.

Building Credibility

The presentation of the manager's effort must be as first class as the analysis. This means that the report must be word processed, use visual representations of the data, demonstrate logical flow of material, and include all options that were considered before making the recommendation (Table 14-2).

Format is important, but it cannot substitute for thorough data analysis, and critical thinking will not be apparent in a report that is hastily put together in an unpolished manner. Be mindful of the audience's time. Keep the report concise, clear, and concentrated. By concentrating on the main issue and not getting sidetracked, a more compelling case is built. The audience must believe in the data and respect

Table 14-2 • **Topical Listing of Report Format**

Report	Title
I.	Executive Summary (Written last, placed first)
II.	Issue Definition
III.	Historical Perspective
IV.	Potential Solutions (Options)
V.	Risk Analysis
VI.	Recommendations
VII.	Operation and Evaluation Plan
VIII.	Conclusion
IX.	Appendix/Reference

the data refinements, alternative strategies, and risk analysis. If they do, the manager will be able to jointly arrive at a workable solution with a reasonable risk.

SUMMARY

Computer-supported decision making enhances the nurse manager's credibility and improves decision making. In today's high-stakes, fast-changing healthcare environment, all decisions must be supported by data, data analysis, and critical thinking. This process is facilitated through the use of various computer software applications. These are powerful tools to generate alternative scenarios before making recommendations, as well as to present them to others in a polished format. Nurse managers who learn to use these tools, and speak the language non-nurse managers rely on, will have a higher probability of garnering scarce resources.

REFERENCES

Angehern, A.A., & Luthi, H.J. (1990). Intelligent decision support systems: A visual interactive approach. *Interface, 20*(6), 17–28.

Mills, A.C., Blaesing, S.L., & Carter, J.H. (1991). Preparing nurses to use microcomputers for the work of management. *Computers in Nursing, 9*(5), 179–183.

Mintzberg, H. (1989). *Mintzberg on management: Inside our strange world of organizations.* New York: Free Press.

Simpson, A.L. (1993). The executive information system's basic eight. *Nursing Management, 24*(2), 32–33.

Turban, E. (1982, Summer). Decision support systems in hospitals. *Health Care Management Review,* 35–43.

Zemke, R. (1988). Decision support technology, can computers harness the power of the irrational? *Training, 25*(8), 65–67.

Part III

Applications in Clinical Practice

Teresa A. Long
Sandra M. Gomberg

CHAPTER 15

Critical Care

Lead, follow, or get out of the way.
—*Anonymous*

INTRODUCTION

Critical care is a term used to describe a hospital setting where aggressive, acute, and extraordinary nursing and medical care are practiced. The units usually providing critical care are often called *intensive care units* and can include the *emergency unit* and *recovery room* as well. Clients are admitted or transferred into the critical care setting based on a defined criterion for what is planned as a short-term stay within the overall hospitalization. Neonatal, pediatric, or adult critical care clients require extensive and ongoing nursing assessments, comprehensive nursing plans of care, and minute-to-minute nursing management of life-threatening illnesses or conditions. Critical care nurses are expert clinicians charged with practicing within advanced standards of practice and regulatory, legal, and ethical guidelines. Decision making and communication challenges loom consistently within their clinical leadership role responsibilities. Nursing leaders must recognize the unique experiences created by the critical care setting and move to consistently and creatively support the nursing staff.

REGULATORY BODIES GOVERNING DECISION MAKING

Regulatory bodies, such as the State Board of Nursing and Joint Commission on Accreditation of Healthcare Organizations (JCAHO), and specialty organizations, such as the American Association of Critical Care Nurses, establish rules and regulations to which special care units must adhere in order to insure safe care of their patients. Hospitals create policies and procedures that address the special care needs of patients in these units. Nurses utilize all of these rules created by regulatory bodies and hospitals in order to guide the decisions they make on a daily basis.

In the critical care setting, the practice of nursing is governed by the Nurse Practice Act set forth by the State Board of Nursing. The Board regulates the practice of nursing by establishing rules and regulations. (State Board of Nurse Examiners, 1983). Nurses need to make decisions about their practice based on these rules. Scope of practice issues are challenged in critical care settings due to the advanced practice of critical care nurses. Critical care nurses often practice autonomously and make independent decisions regarding the care of the patient. Conflict can arise when nurses step outside of the practice constraints of the "professional nurse." The critical care nurse is often faced with these challenging situations and needs to make appropriate decisions in order not to jeopardize his or her job and/or nursing license.

Scenario 15-1

A nurse was caring for a patient, status/post myocardial infarction, in a coronary care unit in a small community hospital. The patient had been in a stable condition, maintained on a nitroglycerin drip, then suddenly developed ventricular tachycardia, lost consciousness, and ceased respirations. A "code blue" was called and the code cart was quickly brought into the patient's room. The patient's nurse began hyperoxygenating the patient with a mask/manual bag-valve resuscitation device. Another nurse felt a weak femoral pulse so immediately cardioverted the patient with 200 joules, per the unit's protocol. The patient subsequently developed ventricular fibrillation and was defibrillated by the nurse with 300 joules, per protocol, followed by chest compressions. Five minutes had elapsed from the time the patient developed ventricular tachycardia, and the house physician had not yet arrived at the patient's room. The nurse, who was "bagging" the patient, recently had successfully completed an advanced cardiac life support course and felt confident to intubate the patient. The patient was intubated by the nurse using the laryngoscope and a size seven centimeter endotracheal tube. The nurse then securely taped the tube in place.

The physician, whose arrival had been delayed due to a crisis situation in the emergency unit, arrived at the patient's room shortly after the nurse had intubated the patient. Although the physician was shocked by the nurse's decision to intubate the patient, an order for drug therapy for the patient was begun, and the doctor continued attempting to defibrillate the patient out of the deadly rhythm. After ten minutes of attempted resuscitation, the patient converted to sinus rhythm and began to regain consciousness.

The following day, the nurse was called to the director of nursing's office and was informed by the nurse manager and director of nursing that the actions taken were clearly outside of the Nurse Practice Act and the hospital's policies and procedures, and therefore, her position was being terminated. The nurse had completed advanced cardiac life support certification and therefore possessed the knowledge and skills to perform the procedure; however, performing this act was not within the acceptable standard of care that would be provided in similar circumstances by reasonable and prudent nurses who have similar training and experience (Pennsylvania Nurses Association, 1992).

The nurse was informed that the actions would be reported to the State Board of Nursing who could potentially suspend or revoke the nurse's license.

Along with the State Board of Nursing, the JCAHO also has specific nursing care standards that critical care units and hospitals as a whole must meet in order to maintain proper accreditation. These standards require that nursing units and departments demonstrate written mechanisms, policies, and procedures that guide hospital nursing staff members in understanding and fulfilling their patient care responsibilities (Joint Commission on Accreditation of Healthcare Organizations, 1992).

In addition to meeting general nursing care standards set forth by JCAHO, critical care units must also meet special care unit standards designed to ensure appropriate decision making by practitioners and proper care of the critical care patients in these units. Failure to adhere to these standards could jeopardize JCAHO accreditation of the hospital.

Scenario 15-2

Mary Jones, RN in the Cardiac Care Unit (CCU), was caring for a stable postoperative open heart surgery patient who was being maintained on an intraaortic balloon pump (IABP). Suddenly, the machine became nonfunctional and was no longer augmenting the patient's heart. Mary contacted the charge nurse in the unit and together they began troubleshooting the IABP, based on the procedure set forth by the CCU on care of the patient on an IABP. Still unable to get the pump to work, the charge nurse contacted the hospital supervisor for guidance. Because the supervisor was unable to find a policy on how to procure another IABP, a biomedical engineer was called who came in from home (since it was the weekend and the employee was not in the hospital). The biomedical engineer was unable to repair the IABP. After searching other units in the hospital, the supervisor located an IABP in the cardiac catheterization laboratory.

In this situation, the staff and supervisor used good judgment and made appropriate decisions in order to provide the necessary care for the patient. They would have been able to make quicker, more systematic decisions had they been able to obtain a written procedure to guide them.

On the following Monday, the CCU charge nurse and the supervisor contacted the nurse manager of the CCU to discuss the lack of an appropriate written procedure guiding the procurement of specialty equipment such as an IABP. Realizing that this was a JCAHO requirement for a special care unit, the nurse manager of the CCU collaborated with the director of biomedical engineering to create a written procedure.

FACTORS AFFECTING CLINICAL DECISION MAKING

Critical care nurses use decision making in the clinical setting to gather and evaluate information and make judgments, all of which result in the provision of patient care (White, Nativio, Robert, and Engberg, 1992). This clinical reasoning is used by nurses to review and analyze patient data and form relationships between the data and the patient's plan of care (Fonteyn, 1991). The nurse's ability to gather the correct information, make appropriate considerations, and act in the patient's best interest is contingent on many factors. First, the critical care nurse must be clinically competent in order to recognize pertinent facts and act accordingly. Second, the critical care nurse must refine decision-making skills in a variety of situations, especially emergency situations. Third, critical care nurses must be adept in negotiating many types of relationships during the course of caring for the critically ill patient; specifically, the collaborative relationship between the nurse and the physician will best serve quality decision making. Finally, the critical care nurse must nurture and perfect the ability to perceive faint subtleties that prove to be essential and often lifesaving in the context of critical clinical decision making.

Competency

The critical care patient population poses multisystem health problems of an everchanging severity. Critical care nurses are required to command a complex body of knowledge and to utilize a wide variety of technology in the expert care of these patients. Clinical experience affects decision-making ability; therefore, prior experience with specific clinical cases supports decision-making proficiency in that clinical situation (Benner, 1984). The nurse then could be an expert in one clinical situation and make appropriate decisions on behalf of the patient; however, that same nurse could be a novice in a different or unfamiliar clinical situation and therefore demonstrate less decision-making proficiency. Clinical and decision-making competencies must be defined and regularly evaluated in both the expert and novice critical care staff nurse group.

Entry-level competency in the critical care setting must be clearly defined and supported. Nurses just entering the critical care specialty often have limited prior experience with such multivariable, time-sensitive, crisis-oriented decisions (Baumann and Bourbonnais, 1993). Feeling overwhelmed by the complexity and instability of a patient can prevent an appropriate scope of consideration of the details needed to make the best decision. Entry-level competencies then may include documentation of general medical/surgical experience, a critical care course that includes advanced pharmacology, basic cardiopulmonary resuscitation, and intravenous access certification. Additional proficiencies in both clinical performance and decision making will develop within a competency-based orientation program orchestrated by an expert preceptor.

Clinical competency and exposure to and observation of an expert practitioner provides the novice with an invaluable frame of reference for decision making. Decision trees could be useful tools for the novice and expert preceptor to utilize in the critical care setting. Decision trees are step-by-step models that assist in directing the thought process in problem-solving situations. The nurse using a decision tree ideally eliminates unnecessary data and focuses on the most pertinent data available in reaching a decision (Baumann and Deber, 1989).

Ongoing competency of the expert critical care nurse is paramount. Advanced clinical competence best supports the professional nurse in making independent decisions within the critical care setting. These competency expectations may include advanced certifications—such as advanced cardiac life support or neonatal and pediatric advanced life support—national clinical certifications, and attendance at defined unit-based or organizational inservices.

The expert critical care nurse must also demonstrate the ongoing ability to identify and consider a variety of information cues about the patient's condition (Bourbonnais and Baumann, 1985); therefore, competency evaluation must include communication skills, assertiveness, and actual decision-making exercises. Strategies such as mock codes and simulated case studies using audiovisual or actual role plays are interactive ways to measure staff performance.

Additional forums must be provided to support the development and improvement of decision-making skills. Staff nurse advisory groups, for example, may provide the vehicle by which staff nurses can identify problems related to some aspect of their decision making and the provision of quality care. Through unit-based quality assurance and improvement programs, staff can monitor patient outcomes and evaluate if the current quality and level of decision making are meeting the complex needs of the critically ill patient. The use of team conferences is helpful to process complex situations and improve interdisciplinary collaboration as well.

Stress

The critical care area demands rapid decision making. Baumann and Bourbonnais (1993) identify stress as an important factor in rapid decision making. Stress comes in many forms: noise from equipment, family anxiety, professional relationships, personal exhaustion, or worsening patient condition (Baumann and Bourbonnais, 1993). One or more of these and other stressors can impact on a nurse's ability to make a decision. Stress can have a positive influence on rapid decision making. The stress can cause the nurse to be more alert and aware of the important data needed in the decision-making process. The nurse will demand accurate responses to questions. Nonessential facts will automatically be disregarded. The nurse then will focus only on relevant issues and make a prompt decision in an effort to prevent or manage a disaster.

Scenario 15-3

A ten-year-old boy is admitted to the pediatric intensive care unit after a near-drowning incident. The child was submerged underwater for over 20 minutes, so there is little hope for neurologic recovery. The child's heart rate is irregular and episodes of bradycardia occur over and over. Hypotension has demanded aggressive pharmacologic management with multiple medications, each requiring ongoing titration. Rapidly increasing intercranial pressure forces the nurse to stop frequently to manually hyperventilate the child and administer additional medications. His parents have been notified of the accident, but are unaware of his extremely critical condition. The nurse masterfully addresses each critical change in the child's status while monitoring all labile body systems. The undivided attention of the physician is demanded to assure that the nurse is able to act on observed data and make decisions in the child's best interest.

Stress in this circumstance forced the nurse to remain alert and aware of important clinical data. The nurse is motivated to focus only on relevant issues and make decisions that will best avert a clinical crisis.

Conversely, stress has been documented to decrease the quality of the critical care nurse's decision making as measured by the rate of error (Baumann and Bourbonnais, 1993). This occurs when the nurse feeling stressed is distracted from considering all of the available pieces of data. This cognitive rigidity limits creativity and the ability to manage a complex situation well (Bourbonnais and Baumann, 1985). Such a narrowed focus will immobilize even the most experienced practitioner, guaranteeing that valuable cues are overlooked.

Scenario 15-4

A term neonate is admitted to the NICU after failing to breathe spontaneously at birth. The child's status stabilizes with ventilatory support. After numerous tests and failed attempts to wean the child off the ventilator, the infant is diagnosed with a rare neurologic condition causing ongoing seizures and respiratory failure. The physicians present the parents with the sad diagnosis. They introduce the discussion of a "do not resuscitate" status in the event of another turn for the worse.

The primary nurse has become increasingly frustrated with the lack of clinical progress this child has shown. The nurse is overwhelmed by the life-threatening diagnosis and resists accepting it as true. When the mother approaches with the parents' decision to ask for a DNR status, the nurse is shocked and questions the mother about their decision in an unintentionally critical way. The mother leaves the child's bedside confused and upset.

The ability to manage this complex psychosocial clinical case correctly is inhibited by the nurse's cognitive rigidity. The nurse is blinded to important clinical cues in the child's condition and valuable emotional cues in the parents. Stress has caused this nurse to fail to make decisions in the best interest of the child, the family, and the healthcare team.

The critical care nurse must identify how stress regularly presents in daily practice. Recognition of how stress is received and utilized within the context of patient care will aid the nurse in maximizing the potential positive influences of stress while minimizing the negative influences.

Nurse/Physician Relationships

The mutually supportive nurse/physician relationship in the critical care setting is paramount to the nurse's decision making. Most nurses enter the critical care specialty anticipating a collegial relationship with the physician; however, the contrary can occur and critical care nurses do report adversarial relationships with physicians (Bourbonnais and Baumann, 1985). Inconsistent levels of communication and collaboration in decision making frustrate nurses. Distraction to details soon develops as nurses experience feelings of lack of control in managing a clinical situation or influencing the final decision (Bourbonnais and Baumann, 1985). Often, it is not clear if the nurse's poor clinical reasoning breeds a lack of confidence by the physician or that the physician's behaviors prevented full participation in decision making by the nurse.

In either case, the critical care nurse cannot afford another avoidable distraction to interfere with decision making. Knaus, Draper, Wagner, and Zimmerman (1986) found that the interaction and mutual decision making that occurs between physicians and nurses within the critical care setting directly influence patient morbidity and mortality. In the intensive care unit where nurses had maximized decision making and autonomy, mortality was significantly less than in units where nurses did not enjoy decision-making autonomy (Knaus et al., 1986).

Intuition

Intuition is an individual's ability to make a decision on the basis of what appears to be limited information (Reu, 1988). Benner and Tanner (1987) describe it simply as understanding without a rationale. While there is limited investigation of and discussion about intuition in the nursing literature, some common observations are pertinent to decision making.

Intuition is understood to be the mastered skill of the expert and the coveted goal of the novice (Benner and Tanner, 1987; Reu, 1988; Scherubel and Carlson, 1991). While the novice and expert use similar decision-making strategies in managing clinical problems, the experts maneuver the process more proficiently (Benner, 1984). Carnevali and Thomas (1993) suggest that experts cluster information in ways that allow them to move quicker, monitor progress better, and use time well when negotiating the decision-making process. It is this superior skill that supports the expert's development and use of intuitive judgment.

Benner and Tanner (1987) studied twenty-one nurse experts with at least five years' experience. Interviews and observations were used to study intuitive judgment. Clear patterns of intuitive judgment were validated throughout. Additionally, a recurrent devaluation of intuitive abilities by other nurses, physicians, and, at times, the sample subjects themselves was obvious. Reu (1988) studied fifty-six professional nurses with an average of 12.7 years' experience in clinical practice; twenty-five of the nurses were critical care nurses. Subjects were interviewed regarding the nurses' individual definition of an experience in using intuition in their practice. The responses were evaluated in regard to the stages of the nursing process.

The results showed that these experienced nurses described intuition in both global and specific terms. The subjects clarified that intuition was used in various steps of the nursing process, yet was primarily present in the assessment and intervention stage. Considering the subjects' responses, it was concluded that the strength of the nurses' intuition urges them to act on behalf of the patient. Intuition then was demonstrated to be an important stimulus in clinical decision making for these critical care nurses.

Benner and Tanner (1987) in a pilot study also found that critical care nurses described experiences of intuition that fit consistently within Dreyfus and Dreyfus's (1985) key aspects of intuitive judgment: pattern recognition, similarity recognition, common sense understanding, sense of salience, and deliberate rationality. For example, the critical care nurses related scenarios where patients acted unlike others do in the same clinical situations. This ability to connect with warning signs in the patient allowed for a quick inquiry and accurate clinical decision, saving the patients' lives.

Validation

The critical care setting is intended for the short-term stay of patients who will move on to different settings for full convalescence. Nurses in the critical care setting begin a complex plan of care that focuses on immediate short-term goals for the patient. Goals for long-term recovery are defined, but are rarely ever actualized during the patient's ICU stay. Some patients, because of debilitating chronic illnesses, experience repetitive stays in the ICU. Over time, close relationships develop between the nurses and the patient and family. In these cases, short-term goals are often the same for each admission. Realistic long-term goals are difficult to define.

Nurses validate the impact, and at times value, of the clinical care decisions they made by evaluating the patient's final outcome. While the nurse recognizes the tremendous accomplishments made by the patient who achieves the goals set, the repetitive lack of opportunities to observe long-term recovery can be frustrating.

Critical care nurses must continue to develop realistic plans of care that address both short- and long-term goals. Clinical decisions should be made and based on the patient's clinical needs and outcomes, both immediate and long-term. Informal discussions with interdisciplinary colleagues and collaborative team meetings provide regular forums for review of clinical decisions made. Nursing conferences with the nurses caring for patients successfully transferred out of the critical care setting for recovery and rehabilitation can help to bring closure to the initial plan of care.

LEGAL ISSUES

Many legal issues exist that affect decision making in critical care nursing practice. The ability to decide or consent to treatment is a major issue impacting on critical care patients. Consent must be voluntary, competent, and informed (Rakich, Longest, and Darr, 1985). Many critically ill patients are unable to give consent because they are unconscious. In a life-threatening situation in an unconscious patient, consent is implied and treatment is rendered.

Patients having advance directives can specify the extent of medical treatment they want should they be determined as incompetent and in a terminal condition or in a state of permanent unconsciousness. The Patient Self-Determination Act of 1990, which became effective December 1, 1991, provides patients with the formal mechanism to make advanced decisions about medical treatment should they become unable to speak or decide for themselves (Johanson, 1990). The nurse is legally required to give the patient information about the purpose, advantages, and limitations of advance directives in collaboration with the attending physician.

Even if advance directives outlining treatment desires have been established, critical care nurses must allow the patient to take part in decision making regarding the plan of care (Reigle, 1992). Nurses should assume that the patient desires to participate in the treatment process. Nurses have an obligation to provide the patient with an open supportive environment in which the patient can make good decisions.

Due to the unstable nature of critical care patients, many lack decision-making capacity. In this situation, the next of kin should be included in decisions affecting the care of their family member. For the adult patient, this person may be a spouse, child, parent, or significant other. In the case of a pediatric patient, this person could be a parent or designated legal guardian. Nurses have a legal and moral obligation to involve the patient's next of kin in planning treatment options. With a comatose or incompetent patient, family members of the patient often disagree on treatment modalities.

Scenario 15-5

A 21-year-old woman is in a motor vehicle accident, resulting in severe head trauma, and is in a comatose state. The patient's spouse wants everything medically possible to be done in order to maintain her life. Prior to the accident, the spouse and patient were having marital problems and were considering divorce. The patient's parents are pessimistic about their daughter's condition and do not want any extraordinary measures done to sustain her life. They feel strongly that she be able to die with dignity.

In this situation, the nurse is challenged to provide support to the spouse and the parents, while recognizing that the spouse is the only one who has the legal right to make decisions for the patient. Since the patient and her spouse had only been considering divorce, the spouse is considered next of kin and has the legal right to choose options regarding life-sustaining treatment for the patient. A nurse is challenged when a black-and-white legal decision quickly becomes gray.

Scenario 15-6

A 53-year-old awake and alert male patient has an advance directive stating that no extraordinary measures be done to sustain life. The patient develops a rapid ventricular tachycardia but is awake and alert. Pharmacologic anti-arrhythmic therapy is administered per physician order, but without change in the heart rhythm. The nurse knows that the patient needs to be cardioverted in order to interrupt this rhythm and save the patient's life. The patient, having experienced the discomfort of cardioversion in the past, states, "Do not shock me with that evil weapon."

The nurse knows that if the patient does not convert to a normal rhythm soon, the hemodyamic status will be compromised and ventricular fibrillation or asystole may develop. The physician must determine the patient to be competent or incompetent and collaborate with the nurse on treatment efforts accordingly. The nurse must recognize the boundaries of legal responsibilities and the patient's ability and right to determine treatment.

ETHICAL ISSUES

Ethical issues surrounding decision making in critical care nursing are viewed differently by critical care nurses, depending upon their level of moral development, religious and cultural background, and past experiences. Past positive or negative experiences with an ethical dilemma will predict a nurse's approach to a similar situation. A nurse coming from a certain religion or culture may view death as a revered state that must occur without interference, while another's culture or religion may lead the nurse to feel that life is to be preserved at all costs. Critical care nurses need to make decisions that may cause conflict between opposing moral responsibilities; that is, promoting a peaceful death versus prolonging life (Rushton, 1992).

Critical care nurses are educated and trained in advanced life support to help save lives and, as such, many nurses have difficulty with "no code/do not resuscitate" orders. Nurses must realize that a decision regarding resuscitation is a moral decision to be made by the patient, not a medical, nursing, or legal decision (Feutz-Harter, 1991). Nurses accept a common premise that nurses help patients to live; however, at times, the nurse must respect the patient's desire to die with dignity. To this end, nurses should support patients as they make important life-choice decisions.

At times, a patient makes a decision to refuse further treatment, despite the fact that his or her condition is not terminal. The patient maintains the right to make that decision, and there is no duty to seek input from family members or next of kin (Feutz-Harter, 1991). A critical care nurse may struggle with this patient's decision, given that the patient is not in a terminal state.

Conversely, and more frequently, nurses undergo tremendous stress when the decision by the patient and family to "do everything" is understood to be futile and perhaps torturous. Critical care nurses possess the expertise to know clinically that there is little hope for a patient's successful recovery; still, the nurse must support the patient/family's resuscitation wishes although he or she may harbor resentment towards the decision maker.

Many times physicians persuade families of incompetent or terminally ill patients to aggressively revive them should life-threatening situations arise; however, it is the nurse who begins resuscitation measures and continues to care for the patient who is dying without a shred of dignity (Bourbonnais and Baumann, 1985). Conflicting ethical beliefs between code classification categories and patients' and families' wishes may impact the nurse's decision-making ability.

Although the critical care nurse is the constant caregiver, sometimes the nurse has little say in the patient-physician interaction concerning decisions about a patient's resuscitation status. Because of extensive knowledge and experience, critical care nurses often feel certain that they would be the caregiver to guide the patient and family in making the best decision, given the opportunity. Frustration often arises due to a nurse's perceived lack of input into patient-physician resuscitation decisions that are made. This perceived powerlessness can lead a nurse to experience suffering, and can therefore cloud decision making (Rushton, 1992). The manner in which a critical care nurse responds in a code blue/resuscitation situation is sometimes colored by ethical beliefs.

Scenario 15-7

An 88-year-old man is admitted to the coronary care unit with end-stage cardio myopathy. He is in severe congestive heart failure and is being maintained on a ventilator and on three different intravenous vasopressive drips. Although the patient is unresponsive with little chance of successful recovery, his family wants to do everything possible to save him. The patient begins to have frequent ventricular ectopy on the monitor, which rapidly develops into ventricular fibrillation. The patient's nurse is ethically opposed to having a code team jump on his chest, and so defibrillates him, and pushes more life-sustaining drugs into him. The nurse could purposefully react slowly in calling a code or intervening, but knows legally that this patient must be treated as a full code as per the family's wishes. The nurse calls the code and responds promptly in performing appropriate nursing interventions. In this scenario, a nurse is placed in a situation in which the actions of other healthcare team members compromise the nurse's ethical beliefs.

Scenario 15-8

A 90-year-old woman with a history of metastatic lung carcinoma is admitted to the intensive care unit with septic shock. She is on a ventilator and on a dopamine drip. Her code status is "full resuscitation" as per her family's wishes, although her physicians have informally indicated that she would be a "slow code" given the situation.

During her third ICU day, she has a cardiac arrest and two resident physicians enter her room and close the cubicle curtain around her bed. The nurse begins chest compressions while a respiratory therapist hyperoxygenates the patient with an ambu bag. One resident says, "Give one milligram of epinephrine IV." The other resident shoots the medication into the trash can and says, "One milligram of epinephrine given."

The nurse is appalled at the resident's action, knowing that it is not only morally and ethically wrong, but legally wrong. A second nurse walks into the room and the nurse doing compressions asks the nurse to relieve. The first nurse leaves the room, calls the chief resident to come to the code, and tells about the "trash can drugs." The code proceeds appropriately after the chief resident enters the room, but ultimately the patient is pronounced dead after a 20-minute code. Although the nurse may not agree with aggressive resuscitation on a terminally ill patient, ethical beliefs will not support the nurse's being witness to taking deliberate action *not* to treat the patient. In this situation, a nurse needs to support the patient and or family in the decision-making process without sharing personal beliefs which may influence the patient's or family's decision.

Scenario 15-9

An 85-year-old man admitted to the coronary care unit for unstable angina is told by his physician that he needs to have open heart surgery to bypass his obstructed coronary arteries. His other option is to be treated medically, but risk the chance of a heart attack that could be fatal. The patient asks what his nurse's grandfather would be told if he was in this situation. Although the nurse does not believe that surgery is in his best interest, it would not be appropriate to express this to the patient. Instead, the nurse tells the patient about the pre-, peri-, and post-operative open heart surgery experience in simple terms. The nurse also tells him about the risks of open heart surgery, as confirmed by his physician, and tells him about the benefits of medical management.

The nurse is not solely responsible for making a judgment regarding a patient's treatment decision; however, the nurse can be the best advocate by giving factual information to the patient and family without trying to make the decision. The nurse can support the patient as he or she independently, or with family, makes important decisions about future medical treatment.

LEADERSHIP FACTORS

Doing the right things right is the product of the ideal relationship between leadership and management. It is the result of decisions made with skill and insight. The highly sophisticated environment of the critical care unit demands that such an ideal relationship and decision-making prowess exist at all practice levels from the bedside to the board room.

Administrative leadership, demonstrated by commitment to quality patient care, facilitates independent nursing practice (Prescott, Dennis, and Jucox, 1987). In their research, Prescott et al. (1987) identified five organizational factors influencing independent nursing practice and decision making:

1. Type of hospital—university, community, or municipal
2. Strong top-level administrative support of nursing
3. Type of nursing unit—small, specialized, or critical care
4. Type of nursing practice model used—primary, functional, or team
5. Organizational value of clinic nursing practice

These organizational factors influence the types of opportunities nurses have to demonstrate leadership and decision making.

Nurse administrators must acknowledge their role to create a work environment that welcomes nurses to participate in a variety of leadership and decision-making opportunities. While some organizational structures more readily support staff nurse leadership, each has or can create such experiences. Similarly, nurses must recognize their responsibility to identify and maximize opportunities to make contributions to the unit and organization by exercising leadership and decision-making skills. Both critical care staff nurses and nurse administrators have the responsibility to consider and recommend new and creative approaches to decision making.

Scenario 15-10

Shared governance is an organizational philosophy which places decision-making responsibility and authority regarding issues impacting on clinical care with the professional nurse at the bedside. The staff nurses of a small eight-bed cardiac post anesthesia recovery room worked well as a clinical team. They were highly respected for their expert and super specialized clinical skills. The nurses recognized the benefits of greater participation in unit management. Nurse administrators recognized the benefits of implementing a creative management model in this unit.

Four initial committees were developed: scheduling, education, budget, and quality assurance. Later the fifth, and most important, peer review committee was developed. A nursing council was begun. It included each committee chairperson and a staff member at large. This autonomous structure worked so well that the unit staff nurse council chairperson participates in all nursing management meetings and functions.

The role of the nurse manager of this unique unit functions like a coach and consultant. Decisions are always made in a collaborative format. This nurse manager has focused on teaching these staff nurse groups aspects of leadership decision making in which they would not traditionally participate. This unit functions as successfully as other hospital units that are organized in traditional structures.

STAFFING ISSUES

Staffing decisions are made to be sure that appropriate staffing patterns exist to insure quality care is provided. A variety of factors pressure the decisionmaker into defining for this instance what appropriate staffing means. For example, unpredictable admission patterns and regular fluctuations in acuity challenge the planned staffing decisions. The critical care staff nurses are the best candidates to participate in day-to-day staffing decisions. By exercising clinical expertise, the critical care staff nurse provides invaluable insight and creative suggestions to respond to staffing problems.

Leadership must be exercised to define the potential resources for the critical care nurse. Often, there are limited line units in the organization. This leaves few opportunities for cross-coverage or reassignment. When more than one critical care unit does exist, issues regarding competency with reassignment must be adequately addressed.

Decisions to augment or reduce staffing patterns are made on the basis of recognized organizational standards. Skill in utilizing an acuity system or classification system cannot rest with the nurse manager alone. Critical care staff nurses should be able to utilize the tools available in making staffing decisions.

Nurse Extenders

Changes in clinical practice, patient needs, and financial resources have prompted the hiring of different categories of caregivers in the critical care setting. The responsibility to assess, plan, and evaluate the nursing plan of care remains the responsibility of the professional nurse. The professional nurse has other colleagues who assist in the execution of this nursing plan of care.

On one critical care unit the following staff may function like this: Monitor technicians read, interpret, and report to the nurse the cardiac rhythms of patients requiring telemetry; critical care technicians perform phlebotomy, change dressings, and suction patients; nursing assistants perform personal care basics such as baths and back rubs; and unit assistants obtain equipment, prepare vacant rooms, and run necessary errands.

The professional nurse on this critical care unit has the role of clinical leader. The professional nurse is accountable to assure the client's nursing plan of care is managed properly. The role includes assigning the appropriate clinical tasks to the appropriate caregivers. Responsibilities also include monitoring outcomes to measure the quality of care delivered and progress towards the goals of that plan of care.

Energy

The nursing leaders of a critical care unit must recognize the staff's energy potential. The clinical environment and pace of work in the critical care unit requires tremendous energy on an ongoing basis. Nurses must learn, though, to tap their personal energy stores as needed. Wasting energy when not required places the nurse, patients, and coworkers at risk. Soon, the nurse will burn out and be unable to appropriately manage the patient's care. Coworkers will be asked repetitively to step in to help colleagues when personal energy stores may be low as well.

Leadership decisions about how staff use energy begin with the staffing schedule. Multiple days worked in a row, double shifts, and frequent rotation can deplete personal energy stores. Assignments for very busy or stressful patients must be shared. The critical care staff nurse can do these things by participating in a self-scheduling, self-assignment program. Nursing administrators should monitor such programs and provide guidance and support as necessary.

Unit leaders should recognize the need to assist staff in reviving low energy stores. Each individual and staff group is different, so strategies must be personalized to the unit. Staff nurse participation is essential to assure appropriateness and timeliness of the plans.

Energy is often restored during gatherings where the staff can have open discussion about both work and nonwork topics. Unit staff meetings, monthly birthday celebrations, committee meetings, or informal group outings can provide the forum needed. Letters of thanks from patients and families can be posted. Regular recognition of staff accomplishments may be shared by nurse administrators. Staff utilization of holiday and vacation time provides staff with necessary personal distance from the workplace when needed.

COMMUNICATION SKILLS AND DECISION MAKING

One of the valued attributes of a true leader is communication skills. This includes the nurse administrator as leader as well as critical care staff nurses. Communication includes the general sharing of pertinent information so that good decisions can be made or the appropriate feedback given about the outcome of a decision made.

Nurses in the critical care unit communicate in a variety of leadership forums. The primary nurse as clinical leader communicates a plan of care to guide bedside decisions for the patient. The charge nurse communicates to the oncoming shift a review of the unit's activity so that assignment decisions are made accurately. The unit-based scheduling committee communicates staffing concerns by denying schedule requests that bring the number of staff scheduled below what is safely required.

Communication is an expected and key skill involved in any leadership decision making. The skill does not come naturally, but must be developed. Both critical care staff nurses and nurse administrators need to work together to monitor and improve communication skills involved in leadership decisions.

SUMMARY

Critical care nursing is practiced in a variety of clinical settings where clients suffer complex multisystem disease processes. Critically ill clients require extensive and ongoing nursing assessments and expert clinical decision making to manage the plan of care. Critical care nurses practice within advanced practice standards and regulatory and ethical frameworks to assure that nursing practice is safe and appropriate.

Clinical decision making is the primary task of the critical care nurse. Advanced clinical decision-making competency must be validated and consistently strengthened to assure critical care staff nurses are able to practice safely. Critical care nurses should acknowledge workplace stressors and how they impact on practice decisions as a key goal in ongoing decision-making proficiency.

Nurses and physicians in the critical care specialty need to find ways to work as colleagues to insure that open communication and collaborative clinical decision making occurs. Intuition is a frequently mastered skill of the critical care nurse and plays an essential role in the nurse's relationship with professional colleagues and ability to make expert clinical decisions.

The critical care setting demands expert leadership and management at all practice levels to insure that quality care is provided. Nurse administrators and staff nurses alike must use their personal and professional energy to optimize an organizational environment conducive to advanced practice nursing decision making. Finally, communication is the most valuable vehicle used by critical care nursing leaders to mobilize decisions in the best interest of both clients and colleagues.

REFERENCES

Baumann, A., & Bourbonnais, F. (1993). When the chips are down; decision making in a crisis situation. *Canadian Nursing, 79*(5), 23–25.

Baumann, A., & Deber, R. (1989). The limits of decision analysis for rapid decision making in ICU nursing. *Image, 21*(2), 69–71.

Benner, P. (1984). *From novice to expert: Excellence and power in clinical nursing practice.* Menlo Park, CA: Addison-Wesley.

Benner, P., & Tanner, C. (1987, January). Clinical judgment: How expert nurses use intuition. *American Journal of Nursing,* 23–31.

Bourbonnais, F., & Baumann, A. (1985). Stress and rapid decision making in nursing: An administrative challenge. *Nursing Administration Quarterly, 9*(3), 85–91.

Carnevali, D. & Thomas, M. (1993). *Diagnostic reasoning and treatment decision making in nursing.* Philadelphia: J.B. Lippincott Co.

Dreyfus, H., & Dreyfus, S. (1985). *Mind over machine: The power of human intuition and expertise in the era of the computer.* New York: Free Press.

Feutz-Harter, S. (1991). Nursing and the law. Eau Claire, WI: G Publishing.

Fonteyn, M.E. (1991). Implications of clinical reasoning studies for critical care. *Focus on Critical Care, 18*(4), 322–327.

Johanson, W.R. (1990). Making a critical decision before it becomes critical. *Heart & Lung, 19*(2), 15a.

Joint Commission on Accreditation of Healthcare Organizations. (1992). *Accreditation manual for hospitals* (Vol. 2). Oakbrook Terrace, IL: Author.

Knaus, W., Draper, E., Wagner, D., & Zimmerman, J. (1986). An evaluation of outcome from intensive care in major medical centers. *Annals of Internal Medicine, 104,* 410–418.

Pennsylvania Nurses Association. (1992, June 8). Perspectives on practice: State board adopts a decision tree. *Pennsylvania Nurse.*

Prescott, P.A., Dennis, K.E., & Jucox, A.K. (1987). Clinical decision making of staff nurses. *Image, 19*(2), 56–62.

Rakich, J.S., Longest, B.B., & Darr, K. (1985). *Managing health service organizations.* Philadelphia: W.B. Saunders.

Reigle, J. (1992). Preserving patient self-determination through advance directives. *Heart & Lung, 21*(2), 196–198.

Reu, L. (1988). Intuition decision making. *Image, 20*(3), 150–153.

Rushton, C.H. (1992). Care-giver suffering in critical care nursing. *Heart & Lung, 21*(3), 303–306.

Scherubel, J., & Carlson, E. (1991). Nurses use of cues in the critically ill. *Heart & Lung, 20*(3), 296–302.

State Board of Nurse Examiners. (1983, September 16). *Rules and regulations of the state board of nurse examiners for registered nurses* (PAB Doc. No. 83-1257). Harrisburg, PA: Commonwealth of Pennsylvania.

White, J., Nativio, D., Robert, S., & Engberg, S. (1992). Consent and process in clinical decision making by nurse practitioners. *Image, 24*(2), 153–158.

Luann K. Lavin
Susan M. Low

CHAPTER 16

Acute Care

"Decision makers can turn opportunities into realities."
—*Anonymous*

INTRODUCTION

Acute care, for the purposes of this chapter, is defined as healthcare provided in a hospital setting. The patient population is over the age of eighteen years, and may be either male or female. The patient is usually considered able to participate in decisions regarding his or her healthcare, and when it is required, able to give legal consent. Exceptions to this rule are patients, who as a result of a congenital process, a physical or mental disease process, or a traumatic process, are legally incompetent. The incompetent population requires an advocate to intercede on its behalf. Often this advocate is the professional nurse.

The physical setting for acute care nursing occurs on what is referred to as a general medical-surgical floor. The nursing unit is usually a combination of private and semi-private rooms averaging twenty to fifty beds. In smaller hospitals the units tend to have a more diversified patient population than the larger hospitals, where the populations are often clustered according to medical diagnoses. The acute care specialty units may include a number of different patient cohorts grouped by medical specialty, such as orthopedics, urology, renal, trauma, endocrinology, oncology, pulmonology, cardiology, or infectious diseases. Some populations, such as gerontology, are found across all units.

The caregivers on these units are from various skill levels. All units will have registered nurses (RNs); depending on the state or regional area, there will also be licensed vocational nurses (LVNs), licensed practical nurses (LPNs), nursing assistants (NAs), care technicians, monitor technicians, and others. Nursing care is planned by the RN. The caregiver to patient ratio is frequently 1:4 to 1:12 depending on the acuity levels, shift, and staffing mixture.

Several types of support staff may be available to assist the individual nurse with the decision-making process. Support staff positions may be nurse administrators, staff development personal, and clinical nurse specialists. Availability of support staff will depend on the organizational structure of the hospital nursing department, the nursing philosophy regarding education, and financial resources for support staff.

Typically, the acute care population differs from the adult critical care patient population, because the acute care patient is hemodynamically stable. The acute care patient does, however, require intervention and monitoring that cannot be received in an out-patient setting. Intervention may involve nursing activities dependent on physician orders for diuretics, anticoagulants, antibiotics, antihypertensives, antianginals, vasodilators, narcotics, insulin therapy, or any number of other medications. Patients are also admitted to undergo diagnostic procedures that assist in identifying appropriate medications and interventions. Medical and surgical treatment is often administered along with physical therapy, speech therapy, and repetitive diagnostic procedures. Patients may also require nursing interventions that include assistance with maintaining and promoting activities of daily living, support in making healthcare decisions, and education and psychosocial support in dealing with various responses to illness. The nurse may also intervene as a patient advocate in assuring that the patient's wishes are adhered to.

The following chapter is organized to include both clinical and administrative decision making in the acute care setting. Legal and ethical issues are first discussed with examples of patient advocacy, the competent versus incompetent patient, restraining patients, and advanced directives. Administrative scenarios are then reviewed, including allocation of beds, room changing, nursing care hours versus bed allocation, and the decreasing length of stay dilemma. Last, clinical decision making is discussed, using examples of nursing delegation, working with difficult people to formulate opportunities, and intuitive decision making.

PATIENT ADVOCACY

The professional nurse is in a unique position as a healthcare provider. He or she must advocate continuously on the patient's behalf. At times, this patient-directed advocating can lead to conflict with the nurse's personal beliefs. This challenges the nurse to put aside personal thoughts and instead sincerely listen to the patient and his or her family. Patients who experience normal deterioration due to the aging process, primarily the elderly, are a group in which this dilemma is often observed.

Scenario 16-1

A patient comes to the hospital from a nursing home, and she is no longer able to control her elimination. Her musculoskeletal system has weakened, thus position change is difficult. Ambulation is impossible for this patient.

This once-active person now depends on others for basic life functions. Food and meal times, which once brought her such pleasure, now only serve to remind the patient of her debilitation and loss of body functions.

This patient has been admitted to the hospital for the treatment of pneumonia. She is oriented and able to make decisions. Antibiotics and intravenous fluids will be administered. Upon further assessment of the patient's nutritional status, the physician may feel it necessary to place a feeding tube.

The physician approaches the patient and her family to gain consent for a feeding tube placement. The patient states that supplemental feeding is against her wishes and refuses consent for feeding tube placement. The daughter of the patient is not in agreement with this decision. When the patient goes off the floor for a chest x-ray and her daughter asks for advice, how should the nurse respond?

There is often a temptation for the nurse to base her response on past experiences. When the problem in this scenario is accurately identified, it can be understood that the nurse is searching for the correct manner of assisting the patient to receive the treatment that she really desires. The family and their existing relationship plays a big part in assisting the patient to make a decision. However, the family is not the party for which the nurse is advocating.

The nurse has various alternatives available to her in this situation. The nurse can voice her opinion of what should happen based on her past experiences. The nurse may share the daughter's concerns with the patient. Or, the nurse can encourage the patient to communicate with her daughter regarding her wishes.

While imposing solutions based on past experiences may be the simplest approach for the busy nurse, each patient and family must be treated individually. Sharing the daughter's concerns with the patient may be interpreted as siding with the daughter and not advocating for the patient. According to the patient's bill of rights, the caregiver's primary loyalty belongs to the patient. The nurse must instead encourage mother and daughter to communicate with each other and support a healthy relationship in order to promote an outcome that the patient truly desires.

The patient later explains to the nurse that she eats as much as she can, and to receive tube feedings would go against nature. The patient continues to explain that she understands what the doctor is saying, that she will get sick easier if she does not eat more; however, this she is able to accept. The patient states that her husband died of pneumonia and it was not so bad. The patient thinks she will be all right if her daughter is with her. Evaluating the above decision, it seems the patient was assisted to make the decision she truly desired.

COMPETENT VERSUS INCOMPETENT

In some situations, it may become necessary to decide whether the patient is competent to make decisions. Competency is a legal concept, which, according to Campbell's (1989) *Psychiatric Dictionary*, is the ability to perform or accomplish an action or task that another person of similar background and training, or any human being, could reasonably be expected to perform. Almost always the term refers to mental capacity. Ordinarily a person is not deemed incompetent on the basis of a physical defect that impairs performance (Campbell, 1989). A psychiatrist will be consulted to determine if a patient is competent to make his or her own decisions. (See Scenario 16-2).

Scenario 16-2

A 70-year-old quiet and introverted gentleman who has been able to live by himself is admitted to the hospital. He is diagnosed with cancer of the lung. He wishes no treatment. The physician feels the benefits the patient would gain from chemotherapy treatment would greatly outweigh the side effects. A psychiatric consult is requested to insure the patient is able to accurately comprehend the physician's recommendations. The psychiatric consultant finds that the patient is not at all hindered in his decision-making ability. The patient verbalizes to the nurse that he knows exactly what the doctor said to him and that he feels that if he does not get treatment he will die sooner. The patient also goes on to tell the nurse that he has lived a good life and that he is all alone. The patient states that the agony of chemotherapy is not worth the limited improvement in the length of his life.

The nurse has no options in view of the patient's statement but to support the patient in his decision. If the physician is uncomfortable with this decision, he may consider consulting the hospital ethics committee for further advice.

Deciding to Restrain Patients

As a group, nurses and physicians most often restrain patients to prevent falls from bed. Restraints are frequently utilized to prevent patients from wandering, as well as to subdue agitation. Restraints are also utilized to protect the patient from harm he or she might incur if medical devices, including intravenous lines (peripheral and central), foley catheters, nasogastric feeding tubes, and chest tubes, were removed.

Alternatives to using restraints should be employed whenever possible. The decision to use restraints involves the nurse, physician, staff, patient, and family members whenever possible. Restraints should also be utilized only on a short-term basis (Evans and Strumpf, 1989). When applying restraints to a patient, always be wary of the potential dangers of unintended removal of medical support equipment and implement a plan that will without a doubt ensure the patient's safety.

Scenario 16-3

Mr. Gregory was admitted to the hospital for a transurethral resection of his prostate gland (TURP), and has a past medical history of Alzheimer's disease. He returned from surgery, after having a local anesthetic, with an indwelling foley catheter and a continuous bladder irrigation. Upon return to the floor, Mr. Gregory asks the nurse to remove his catheter, since he does not feel he needs it anymore. The nurse explains to Mr. Gregory that he must continue to have his urinary tract irrigated in order to prevent any blood clots from forming.

When the nurse returns to assess Mr. Gregory's output, she finds Mr. Gregory attempting to pull out his foley catheter. There are no visitors to assist the nurse in monitoring Mr. Gregory. The nurse speaks with his physician and an order is obtained for soft wrist restraints. Mr. Gregory refuses to allow the nurse to place them on him.

The real problem here is that the nurse cannot insure that Mr. Gregory will keep his catheter in place. And he may cause further damage by attempting to remove it. The nurse may also feel that the problem consists of Mr. Gregory not allowing her to place the restraints. Maybe restraints are not the right answer to the real problem of trying to maintain Mr. Gregory's catheter. Possible alternatives for the nurse include:

1. Discussing the need for the catheter with Mr. Gregory
2. Contacting the physician for a psychiatric consult to determine if it is legitimate to restrain Mr. Gregory against his will
3. Contacting the physician for a mild sedative to help the patient to be more relaxed regarding the catheter
4. Calling security and asking for assistance in applying the restraints

Force is usually the last resource the nurse chooses. A psychiatric consult could take hours and the potential for harm to the patient is more immediate. A mild sedative may allow the short-term relief the patient needs to cope with the catheter placement. The purpose of this choice is not to "snow the patient," but to help him relax so that he is better able to tolerate the foley.

Simple nursing interventions such as placing Mr. Gregory's hands above his sheets and taping his catheter securely to his leg could also provide additional support to the patient. Restraints should never replace direct observation of the patient by the nurse.

Advanced Directives

The 101st Congress, in the Omnibus Budget Reconciliation Act of 1990, Section 4206, mandates what is referred to as "Advance Directives," or self-determination. The law requires that all adult patients receive the following information: "Individuals' rights under state law to make decisions concerning medical care, including the right to accept or refuse medical or surgical treatment and the right to formulate advance directives and the written policies of the provider or organization respecting the implementation of such rights" (Congressional Quarterly, 1990, p. 146).

The law's intent of educating the populace will bring about an increase in the number of patients entering the hospital who have made decisions regarding their healthcare preferences should they become unable to communicate. The law also allows that the decisions be written, and that a durable power of attorney be chosen prior to a crisis situation.

Healthcare providers have a great opportunity to benefit from this law. Now there is an acceptable mechanism for the patient to communicate his or her wishes, alleviating the need for the nurse to guess or interpret information gleaned at a time of crisis.

Because "Living Will" laws may differ by state, each nurse must be aware of the laws in the state in which she or he practices. The hospital legal department should be able to assist the nurse in finding this information for his or her respective state.

When referring to a patient who is making a decision contrary to the physician's recommendations, it is clear that the patient does have a right to choose the healthcare alternative he or she wishes. The nurse's responsibility now becomes one of a support person and educator. If ever an individual nurse cannot support a healthcare decision a patient or his or her family has made, the nurse must remove him- or herself from the care of the patient. The wishes of the patient can never be denied in favor of the wishes of the nurse.

Scenario 16-4

A patient who is 27 years old and diagnosed with lymphoma presents an advanced directive stating he does not wish to be resuscitated. The nurse will need to make her decision as to whether she can accept the patient's direction on a professional as well as personal level. Knowing one's self and identifying one's true feelings will enable the nurse to make a decision, and more importantly, implement the decision.

Once the nurse has decided, the patient will certainly benefit by receiving care from a provider who is comfortable and can work with his decision. A good relationship can be established as well as therapeutic communication. Evaluation of this type of decision should result in the nurse's feeling comfortable with the decision she has made.

ALLOCATION OF BEDS

One issue that is consistently debated on the acute care unit is the allocation of patient beds. Oftentimes hospitals have subspecialties that necessitate geographical placement in order to promote optimal patient care.

Scenario 16-5

What happens when the nurse gets a call that a patient is in need of peritoneal dialysis and has a fractured hip? Does the patient need to be placed on the orthopedic unit or on the unit that is able to provide peritoneal dialysis?

Depending on whether the hospital management structure is centralized or decentralized, the decision will be made differently. In a centralized system most of the decision making authority is held by a few people. Each person who has some authority is responsible for only a few subordinates. This is termed a **narrow span of control** (Ellis and Hartley, 1991). There may be many levels of management through which communication must travel. A charge nurse will have little authority for autonomous decision making in this type of structure, and may need to await instructions from her supervisor.

In a decentralized system, there are fewer levels of management with a **broad span of control.** There cannot be close supervision when the supervisor is responsible for many people; therefore, the supervisor relies on individuals to make independent decisions (Ellis and Hartley, 1991). Nursing management will typically assist the charge nurse in problem solving as needed and delegate the implementation. Autonomy and independent decision making is promoted in a decentralized system, and the charge nurse will become more involved in decision making.

In addition, there is a spectrum of systems ranging between what we have defined as true decentralization and centralization. Upon entering a new institution, each RN will need to learn in what type of system he or she is practicing. The climate in which this is learned or taught may be formal, informal, or a combination. Frequently, the system diversity is not identified immediately, but learned through interactive experience with peers.

Regardless of the type of the structure, when gathering the information on which to base a decision, a variety of resources are available. These resources include, but are not limited to the nurse manager, nursing supervisor, bed facilitator, physician, and admissions office. The nurse participates in the decision-making process, however, but does not make an isolated decision.

In order to make an appropriate decision, the nurse will need to communicate with the involved departments and decide on the best possible alternative. The best alternative will provide quality patient care and work within the hospital system. It is important to remain patient-focused at all times. The patient must not become the victim. Providing effective communication when dealing with other departments will help ensure the desired outcome.

In reference to the situation involving the peritoneal dialysis patient with a fractured hip, the decision will need to be based on which patient problem is most acute. Keeping in mind the hospital structure in which the nurse is operating, the nurse will need to insure that the resources are available to provide optimum outcomes. For example if the patient is to reside on the peritoneal dialysis floor, the nursing staff will need to insure that the orthopedic needs are met. In this decision-making process the implementation phase is critical.

ROOM CHANGING

There are times when patient rooms will need to be changed in order to facilitate quality patient care. Utilizing effective communication skills, showing empathy, and being supportive of patient feelings will help smooth out this process. Patients are usually not pleased when they are being asked to move, but oftentimes do not have a choice in the matter.

It is important to be knowledgeable of hospital policy on room designation. Once the nurse knows this information he or she is ready to implement the patient move.

> ***Scenario 16-6***
>
> Mrs. Miller is in a single-patient room, though she has not requested the room. She is not paying for a single room and her medical condition does not indicate a need for a single room. At the time of her admission it was the only room available. Tonight the floor is receiving a patient with weeping infected sacral wounds and a hacking cough. This patient needs to be isolated from other patients until the infection is under control. The nurse must now discuss with Mrs. Miller the need for her to move to a semi-private room. Mrs. Miller has grown accustomed to the single room and her multiple family members have her phone number.

The nurse is faced with limited alternatives. The nurse should contact the admissions office and the nurse facilitator to be sure that no other beds are available for the new patient. When all other options are exhausted, the nurse must firmly but kindly insist that Mrs. Miller move. The nurse can offer to phone her family members and inform them of her new room and number. She also can contact the hospital's patient representative to see Mrs. Miller in the morning to help support the patient through the transition.

NURSING CARE HOURS VERSUS BED ALLOCATION

An additional bed allocation issue occurs when the patient who requires nursing care hours (NCH) above what is normally delivered on a given unit cannot be reallocated. **Nursing care hours** are defined as the average number of hours of care that the average patient will receive over a twenty-four-hour period. Nursing care hours are greater on intensive care units than acute care units. It is necessary to realize that the patient accepted into the intensive care unit must meet certain criteria. In other words, increased complexity of care does not always coincide with intensive care acceptance criteria.

This typically happens on the acute care unit, when a patient has a poor prognosis and is receiving multiple treatments that are not resulting in a positive response. While the patient is requiring an increased number of nursing care hours, he or she is still not a candidate for transfer to a floor that delivers more intensive nursing care hours. This truly can be a challenge for the nurse caring for the patient, as well as the entire nursing staff on the unit. Assignments often need to be altered in order to accommodate the elevated acuity level and all staff members may have a more challenging assignment.

Various hospitals have different ways of dealing with this type of acuity crisis. If the situation is short-term due to imminent death, the other unit personnel are often able to reassign themselves temporarily. If the situation is going to be longer in duration, the nurse manager may need to become involved to procure additional staff for the unit.

Scenario 16-7

Mrs. Long, a 57-year-old obese, black female with a past medical history of hypertension, diabetes mellitus, and peptic ulcer disease, is admitted through the emergency room in hypertensive crisis. After receiving a head x-ray it is apparent that Mrs. Long has had a massive right-sided cerebral vascular accident (CVA). Mrs. Long's condition was stabilized in the intensive care unit. The physician has evaluated her condition to be irreversible.

The physician feels Mrs. Long is no longer a candidate for the intensive care unit and would best be cared for on an acute care unit, because Mrs. Long has irreversible damage and poor quality of life expectancy. The family is approached by the physician and arrangements begin to be made to care for Mrs. Long at a nearby nursing home.

The family decides Mrs. Long is not to be resuscitated should she have a respiratory or cardiac arrest prior to transfer to the nursing home. Mrs. Long continues to be on intravenous fluids, antihypertensive medications through a central line, as well as frequent blood glucose monitoring. In the second day out of the intensive care unit, Mrs. Long develops a gastrointestinal bleed as evidenced by black bowel movements. The doctors believe Mrs. Long still is not a candidate for the intensive care unit. Care for Mrs. Long now includes close blood pressure monitoring, multiple intravenous fluids, blood products, turning, cleaning, and family support.

The charge nurse has an opportunity to intervene with the critical decision making and to assist the staff to provide optimal care for all patients on the unit. The charge nurse can request that an evening staff member come in early, plan for additional help for the next shifts, adjust the present assignment so that the team caring for Mrs. Long gets additional support, or suggest that Mrs. Long be transferred back to the intensive care unit.

The charge nurse chose to divide the assignments to assist the team caring for Mrs. Long and to make arrangements for additional help on future shifts. The option provides immediate assistance while at the same time allowing for optimal care for all patients on the unit.

The decision not to lobby for a return to the intensive care unit is the appropriate alternative given that Mrs. Long's prognosis is poor and the intensive care unit beds are reserved for those who can most benefit from that level of care. To the busy and challenged acute care nurse, this is not always the easiest rationale to understand. Education regarding the goal of care for Mrs. Long may assist the staff to understand the rationale for keeping her on the unit.

DECREASING LENGTH OF STAY

Proactive reimbursement and quality of patient care have been the recent driving force for healthcare practices. Hospitals are constantly needing to do more with less. By decreasing the length of patient hospitalization stay, the hospital is able to regain reimbursement that is necessary to recapture their costs of servicing the uninsured.

This philosophy is not new for practicing healthcare workers; however, it poses problems in every area of the acute care facility. As community health resources struggle to get into place, the acute care nurse is struggling to provide all necessary treatment, education, and documentation that is essential for basic patient health maintenance upon discharge. At one time the hospital had the luxury of a longer hospital stay and stabilizing a patient in diabetic ketoacidosis in the critical care unit and then moving the patient to the acute care unit to begin diabetic teaching. Now the hospital must stabilize and teach the patient concurrently on the acute care unit.

Nurses are no longer able to complete all educational and rehabilitational goals prior to discharge. An invaluable resource for the nurse in assisting with patient discharge is the nurse case manager. For example, if the patient is a new diabetic and requires thorough diabetic teaching, the only thing holding up discharge may be essential education. The case manager may assist with education and arranging for appropriate placement on discharge with adequate community nursing and family supporters. The case manager will need to begin arranging visiting nurse support immediately upon patient arrival to the hospital.

Communication is integral to discharge planning in this type of environment. It cannot be the sole responsibility for any one particular shift. Time is money, and facilitation of timely discharge is essential. A good philosophy to incorporate is upon patient arrival to the floor, plan for discharge!

Scenario 16-8

Mrs. Allen is admitted through the emergency room to the intensive care unit on an insulin drip. Her blood sugars are quickly stabilized and her ketoacidosis resolved. She is now ready for transfer to the floor. Ideally, the emergency room staff should refer Mrs. Allen to social services for community referral as soon as she is assessed to be a new diabetic. Now in the intensive care unit, Mrs. Allen is visited by the social worker and evaluated for her potential needs.

The social worker finds that Mrs. Allen is 66 years old and lives with her 66-year-old husband. Mr. Allen is still working and Mrs. Allen is responsible for all meal preparation. Mrs. Allen states that she gave shots to her mother-in-law for three years before she died of renal failure, and she believes she can give them to herself. When asked if she would like to see a visiting nurse at home, Mrs. Allen states she is interested if Medicare will pay for it.

The social worker assures Mrs. Allen that Medicare does pay for home care. The nurses in the intensive care unit begin teaching Mrs. Allen how to perform finger stick glucose monitoring using one of the home testing products. The instructions are continued on the acute care unit when Mrs. Allen is transferred. The patient is mastering the insulin injection also. Mr. Allen receives one educational period during visiting hours on the third day of Mrs. Allen's hospitalization.

Plans are made for Mrs. Allen to go home on ten units of NPH insulin in the morning of the sixth day of her hospitalization. Mrs. Allen is able to give herself her insulin shot for three consecutive days before she is discharged. The visiting nurse will visit the patient at eight in the morning on the first two days she is at home and then reassess how much additional education Mrs. Allen and her husband need.

As outlined above, it appears that Mrs. Allen is a positive person who learns quickly. Even this very optimistic woman will need instructions regarding multiple issues such as sick day care, foot care, hypo- and hyperglycemia reactions, and exercise. This is a great deal for a recovering individual to absorb. The acute care nurse must assure that there are resources for this patient once she is discharged.

DELEGATION

Nursing on an acute care unit involves working with a variety of skill levels. Each skill level has different accountabilities and responsibilities, determined by an associated job description. Patient care assignment is the responsibility of the professional nurse. When making a patient care assignment, the professional nurse will delegate certain aspects of care to the LVN, the LPN, the NA, care technicians, monitor technicians, and others.

The professional nurse is responsible for ensuring a plan of patient care. Care that is planned and delegated appropriately and is within the job expectation, is the responsibility of the direct caregiver. It is the professional nurse, however, who will need to ensure that the assignment is adequately completed.

The professional nurse may accomplish patient care through delegation and continually assess her coworkers for completeness. Whenever new techniques or equipment are instituted, the professional nurse has a responsibility to ensure that proper supervision is provided and that utilizing the technique or equipment is delegated to the appropriate skill level.

Scenario 16-9

Visualize the situation of an RN caring for eight patients with an NA. One of the patients the nurse has assigned to the NA requires continuous tube feedings. The NA tells the RN that while she attended the inservices on the new feeding pumps yesterday, she has not had the opportunity to use one, and asks the RN to feed the patient for her.

The nurse could acquiesce and feed the patient for the NA Or, she can plan with the NA how she will facilitate gaining the necessary comfort level with this skill. While it may be easier today for the nurse to just feed the patient, it would not address the problem of the NA's not knowing how to use the pump. It is clear to achieve optimal patient outcomes in the future and for today, that the nurse will need to plan the time to observe the NA performing the feeding procedure.

Factors Contributing to Delegation

Organization is the first key to successful patient care when delegating. When a patient assignment is determined, and patient reports are given, it is essential to gather all data in order to make an informed decision on who will be needed to do what. It is important to note that no decision is ever final. What seems necessary and likely to work at the beginning of the shift may not be feasible by the middle of the shift, depending on what changes have occurred. A good motto on the medical-surgical nursing unit is to "always expect the unexpected." Flexibility and the ability to change at a moment's notice, make a good nursing team.

Scenario 16-10

At the beginning of day shift, on a unit that assigns nursing care in districts, there are twenty patients and four empty beds. There are four patients in the first district, eight patients in the second district, and eight in the third district. The district with only four patients has one RN, and the districts with eight patients have one RN and one nursing assistant. At 10:00 AM, the RN with four patients receives notification that her district will be receiving three admissions. The nurse determines that she will not be able to care for the three new patients and the four patients she has already.

When exploring her options, the nurse would need to evaluate available alternatives. The nurse must first assess her available resources. The nurse may need to involve her nurse manager or assistant nurse manager in the problem solving, depending upon the structure in which she works. Or the nurse may independently consult her peers to jointly assess their patient load and make the changes necessary to provide positive patient outcomes. There may be staffing resources available from outside the unit itself, for example, from other units or from the nursing office. If there are no additional resources, assignments will need to be rearranged to insure that all patients on the unit receive optimal care.

Prioritization is the second most essential key for successful delegation. The nurse will need to have a good knowledge base and assessment skills to know which patients she will need to provide with immediate attention and which patient needs she can delegate to other members of the healthcare team. For example, if the nurse has a district of eight patients for which she is responsible, and one patient is unresponsive with a blood pressure of 60 systolic, it is not very difficult to decide who will need immediate attention. However, if the nurse has a new admission, a pre-op patient to prepare for the operating room, a post-procedure cardiac catheterization patient, and a patient who needs to be placed on the bedpan, she will need to prioritize where her energies are needed and what she can delegate to other team members.

In the above example, if the RN had received report from the emergency room that the admission coming was stable, she might delegate greeting and initial vital signs of this patient as well as the patient needing the bedpan, to the NA. The nurse would instruct the patient for the operating room to void and remove all undergarments and dentures, while she attended to the initial assessment of the post-cardiac catheterization patient for post-procedural bleeding or changes in vital signs and peripheral pulses. Once this was done, the nurse could complete the preparation of the patient for the operating room.

Delegating to difficult people can be one of the biggest challenges in acute care nursing. Once the nurse has mastered this skill, she will be able to use it not only on the job, but in all challenging situations throughout life. Some nurses seem to have a natural talent for developing relationships; for others it seems more difficult. However, it is believed that this skill can truly be learned and mastered if the nurse perseveres.

One guideline for the nurse is never to delegate something she would not do herself. If the situation looks difficult or utterly impossible, it is a job for a team and not one individual. Compromise is a very powerful skill to learn to implement with coworkers. If the coworker decides that the assignment delegated is too difficult, it can be negotiated.

Providing coworkers with options is another useful skill. If the workload is complex, or if coworkers prefer not to work with certain types of patients, providing options that are an even exchange will facilitate a compromise.

Enthusiasm, motivation, and an understanding that the job will get done are all important characteristics to display when the nurse is delegating. If the nurse is able to bring enthusiasm into the workplace, she will foster creative thinking in order to promote effective solutions for patient care. Motivation and an understanding that the job will get done will paint a picture of a nurse who provides quality care.

FORMULATING OPPORTUNITIES

Converting a losing situation to a winning situation is a technique you can easily put to work for you.

Scenario 16-11

The nurse receives a call from a physician regarding a medication error that happened to his patient while she was providing care. The physician is extremely upset and continues to voice complaints about many other situations that have nothing to do with this isolated incident. The physician ends his lecture by stating that all nurses working at this hospital should go back to school.

The nurse's first inclination would be to stick up for herself and tell the physician that he is wrong and that he has no right speaking to her this way. However, is that really going to influence his behavior? By giving this type of reply, you will most assuredly add fuel to the fire that is already burning, and potentially make a bad situation even worse.

Consider for a moment if the nurse were to reflect what the physician has said, recognize his frustration, and allow him to ventilate. What does that physician really want to hear? Most likely he wants to hear that proper measures are being taken to insure patient safety, and that the appropriate people are being notified to prevent this mistake from happening again. By questioning what the physician really wants, the nurse will gain insight as to how she can turn this situation into a positive one. Quite obviously the physician needed to ventilate his frustrations. By choosing to react calmly and focus on patient safety, the nurse will make an impression as a professional and provide the opportunity to establish a good rapport with this difficult physician.

Utilization of a common denominator will also assist the nurse in therapeutic conversation with her coworkers. A good philosophy to keep in mind is that all work done on the unit is for one benefit—quality patient care. Instead of looking at an assignment as something to do in order to get a paycheck, the nurse will benefit most by developing an attitude that the assignment is a method for the patient to receive optimal quality care.

INTUITIVE DECISION MAKING

Scenario 16-12

Mr. Smith was admitted to the hospital with an acute change in mental status consistent with that of a cerebral vascular accident (CVA). The nurses assessed that the most frustrating part of his symptoms was the expressive aphasia. The nurses, with the assistance of the neurologist, have recently concluded that Mr. Smith does not demonstrate receptive aphasia since he is able to appropriately nod his head for yes and no answers. On the third day of his admission, Mr. Smith's nurse performed her routine assessment and felt there was something that just looked out of place. Mr. Smith looked more fatigued and had a pale color. Vital signs were stable and the neurological assessment was within normal limits for Mr. Smith. When escort arrived to take him to physical therapy, Mr. Smith got a sad look on his face. The nurse asked Mr. Smith what was wrong. Not being able to answer this question, the professional nurse proceeded to call the physician. The nurse was not really sure what was bothering Mr. Smith, but he knew that physical therapy was not the best thing for him right now.

The nurse acted intuitively and intervened to provide what she thought was necessary quality care for Mr. Smith. Unfortunately, Mr. Smith had a seizure later that morning while sitting in his chair. However, the nurses and doctors were able to provide immediate interventions that Mr. Smith would not have received in physical therapy, thus preventing him from having any further damage.

At times, it is the responsibility of the nurse to be assertive in guiding a patient in a particular direction. Nurses should use their knowledge, skills, and intuition to assume responsibility for the patient when their abilities tell them to do so. Greater consumer awareness has recently made nurses more reluctant to take responsibility away from the patient, because patients want to maintain control of their care (Wondrak, 1992). However, there is a time when the nurse needs to articulate what the patient may be unaware of, or may have difficulty putting into words.

In the above situation, the nurse reacted to the situation much in the way you would expect a proficient or expert nurse to respond. A nurse who has been in practice for only a few months or even only a few years, may not have developed the skills to exhibit this type of autonomous behavior. Intuitive decision-making skills may not be developed according to the number of years of practice a nurse possesses, but rather the experience gathered from other role models in the profession, as well as continued formal and informal education.

Referring to the above situation, the novice nurse might be expected to react by sending Mr. Smith to physical therapy, without further questioning. The advanced beginner may perform further assessments and conclude that Mr. Smith should go to physical therapy. The competent nurse may contact the physician and share his or her assessments in order to let him make the decision. The proficient nurse may perform some additional research of recent lab values and contact the physician to assist in the decision making. The expert nurse would most likely perform an assessment, including research of recent lab values, and make a decision based on her past experiences with similar cases of patients. The expert nurse would most likely contact the physician to share his or her recommendations. All in all, the different experience levels of nurses may account for different decision-making skills on the acute care unit.

SUMMARY

Decision-making scenarios as they apply to acute care for the adult patient on a general medical-surgical floor in the inpatient setting have been reviewed. Legal and ethical issues in examples of patient advocacy, competency, use of restraints, and advanced directives were explored. Scenarios involving administrative decisions about bed allocations, room transfers, required nursing care hours, and decreased lengths of stay were shared. Clinical examples with delegation of workload, working with difficult people, and use of intuitive decision-making processes were provided. The intent of the authors was to assist the novice decisionmaker in the acute care setting to generate appropriate decisions and in the midst of difficulty to turn opportunities into realities.

REFERENCES

Campbell, R.J. (1989). *Psychiatric dictionary* (pp. 139, 363–364). New York: Oxford University Press.

Congressional Quarterly. (1991). *Congressional quarterly almanac* (p. 146). 101st Congress 2nd Section Volume XLVI. Washington, DC: Author.

Ellis, J., & Hartley, C. (1991). *Managing and coordinating nursing care.* Philadelphia: J.B. Lippincott Co.

Evans, L.K., & Strumpf, N.E. (1989). Tying down the elderly: A review of the literature on physical restraint. *Journal of American Geriatric Society, 36,* 65–74.

Wondrak, R. (1992). Intuitive actions. *Nursing Times, 88*(33), 41.

Susan L. McCulley
Sandra M. Gomberg

CHAPTER 17

Maternal and Child Health

Don't be a part of the problem, create solutions.
—*Anonymous*

INTRODUCTION

Maternal child health includes the clinical issues of the pregnant and postpartum woman and of the neonate. **Pediatric healthcare** includes the infant and growing child. The clients in these settings must always be appreciated as members of a family unit. At a minimum, obstetric and pediatric nurses address the mother/fetus or mother/child dyad in planning nursing care. Ideally, family units are well-defined, and the father of the fetus or child is welcomed in a family-centered approach. Each pregnant woman or parent of a child may, however, define her immediate family by including a significant other, longtime friend, or extended family members.

All areas of healthcare delivery are subject to scrutiny by regulatory agencies. Regulatory agencies work to insure that public safety is guaranteed through the delivery of quality health care. Maternal child and pediatric nursing is subject to additional regulatory requirements. These additional standards work to support the practicing nurse in clinical decision-making strategies.

The specialties of maternal child and pediatric nursing demand careful delineation of clinical competencies and standards of nursing practice. Critical behavior, including decision-making skills, must be evaluated during the initial orientation period and on an ongoing basis. The maternal child and pediatric clinical nursing process requires expert assessment and communication skills with clients and professional colleagues. A variety of barriers, such as language barriers and time restrictions, challenge the maternal child and pediatric nurses. By focusing on communicating with the client and the family unit, the nurse will be able to make accurate decisions and negotiate a plan of care to meet even the most complex demanding clinical needs. In the obstetric and pediatric settings, nurses must assure that the child's parents are fully involved in the healthcare issues and decisions pertaining to their child. The pediatric nurse is challenged when the family unit is not so easily defined. Social and economic struggles have shattered traditional family units. Nurses thus look to regulatory agencies or the court system to define and direct guardianship and the process of obtaining proper consent. Nurses in the obstetric and pediatric settings must remain expert in supporting nontraditional family structures within legal parameters.

Maternal child and pediatric nurses participate in ethical clinical situations. Complex social and economic decisions can prompt difficult decisions about discharge readiness and client/family compliance with an urgent nursing and medical plan of care. The right to refuse treatment surfaces in both obstetric and pediatric settings. Nurses must be well prepared to address ongoing ethical decisions in maternal child and pediatric settings.

Leadership in maternal child and pediatric settings surfaces at many different levels. Each time a nurse makes a clinical decision in the best interest of a client, leadership is demonstrated. In the more formal sense, the leadership abilities of the maternal child and pediatric nurse manager and charge nurse provide the organizational structure in which clinical care is delivered. Resource allocation, both personnel and material, requires a fine balance if quality care through expert decision making is to be delivered.

OVERSIGHT BY REGULATORY BODIES

Regulators are the public and private sector groups who, out of concern for the individual and society, have established rules, regulations, and policies to ensure standards of quality in healthcare. In the United States, these include Congress and federal administrative agencies, state and local government entities, private organizations, and healthcare professionals (Berger and Williams-Brinkman, 1992).

There are many regulatory agencies, and depending on the type of facility in which one works, the governing agencies may vary. Maternal child and pediatric nursing as specialties are often subject to additional regulatory requirements. The federal government makes healthcare organizations accountable for the care they deliver. The government mandates the reimbursement for care to Medicare and Medicaid clients, and is responsible for assuring the safety of foods, drugs, and cosmetics made available to consumers.

The Joint Commission for the Accreditation of Healthcare Organizations (JCAHO) requires that standards of care be written and that these standards reflect the needs of the maternal child and pediatric client. State regulatory agencies are responsible for the licensing of certain services by educational and health care facilities and individuals. Each state can determine its own requirements for licensure. Under this licensing organization, usually referred to as the Department of Health, the maternal child and pediatric settings are subject to specific infection control practices, staffing ratios, safety practices, and special requirements.

Private organizations and nurses as healthcare professionals regulate their own practice. The National League for Nursing accredits nursing educational programs.

The American Nurses Association (ANA) and the Organization for Obstetric, Gynecologic, and Neonatal Nurses set standards from which many facilities have developed local policies and procedures.

The Nurse Practice Act defines the legal scope of nursing practice. Nurses should understand the practice act and become familiar with the workings of the agency that enforces the act. All registered nurses, regardless of specialty, place of employment, years of experience, or educational background, must perform nursing duties within the guidelines of a state nurse practice act (Phillips, 1992). The local, state, and federal government can pass legislation that regulates what can be taught to consumers. The passing of living will legislation and advanced directives gives nurses guidance in handling decisions regarding withholding certain life-sustaining measures and cardiopulmonary resuscitation. When decisions arise on the job, the nurse should take into account the regulations that apply to that particular situation.

Scenario 17-1

John Jones, RN, is working the evening shift in the general nursery. He has been working on the mother/infant unit for one year. He is in charge of the nursery this shift. At 7 PM, he receives a call from the admissions office stating that Dr. Katz requested that baby girl Casey who was discharged two days ago be readmitted to the nursery because of jaundice and an elevated bilirubin. In the year that John has been on the unit he has never seen this occur.

John must first identify the problem that needs to be solved. He will need to decide if the infant should be admitted or not. If the baby is not admitted to the nursery, where else would she go?

The next step in the decision-making process is to seek out alternatives from which to select appropriate decisions. He can do this by looking to other staff on the unit to determine the unit's historical norms. Other sources of information available to John would be the unit's policies and procedures and the unit's manager or hospital supervisor.

After discussions with other staff, John has found that infants are not readmitted to the nursery once they have been discharged. They are admitted to the pediatric unit within the institution. Some staff felt that this may be due to a regulation. The unit policies and procedures did not provide him with the information he needed. The nursing supervisor reviewed with John the Department of Health standards for his state; here they found the information necessary to support the admission of the infant to the pediatric unit.

John was able to call Dr. Katz and relay this information to him. The infant was admitted to the pediatric unit later that night. John used the routine decision-making process steps within a bureaucratic organizational model. This is a common model used in healthcare organizations and consists of utilizing standard operating procedures to make decisions.

Regulatory standards play a major role in how we deliver clinical care. They provide the nurse with a valuable framework that enables him or her to move through clinical decision making.

CLINICAL DECISION MAKING

Maternal child and pediatric nursing care is provided in a variety of inpatient and outpatient clinical settings: regional children's centers, birthing centers, large tertiary care centers, or community hospitals. The clinical nursing units providing maternal or pediatric services are highly specialized, and often one of a kind within the medical center. The clear definition of standards of nursing care and clinical competency expectations are paramount to the nurse's ability to make decisions and provide quality care.

Standards of Practice

Standards of practice in the maternal child and pediatric settings must be firmly rooted in sound references. Standards must provide clear options for the professional nurse making clinical decisions. Standards of practice must be readily available on the nursing unit in a user-friendly format. Regular review and revision of standards will assure their consistency with current trends in clinical practice. Standards must remain consistent across clinical practice areas; for example, the infant receiving phototherapy to treat neonatal hyperbilirubinemia in the newborn nursery should receive the same standard of care if treated in the intensive care nursery or on the general pediatric unit. Such consistencies support safe staff sharing as well as a larger pool of resources familiar with the standard when questions arise. Additionally, consistent standards of practice support prompt decision making when acute changes in the patient's condition require an urgent transfer from one unit to another.

Competency

The professional nurse seeking positions within maternal child and pediatric specialties should expect and demand aggressive entry-level position requirements and ongoing support to validate clinical competence. The initial professional orientation plan should include a list of critical behaviors required in the safe delivery of nursing care in the specialty practice setting. These critical behaviors should be ranked in the correct order of priority and assigned a targeted timeframe for their completion (Butts and Witmer, 1992).

Often the preceptor/orientee dyad is the relationship developed to facilitate the achievement of defined competency behaviors. As professional nurses move through the probationary orientation period, progress in mastering critical behaviors is monitored closely. Failure to progress as anticipated is an opportunity to develop individualized action plans for the new employee.

Evaluation of competency for maternal child and pediatric nurses must not end with the initial orientation program. Ongoing competency behaviors must also be clearly communicated in order of priority and have an associated timeframe for their completion. These expectations can be met in a wide variety of ways. Creative peer review systems and annual inservice conferences are two alternatives. Recognition of national specialty certifications or completion of continuing education programs may be creative ways to document ongoing competency.

Professional nurses, nurse educators, and nurse managers find listing necessary clinical competency behaviors an easy task; however, the corresponding decision-making proficiencies are more difficult to articulate. Rational and competent clinical decision-making skills are essential critical behaviors for successful professional nurse job performance. Decision-making competency provides the nurse with the structure to select and implement appropriate and timely clinical options.

Decision-making competency cannot be isolated as a singular behavior to be mastered. It is one of a broad list of intermingled skills that must be mastered and maintained. Demonstrating clinical knowledge, command of the nursing process, technical skills consistent with organizational policies and procedures, the Nurse Practice Act, and regulatory agencies such as JCAHO and the Department of Health are necessary adjuncts to expert decision making.

Communication

Obstetric and pediatric settings are consumed with complex clinical situations in which communication is paramount. These clinical situations are further complicated by the client's inability to verbalize or to accurately direct the nurse to the source of a problem or concern. A mother in active labor cannot alert the nurse to variable decelerations of the baby's heartbeat. The newly postpartum mother, weak and exhausted, is unaware that her uterus remains boggy and the increased vaginal bleeding is the beginning of an acute hemorrhage. The neonate born to a diabetic mother cannot warn the nurse of impending hypoglycemia. The seven-year old seizure patient who reports feeling tired has not clearly signaled the nurse that a grand mal seizure is imminent.

Adolescent mothers are a unique client population that present a communication and decision-making challenge in the obstetric setting as well as the pediatric setting. Research documents the unpredictability of adolescent decision-making abilities (Strauss and Clarke, 1992). Paper-and-pencil inventories, phenomenological studies, and direct interviews are some examples of tools used to measure decision making in adolescents. However, environmental factors, including socioeconomic status and intelligence, have been identified as intervening variables in these studies; therefore, age alone cannot be used as an adequate predictor of maturity of decision-making ability (Strauss and Clark, 1992). Age considerations and comprehensive individualized developmental assessments are imperative in engaging the adolescent in decision-making behaviors. Communication is the key to working with the adolescent population in teaching them decision-making skills and supporting them through difficult decision-making processes.

Scenario 17-2

A 16-year-old mother brings her ten-week old infant to the pediatric clinic with the chief complaint of a fever. The infant is lethargic and pale. The rectal temperature is 103.5. The child is 15% dehydrated. The clinic physician explains to the mother, "Your child is gravely ill and requires intravenous fluids and antibiotics immediately. We must also perform a spinal tap by placing a needle in your baby's back so we can be sure the baby doesn't have meningitis." The physician hands the mother a detailed consent form to sign. The mother begins to cry, refusing both the intravenous line and the spinal tap. She sobs, "Just give my baby medicine to make him better." The physician becomes frustrated and leaves the room. At the desk he states, "If this mother doesn't cooperate, I'll just call the Department of Human Services and get emergency consent."

The experienced pediatric nurse recognizes that the mother of this infant is struggling to act in her baby's best interest. Her ability to process the information presented by the physician is minimal; therefore, she is unable to make an informed decision. While holding the baby, yet sucking her thumb, Mom is demonstrating clear signs of developmental immaturity, another barrier to optimal decision-making behaviors. The nurse must decide on the type of approach that will be most supportive to the mom while assuring that the infant receives the care he needs immediately. The nurse enters the room.

"Miss J, you did a great job by bringing Kenny to the clinic today. You were right. Kenny has a high fever and does need medicine to help him get better." Mom looks up and smiles, listening closely to the nurse. "There are lots of reasons that little babies like Kenny get fevers. Even if you do all of the right things at home, they can still get really sick and need to come to the hospital."

Mom offers, "I always put a hat on him when I take him outside like the nurse told me to."

The nurse replies, "Well, I can see that you have been doing a good job because he has gained weight and is growing well. I would like to go over some of the things we do here at the clinic when moms bring in little babies who are sick like Kenny." The nurse goes on to describe to her why the infant needs an intravenous line and intravenous antibiotics. The nurse explains why almost all of the babies with a fever over 103 and dehydration get admitted to the hospital. The nurse reviews the spinal tap procedure and assures the mom that she does not want her to watch, but that she will stay with Kenny during the procedure. The nurse explains to the mom that the doctor will be back in to go over this information again with her and reminds her to ask any questions she has before signing the consent form.

Mom's interaction with the physician goes much better the second time. She asks appropriate questions and demonstrates a strong desire to do what's best for her baby. She is much better prepared to participate in an informed consent process.

The nurse's intervention both disarmed and supported the mother. By focusing on positive things that the mother had done, the nurse minimized feelings of guilt and frustration that interfered with the mother's ability to listen to the information being given to her. By describing what needed to be done in words and phrases, the mom could understand in her emotional state, the nurse paved the way for a positive rather than hostile second encounter with the physician. Finally, by anticipating other fears common to the mom's current developmental level, the nurse supported her by advising against the mom watching a frightening procedure, yet assured her she would stay with the infant. The mom was able to feel in control and feel that she wasn't letting her baby down.

Death

The maternal child and pediatric setting is usually perceived as one of happiness and exciting new beginnings. Death is not regularly expected, yet it does occur in these practice areas. Death in the obstetric setting is devastating. Complications with pregnancy or the labor and delivery process place both the mother and baby's life at risk.

Scenario 17-3

A 31-year-old woman arrives at the delivery room in active labor. She is 39 weeks pregnant and has had regular prenatal care. Following the birth of a healthy baby girl, the mom developed disseminated intravascular coagulation. The delivery room staff demonstrated expert decision-making skills and provided competent emergency care, yet the mom died as a result of uncontrollable hemorrhage.

Even the most thorough cognitive education does not prepare staff members for the emotional upheaval they feel after the unexpected death of a patient. Anger, guilt, fear, and sadness can quickly overcome the staff. The sharpness of usual clinical decision-making skills is dulled by the emotional crisis.

Scenario 17-4

A 12-year-old child, Tiffany, has been diagnosed with a severe leukemia. With her parents at her side, she has been in the pediatric ICU for over two weeks, yet her condition continues to worsen. The staff recognizes the likelihood of her death and must plan her care accordingly.

A team meeting is planned with the nurses, physicians, social worker, and child psychologist. The case is reviewed and plans are made to begin preparing Tiffany and her family for her death. A developmentally appropriate approach was then implemented to answer Tiffany's questions compassionately and accurately. Small staff meetings occurred regularly to inform nursing staff of changes made in the plan of care.

That afternoon Tiffany stopped breathing. The team moved through the decision making steps for resuscitation with skill just as the family had requested. The staff tearfully ended the unsuccessful resuscitation after conferring again with the family.

In this case, the staff expected death and even planned for it. The opportunity to participate in the plan of care and impact on the quality of Tiffany's last days provided an effective means of coping for the staff. The staff was supported in their need to grieve Tiffany's loss as well. They offered tearful hugs to parents and each other.

COPING WITH DEATH

In some pediatric settings, such as an oncology unit, death is a frequent challenge. The nurse's ability to make individualized patient care decisions over and over weakens when the outcome rarely supports the efforts. Frustration and anger and the limitations of technology place successive decision making at risk. Caution must be used to assure that support mechanisms are evaluated regularly.

After the death of a client, the management team plays a vital role in supporting the nursing staff and assuring competent decision making continues. The management team must recognize the nurses' behaviors and move to support these colleagues.

Adjustment of assignments, time away from the unit, and open forums for discussion can be quickly implemented. The nurse manager can consult organizational experts in the employee assistance program to provide a confidential opportunity for individual support. Interdisciplinary case reviews and educational updates should be planned to reinforce the strength of decision-making skills. Ongoing staff input should be solicited to assure all educational and emotional needs are met.

Time Constraints

Obstetric and pediatric settings are dynamic clinical settings. Movement of clients in and out of the units and their transition through stages of labor or illness to wellness is usual and expected; however, this constant change can be misinterpreted as constant crisis. While clients in these clinical areas regularly experience rapid and unexpected physiologic changes, the nurse must approach clinical decision making rationally and not with undo alarm.

Governmental agencies, insurance companies, and ongoing healthcare legislation have placed recommended timeframes and outcomes on medical conditions. As a result of these regulated constraints, the maternal child and pediatric nurse is forced to make difficult decisions about what information is essential to include in the teaching plan and what, although important, can be left out. Nurses must then be able to make timely and appropriate decisions to refer clients to professional colleagues such as social workers to provide maximum support for the client and families.

Scenario 17-5

Allison G, 12 months old, has been admitted to the general pediatric unit for the third time in six months. Her diagnosis is respiratory distress and reactive airway disease. Allison arrives on the pediatric unit receiving one liter of oxygen via a nasal cannula and an aminophylline drip infusing via a peripheral IV.

The nurse caring for Allison knows the targeted length of stay for reactive airway disease is three days. The nurse develops a teaching plan to begin immediately. The nurse enters the room to discuss Allison's treatment with her parents and finds Mrs. G, Allison's mom, crying. Mr. G describes his frustration with Allison's recurrent illness. Mrs. G describes feeling helpless when Allison has difficulty breathing at home. The nurse recognizes that Mr. and Mrs. G have a knowledge deficit about Allison's medical problem and how it is treated. Based on the assessment, the nurse makes a clinical decision to amend the teaching plan to include a review of the mechanism of Allison's respiratory distress and possible interventions available to Mr. and Mr. G at home.

The nurse identifies that Mr. and Mrs. G's concerns are valid and are important to share with the other members of the clinical team. After reviewing the case with the physician team, it is agreed that a home nebulizer would help maintain Allison's respiratory condition at home and limit frequent emergency visits. Mr. and Mrs. G are appropriate candidates for using a nebulizer at home, and they have verbalized a desire to do more at home to help Allison feel better. The nurse recognizes the opportunity to contact the social worker to coordinate the equipment required at home and provide additional support for Allison's parents. The collaborative interdisciplinary team agrees to request two skilled nursing visits at home to reinforce the in-hospital teaching and review the use of the nebulizer machine at home.

By the third day of Allison's hospitalization, she is breathing easily on room air and is successfully taking oral bronchodilators. The discharge plan includes the coordinated home care services as discussed earlier. Mr. and Mrs. G verbalize feeling ready to take Allison home and are looking forward to learning how to use the nebulizer machine as part of Allison's care at home.

The nurse in this situation was able to revise the anticipated plan of care to assure it met the individualized needs of the family. By strategically assessing the ongoing clinical situation and making appropriate referrals, a productive interdisciplinary team develops. While Allison's medical problem is likely to recur, Mr. and Mrs. G are now better prepared to actively participate in her ongoing care needs.

Focus on the Family

As demonstrated in the above clinical scenarios, the maternal child and pediatric settings focus on the clinical nursing care of an individual as a member of a family unit. The pregnant mother and her unborn child, and the parents of a sick child are examples of clients that receive nursing care. Maternal child and pediatric nurses must be able to make accurate determinations of which members comprise a particular family unit. The initial nursing history usually identifies family members closest to the client. Often, true family dynamics and relationships unfold as the plan of care is executed. Ongoing communication and assessment must direct the maternal child and pediatric nurse in determining the actual patient and family unit in need of nursing intervention and support.

LEGAL ISSUES

Maternal child and pediatric nurses make clinical decisions and implement the prescribed plan of care on behalf of their clients. Ongoing communication is paramount to sharing the clinical progress of the patient and assuring that important teaching is completed. In order to make accurate clinical decisions, the maternal child and pediatric nurse must know who has the legal authority to make decisions for the patient, provide consent for treatment, receive confidential clinical information about the patient, and take responsibility for the patient following hospitalization. Nursing practice decisions in the maternal child and pediatric settings require that systems exist to differentiate minors from adults, and identify the legal guardian for minor clients so that the plan of care is executed safely.

Scenario 17-6

A 17-year old primaperous mother, Ms. P, arrives in the delivery room in active labor. She has had minimal prenatal care and is estimated to be 28 weeks' gestation. Her mother brought her to the hospital and stays with her during the labor and delivery.

A 28-week male infant is born by spontaneous vaginal delivery. The baby's apgars are two at one minute and five at five minutes. Baby P requires intubation and ventilatory support. Baby P is also noted to have peeling skin on his hands and feet and an enlarged liver. The infant is transferred to the NICU with a diagnosis of extreme prematurity, respiratory distress, and presumed syphilis.

Ms. P recovers in the delivery room and is transferred to the postpartum unit. The neonatologists have met with her and her mother briefly and have explained about Baby P's critical condition and the diagnosis of presumed syphilis. The obstetrical team has also met with Ms. P and has begun her treatment for syphilis. The mom is discharged two days later and will be followed in the OB/GYN clinic on an outpatient basis.

Five days later an 18-year-old man comes to the NICU to visit his son Baby P. He asks the nurses why the baby is on a breathing machine and why the baby has a rash. In the obstetrical history, the mom denied knowing the identity of the father of the baby. The NICU nurse must decide what clinical information, if any, should be shared with this man. The nurse is wedged between questions about the baby's legal rights to confidentiality, the mother's rights as the known legal guardian, and the man's potential rights as the reported father of the infant. Additionally complicating the case is the hospital's obligation to report the incidence of contagious sexually transmitted diseases and this man's right to know about his own possible exposure.

These are all complex decisions that the nurse cannot make all at one time or alone. First, the nurse must make the decision about what to tell the anxious man at the sick infant's bedside. The nurse must act in the baby's best interest and tell the man that the mother had not given authorization to release information to anyone.

Caution must be used to defuse a potential hostile interaction. The nurse may decide to generalize that the infant is progressing well and recommend that the man contact the mom directly or contact the NICU social worker in the morning to receive appropriate information. The nurse must then follow through in the decision-making matrix, notify the physician of the situation, and recommend a social service consult if it had not been done already. The nurse must be sure that the decisions made are well communicated to the appropriate shift nursing leaders such as the charge nurse or supervisor. Finally, the nurse must be sure to clearly document the decisions and action in the medical record, as they are extremely pertinent to the infant's future clinical plan of care.

The traditional definition of a minor is an individual under the age of 18 (Rhodes, 1992). Legal exceptions and institutional interpretation to the standard definition can allow any of the following criteria to change the status of a less than 18-year-old client to adult:

- High school graduate
- Current or previous pregnancy
- Living away from parent/guardian and supporting self

Other criteria can allow a minor temporary adult status for purposes of direct access to necessary healthcare services:

- Testing for and treatment of sexually transmitted diseases
- Testing for and treatment of AIDS

Nurses must be well-informed about institutional policies guiding this determination to assure clients or their parents or legal guardians are informed, and consent has been correctly obtained, before treatment is administered.

Once the determination of minor status has been confirmed, clarification of the legal guardian must occur. Parents are the legal guardians of their child; however, when circumstances exist where the parents are not present or are unable to provide for the child's essential needs, another adult must take responsibility (Rhodes, 1992; Weiler and Helmes, 1992). A legal guardian is the legal recognition that one person has the authority to make personal, health, and financial decisions for another person (Weiler and Helmes, 1992). The exact specifics of obtaining guardianship vary from state to state; most, however, include filing a petition within the court system and attending a hearing with a judge presiding.

Once appointed legal guardian, this adult must assure that the child receives care, comfort, education, healthcare, and the opportunity to develop self-reliance and independence (Weiler and Helmes, 1992). Legal guardianship does not always require total financial responsibility for the child. The guardian, once appointed, is required to report to the court regularly to assure that the child's needs are being met.

Scenario 17-7

Weiler and Helms (1992) describe the following scenario. A large university tertiary care medical center performs bone marrow transplants on pediatric clients.

The bone marrow transplant donors are usually siblings of the dying clients. Nurses raised questions regarding the parents' ability to give rational informed consent in the best interest of their child who will be the bone marrow donor when the life of their other child is tentative and dependent on the procedure.

The issue of parental consent for two children participating in a bone marrow transplant was referred to the legal department. The hospital's lawyer, a previous pediatric nurse, drafted an extensive protocol. It included the requirement that parents facing this unusual situation must seek legal guardianship status through the typical court system prior to the hospital's accepting their consent for the procedure to be performed on the donor child. The goal was to help the parents separate the rights of both children. It also moved the perceived burden to judge the parents' ability to give informed consent in the best interest of each child from the hospital and its staff to the court issuing the guardianship.

The nurses acting in this situation were able to question the decision making process in clinical practice in their organization. The nurses recognized their limited role in the process of actually obtaining informed consent; however, they focused on the individual rights of their minor clients and questioned the decisions on which the healthcare team outlined the plan of care for each child involved. They sought consultation from organizational experts. The experts defined a new organizational policy that the nurses were able to utilize in their day-to-day practice in making decisions about the nursing plan of care.

Nurses face a variety of opportunities such as this to participate in some level of legal issues involving the maternal child and pediatric client. Nurses do not obtain informed consent but have the obligation to support clients in this decision-making process. Nurses do not determine legal guardianship or clarify minor and adult status; however, the nurse must raise questions and participate in this social assessment of the patient and family to assure the nursing plan of care is carried out properly and in the patient's best interest.

Busy shifts, clients who do not speak English, hostile family members, and inexperience are some of the barriers to the nurse's full participation in the legal aspects of patient care. Nurses need not know all of the answers, but must know how to access key sources for the information necessary for their clinical decision making. Individuals in clinical leadership roles, such as the charge nurse, head nurse, or shift supervisor, will be experienced in clarifying the organization's policies and procedures pertinent to legal issues. Additionally, nurses must be clear about the hospital's leadership hierarchy when complex situations cannot be solved by routine standing policies. Administrators, in nursing and other disciplines, often serve as the next step resources in the clarification of legal issues.

ETHICAL ISSUES

Berger and Williams-Brinkman (1992) define **ethics** as a branch of philosophy that attempts to discern which actions are right within a given situation. Ethics also deals with the principles that should promote action and the theories that justify these principles.

Ethical decisions are made based on the acceptable principles of right and wrong conduct within a group. As society changes, so do the issues affecting all of us as healthcare providers. In the specialties of maternal child and pediatric nursing, many issues that face all nurses may impact on the well-being of both mother and child (Buchanan and Cook, 1992). These issues include influences from advances in technology and society in general. Pharmacological and technological advances have given way to earlier genetic testing, controlling of preterm labor, and aggressive intervention of low birth weight and previable infants. Societal influences have brought about new ethical dilemmas. Nurses find themselves dealing with issues related to AIDS-infected infants, drug-addicted infants, and child abuse cases.

In order to act ethically, nurses must do what *ought to be done* in providing the best care possible for the client. There are times, however, when it is difficult to determine what ought to be done (Johnson, 1992).

The American Nurses' Association Code for Nurses, with its interpretive statements, and the ANA social policy statement provide a framework for making ethical decisions from the standpoint of the profession. The patient's bill of rights clarifies rights for clients in institutional settings and implies an obligation on the part of the nurse to assist the clients in securing them (Smith and Peterson, 1988).

Ethical and legal issues are often intertwined, making them difficult to separate. This dilemma occurs frequently in the obstetrical suite. Now that these multiple rights are being recognized and identified, questions arise as to the role of the government and the courts in resolving these issues. Nurses and healthcare institutions must develop mechanisms to resolve the conflicting rights that may be raised during a pregnancy. They must recognize their roles in clarifying these rights and issues and their responsibilities for seeking court intervention when necessary for resolution. The pregnant woman is no longer the sole patient (Feutz-Harter, 1991).

Scenario 17-8

Ms. Brown is a 21-year-old who is pregnant for the first time. She presents to the delivery room at 26 weeks' gestation in premature labor. This condition was precipitated by the use of cocaine for the past three days. After failure to control contractions by hydration, the physician places Ms. Brown on tocolytic therapy. After 24 hours of therapy, she complains of restlessness and fluttering in her chest. She has demanded that all medications be stopped. The patient is weaned off the medication but contractions have continued. Ms. Brown pulled out her intravenous access site and refused to have a new one inserted. Upon vaginal exam, cervical dilitation has occurred. Ms. Brown was notified that tocolytics were necessary to prevent the premature delivery and/or possible death of her infant. She refused to take tocolytics in any form. The physician has requested that Ms. Curry, who is assigned to Ms. Brown, reinsert the intravenous access site and tell Ms. Brown that unless she is given the tocolytics that she needs, her baby will die. Ms. Curry is uncomfortable with this approach.

Although ethicists have proposed several ethical decision-making models, Curtain's (1978) model encourages one to examine the relevant data, rights, duties, consequences, and ethical principles involved in the situation before determining a course of action. Curtain's (1978) ethical decision-making model consists of six steps.

The first step is to obtain the information necessary to understand and define the problem. Ms. Curry spends time developing a rapport with Ms. Brown. She asks open-ended questions that encourage continued discussion and information exchange. During this time she finds that Ms. Brown is single and has no permanent place to live. She also is told by Ms. Brown that she is not sure whether she wants this baby and feels the baby would be better off dead.

Ms. Curry needs to identify the ethical components involved in this situation. Ms. Curry must look at both the legal and ethical considerations, because these issues are often in conflict. The components involved in this situation are the right to refuse treatment and the preservation of life. Johnson (1992) notes that every competent adult has the right to refuse treatment for him- or herself and his or her children if informed about the condition and the consequences of his or her refusal. However, as healthcare workers, we are looked upon by society to perform our practice in a way that preserves and protects life. Not only must Ms. Curry look at these components prior to determining how to handle the situation with Ms. Brown but she must also take into account other individuals who may be involved in this process. The main decision-maker in this scenario is Ms. Brown but others are involved—including Ms. Curry, the physician, and other healthcare providers caring for Ms. Brown this evening.

The fourth step in ethical decision making is to explore all options. Ms. Curry must look at how she wishes to approach the situation with Ms. Brown. Does she allow Ms. Brown to refuse all treatment? Does she intimidate Ms. Brown in the hope of providing her the treatment the physician feels she needs? Does she negotiate, listen, and offer other supports to Ms. Brown to help her through the treatment?

Four key ethical principles need to be considered before an option can be selected. These include autonomy: the individual choice; nonmalificence: the duty to do no harm; beneficence: to do good and prevent harm; justice: to treat a patient fairly (Johnson, 1992).

In this scenario, Ms. Brown's right to individual choice is not the only thing that needs to be considered. Nonmalificence tells us that we should do no harm, and thus intimidation should not be an option. Beneficence requires that good is done and harm is prevented. Negotiating with Ms. Brown and enabling her to take the necessary medication is a viable option. Justice requires Ms. Curry to decide whether it is fair to allow Ms. Brown to refuse treatment and possibly have her infant or do what she can to encourage the use of tocolytics. At this point, Ms. Curry can choose an option. Her decision was to negotiate and provide the necessary support to Ms. Brown to encourage the continued participation in her prescribed treatment.

Ethical decisions will continue to confront nurses. The nursing profession, and especially its leaders, must become more active in the political arena to assure a voice in the laws that often position nurses in a situation causing a moral dilemma.

LEADERSHIP

The nurse manager is often placed in a position in which decisions that must be made are unfavorable and controversial. These situations arise most frequently when dealing in the areas of staffing, delegation, assignments, and resource allocation. How often have conflicts been seen among staff members because one individual was given an unfair assignment in relation to the rest? How often have complaints been heard about the number of people the manager assigned to the nursery on a specific day. How many times have nurses compared the support services available in the labor and delivery room to those on a postpartum unit? Decisions are made daily by nurse managers, and numerous factors must be considered in coming to a rational determination.

Many of these factors have been discussed in this chapter. They include upholding regulatory standards and hospital policies, abiding by legal requirements, maintaining clinical standards, and weighing pros and cons of ethical issues.

Scenario 17-9

Jane is the nurse manager for a 20-bed postpartum unit and the general nursery. She has just met with the director of nursing where they discussed the high costs of her unit supplies. Jane must determine a creative way of reducing costs without impeding quality care. Jane realizes that any decision on cost reduction measures will require staff buy-in. Her strategy is to present the situation to her staff and request assistance.

Before this can occur, there is some preliminary work that must be done. Jane requested a list of all the items stocked on her unit along with the pricing and current usage. She reviewed the list and highlighted those items that were not charged directly to the client.

At the unit staff meeting that week, Jane presented the problem she was facing to the staff. She petitioned for help in looking at current practices on the unit that could be changed without jeopardizing care. The highlighted items were to be addressed first if possible. Within one week of the meeting, the staff had come up with multiple rituals they performed that could be eliminated or reductions in allocation of items that could be made. One such reduction was to not give a tube of balmex ointment to each newborn in the nursery. This routine started years ago when lengths of stay were much longer. With the decrease of a stay to one to three days, it was felt this item was not needed for the newborn unless buttocks excoriation was present.

This nurse manager's strategy was to make the staff a partner in decision making. She acknowledged the staff's expertise and need for autonomy in the practice setting. Jane was able to find a means of cost savings and revamping of unit practices by her collaborative approach to problem solving. Nurses as professionals are beginning to take hold of the concept of autonomy. Over the years, shared governance and professional practice models have sprung up throughout the country. Nurses are finding great satisfaction in the opportunity to provide input into decisions affecting the practice setting. Along with the positives associated with autonomy, so too are negatives. Decision making can be frustrating, time-consuming, and con-

Scenario 17-10

Steven is a professional nurse who works on a 20-bed pediatric unit. He has been a nurse on this unit for three years. He has been assigned the role of charge nurse. Steven feels that the staff members on his unit always work together as a team. Whenever he has needed someone to help another staff member or take on additional responsibilities because of the unit need, he has always gotten his peers' and subordinates' support. Today, however, Jennifer, an LPN from the nursing pool, was sent to work on the pediatric unit. Steven reviewed the assignment and made adjustments to accommodate for the addition of the pool nurse. As the day progressed, one of Jennifer's five patients was discharged, and a second child was taken home against medical advice. An hour later, two of Steven's babies began to exhibit significant problems.

Steven found it impossible to care for his three patients effectively. After a quick evaluation of the staff assignments, Steven noticed that all of the staff, except Jennifer, had at least five patients.

Steven then requested that Jennifer take one of his patients. Jennifer felt this was unfair because she had three clients as did Steven. Jennifer accused Steven of dumping on her because she was from the pool.

Steven, at this point, needs to make a decision:

- Should he continue to care for all three of his clients knowing that he cannot meet all of their needs at this time?
- Should he request the assistance from another staff member on his unit and let Jennifer have only three patients?
- Should Steven continue to negotiate with Jennifer for assistance?

Steven must begin to make his decision by asking himself, "What are the risks if I continue caring for my three patients?" Steven realizes that he is unable to provide adequate care to all three of his infants and deal with the increasing problems present with two of the infants. Steven, realizing this, begins to survey alternatives. He begins to gather information about the level of care and number of clients still being cared for by other team members. He begins to weigh these alternatives. If Steven gives an additional patient to someone other than Jennifer, he knows it would be unfair. If he keeps all three patients, he is being unfair to his clients. If he gives the client to Jennifer, he knows he must be prepared to state his rationale for this decision.

Steven realizes that the best alternative is to give one of his patients to Jennifer. He notifies Jennifer of his decision, and after a short discussion, Jennifer accepts what has to be done. Steven utilized the conflict model of decision making to address this issue.

flict-generating. Nurse managers must begin to provide the maternal child and pediatric staff nurse with the education and knowledge necessary to utilize decision making strategies and models.

Although in this scenario the stages in this decision-making process occurred sequentially, this does not need to be the case. This model can be used in a variety of situations in which the maternal child and pediatric nurse is faced with a challenging opportunity or threat.

SUMMARY

Maternal child and pediatric health includes the family-centered care of pregnant and postpartum women and infants and growing children. Regulatory bodies, standards of practice, and ethical frameworks provide essential structure for the professional nurse's clinical decision making. Determination and support of clinical competency and decision-making skill support successful decision making. Nursing leaders in the maternal child and pediatric settings insure that resource allocation, both personnel and nonpersonnel, support that safe quality care is provided. With the proper resources available, professional nurses in these specialty settings will exercise expert decision making with continual improvement and quality care will be provided.

REFERENCES

Berger, K., & Williams-Brinkman, M. (1992). *Fundamentals of nursing: Collaborating for optimal health.* Norfolk, CT: Appleton & Lange.

Buchanan, S., & Cook, L. (1992). Nursing ethics committees: The time is now. *Nursing Management, 23*(8), 40–41.

Butts, B.J., & Witmer, D.M. (1992). New graduates: What does my manager expect? *Nursing Management, 23*(8), 46–48.

Curtain, L.L. (1978). A proposed model for critical ethical analysis. *Nursing Forum, 17*(1), 12–17.

Feutz-Harter, S.A. (1991). *Nursing and the law.* Eau Claire, WI: Professional Education Systems.

Johnson, S.A. (1992). Ethical dilemma: A patient refuses a life-saving cesarean. *The American Journal of Maternal/Child Nursing, 17*(5), 121–125.

Phillips, J. (1992). Regulating nursing practice. *Nursing Spectrum, 1*(18), 10–11.

Rhodes, A.M. (1992, July/August). Parental prerogatives: Newmark v. Williams. *Maternal Child Nursing, 17,* 197.

Smith, P.B., & Peterson, M.F. (1988). *Leadership, organizations, and culture: An event management model.* London: Sage Publications.

Strauss, S.S., & Clarke, B.A. (1992). Decision-making patterns in adolescent mothers. *Image, 24*(1), 69–74.

Weiler, K., & Helms, L.B. (1992, September/October). Who's in charge? Guardianships and children. *Maternal Child Nursing, 17,* 232–235.

Jeanne L. Held
Anne Robin Waldman

CHAPTER 18

Oncology Nursing

Nurses help make cancer livable.
—*Anonymous*

INTRODUCTION

The newly diagnosed cancer patient needs to make one of the most important decisions of his or her life—whether to accept treatment for this life-threatening disease. The result of this decision then influences the clinical decisions made by the nurse during the course of treatment. The patient's decision is influenced by many factors. This chapter will address how the factors crucial to the decision-making process affect the patient during the course of the illness.

The patient's initial decision regarding treatment is the keystone for determining the direction of nursing care. While the patient is the one who makes the ultimate decision whether to accept aggressive, potentially curative treatment or nonaggressive, palliative treatment, it is the healthcare team that is instrumental in assisting in this decision-making process. The nurse can help empower the patient to make this decision by ascertaining the patient's level of knowledge, by determining what additional information needs to be provided by the physician, by reinforcing information provided by the physician, and by helping the patient coordinate his or her thoughts. The patient should be encouraged to include the family or significant others in this process.

At the time of diagnosis, the patient has been subject to anxiety, fear, concern about the future, the possible treatment regimen, and facing his own mortality, possibly for the first time. These stressors interfere with the patient's ability to ask pertinent questions, make decisions, and communicate his or her concerns in an appropriate manner. The nurse can be instrumental in providing the patient with support by being available to listen nonjudgmentally to fears and concerns and by guiding the patient through this paralyzing period of time.

CRUCIAL FACTORS

We have identified six factors crucial to the decision-making process:

- Histologic category
- Stage of the disease
- Patient's physiological status
- Attending physician's personal preference regarding treatment regimens
- Patient's individual preference regarding treatment

Disease Process

The histologic category and stage of the disease are two of the major determinants of the type of treatment the patient will receive. Certain cell types of localized tumors are best treated with surgery. For example, many patients with an early diagnosis of colon cancer will be cured by surgical resection alone because the disease is still confined to the colon. Other types of localized cancers that are usually resectable are renal cell, breast, prostate, gastric, and esophageal. On the other hand, many newly diagnosed patients with cancer of the pancreas present with such far-advanced disease that surgery is not a treatment option. Any patient that presents with metastatic disease is usually not a candidate for curative surgical resection.

Histologic types that are not amenable to surgical management are best treated with chemotherapy, radiation therapy, or a combination of both. For example, hematological malignancies are all treated with these modalities. Other malignancies treated in this manner include any metastatic disease, patients receiving adjuvant treatment for a solid tumor, and for palliation of symptoms such as pain or bleeding.

The patient's physiologic status will influence the physician's decision-making process. Cardiac, pulmonary, and renal status may preclude certain surgical procedures and antineoplastic agents. Physiologic status usually does not preclude treatment with radiation therapy. Nonambulatory patients and those with poor nutrition, as reflected by a low serum albumin, will usually do poorly with chemotherapy (Cohen, MaKuch, Johnston-Early, Ihde, Bunn, Fossieck, and Minna, 1981). They may also experience significant side effects from radiation therapy, such as excessive fatigue and weight loss. No matter what the physiologic status, the patient with potentially curable malignancies such as acute leukemia and the aggressive lymphomas will still be offered aggressive therapy.

Physician's Philosophy

The physician will present the patient with a treatment plan. This plan will include a discussion of the disease process, the treatment options, and the option the physician feels is best for the patient. While most patients will agree to the physician's recommendations, there are occasional patients who feel that the treatment-associated side effects are unacceptable. Reasons cited include religion, cultural background, previous experience with cancer causing a fear of treatment and its side effects, influence from family or significant others, a lack of belief in the healthcare system, and financial issues (Disch and McEvoy, 1991). The patient may make an immediate decision to accept treatment or choose to take time to consider the options. Depending upon the growth rate of the tumor this may or may not make a difference. For example, a patient with acute leukemia only has a day or two to make this decision, whereas someone with a breast lump or colon mass can delay the decision-making process by a week or even several weeks without it making a difference in the treatment process. A patient may be offered an experimental protocol or standard treatment for his disease process, but may choose the latter, because experimental protocols usually require more frequent office visits and diagnostic evaluations that the patient believes will interfere with his or her usual lifestyle. Because of personal needs for the patient's survival, families may exert undue influence in the decision-making process, thereby forcing the patient to accept treatment that he or she may otherwise have refused. Here, the nurse can be most helpful by spending time with the patient explaining the details of both options, clarifying information, and offering emotional support.

Another focus of decision making rests with the physician's individual preference regarding treatment. This surrounds the issues of quality of life versus quantity of life. As a result, a patient with poor physiological status may be influenced to accept treatment that he or she otherwise may not have desired or accepted. These patients may receive treatment for a disease with a poor response rate and potentially severe life-threatening side effects. At the other end of the spectrum, there are primary care physicians who believe that the available treatments for certain malignancies are futile. Therefore, the patient is denied treatment.

Patient's Preferences

The patient's geographical location and financial circumstances may influence treatment availability. For example, the patient may be able to afford to travel miles to a medical facility that is able to provide the needed treatment, or, on the other hand, he may live in close proximity to a treatment center but not be able to afford treatment.

Scenario 18-1

Mr. C. was a newly diagnosed 70-year-old retired avid golfer with asymptomatic, stage 2 large cell lymphoma. The disease involved only one side of the diaphragm. Mr. C's physician presented multiple treatment options to Mr. C. These treatments included three options:

- An eight-drug regimen requiring frequent trips to the physician's office, frequent lab work, and a high number of severe side effects, including bone marrow depression, alopecia, nausea, vomiting, diarrhea, mouth ulcers, and peripheral neuropathy

- A standard treatment with four drugs administered one day per week for a minimum of six months with less severe side effects than the eight-drug option
- Another four-drug regime given one time per week for three weeks, this cycle repeated for six cycles with even fewer side effects

The physician recommended the most aggressive regime, the eight-drug regimen with toxic side effects. The physician's rationale for this option was based on the histology of the disease. This option offered the greatest probability for a cure. The nurse's role in this situation was to discuss the treatment options with the patient to assure understanding of the risks and advantages and then to support the patient in his decision. In this situation, the patient preferred the option that would least interfere with his retired lifestyle and involvement in daily golfing activities.

DECISION MAKING DURING THE TREATMENT PROCESS

Antineoplastic therapy is administered in cycles, most of which range from three to six weeks in length to allow for recovery from side effects such as bone marrow depression and mucositis. The patient entering treatment with a good physiological status generally will tolerate the planned treatment and its side effects better than the patient entering treatment with a poor physiological status. Occasionally, the patient may find that the toxicities of therapy are intolerable and outweigh the potential benefits provided by ongoing treatment. At this time the patient may require hospitalization, intravenous fluids, antibiotics, and other supportive therapies. The patient may determine that this poor quality of life and the time spent away from home and family is not acceptable and drop out of treatment. For patients who make this decision, hospice may be an appropriate option.

There are patients who may initially respond to treatment and then fail to achieve a durable response, and there are those who never respond at all. Patients with chemosensitive tumors may be offered alternate regimens; however, these may be no more effective than the original regimen. The patient may decide that the toxicities of treatment are worse than the symptoms of the disease and opt for palliative measures. The nurse can be instrumental in guiding the patient through this crisis. All the patient's hopes and dreams for a cure, if not at least prolonged survival, are dashed, and it usually is the nurse whose interventions help the patient adapt to the realities of the disease. The nurse can help the patient refocus his or her hopes for cure into those for quality of life through palliation. The nurse can present the hospice concept to the patient and family as one means of achieving this goal.

Scenario 18-2

Twin brothers, Mr. W.T. and Mr. A.T., were age 38, both married, and each had two small children under the age of 10. Both men were in good health until they noticed some weight loss over a period of six months. Mr. W.T. developed some midabdominal pain, which sent him to the doctor, while Mr. A.T. noticed that his eyes were yellow and had generalized pruritis. These unfortunate twins underwent a complete staging workup and were diagnosed with cancer of the pancreas with liver metastases. Both men were advised that there was no curative treatment for this disease, but each was offered palliative treatment with chemotherapy or hospice care. Side effects of chemotherapy were discussed and included diarrhea, mucositis, bone marrow depression, fatigue, and fever. Mr. A.T. opted to accept chemotherapy, with the hope that he would achieve a remission and have prolonged survival with quality in his last few days of life. Chemotherapy involved daily intravenous infusions and subcutaneous injections of medications for one week. Mr. W.T. chose hospice care in the home with his wife and family as caregivers with pain management and relief of symptoms. He died comfortably at home four months later surrounded by his loving family. After three weeks of chemotherapy, Mr. A.T. developed profuse, watery diarrhea with dehydration and hypokalemia requiring hospitalization for hydration and potassium repletion. While hospitalized, Mr. A.T. developed a massive pulmonary embolus and died immediately.

In this scenario, both patients had the same outcome, death, with approximately the same longevity regardless of the treatment option chosen. Thus, the patient hoping for an increased length of survival and willing to undergo the increased toxic side effects did not receive any extra benefits. Both patients were supported in the decision-making process to choose the treatment option with which they felt most comfortable.

SUMMARY

Nursing interventions are crucial to the patient's decision-making process. Factors that influence patient and physician decision making have been discussed. Nurses provide information and support to patients and their families during these difficult periods.

The diagnosis of cancer creates a devastating, emotional dilemma for patients and families. The very fabric and core of the family is destroyed as roles change and stress mounts. The anxiety associated with the word "cancer" and its ramifications produces barriers to learning and understanding the diagnosis, disease process, treatment options, and prognosis. The nurse listens, clarifies, confirms, and validates the patient's perceptions of the disease and the outcomes. Without nursing support and nonjudgmental listening, some patients and families would not be able to make decisions related to treatment options.

REFERENCES

Cohen, M.H., MaKuch, R., Johnston-Early, A., Ihde, D.C., Bunn, P.A., Jr., Fossieck, B.E., Jr., and Minna, J.D. (1981). Laboratory parameters as an alternative to performance status in prognostic stratification of patients with small cell lung cancer. *Cancer Treatment Report, 65*, 187–195.

Disch, J., & McEvoy, M.D. (1991). Factors affecting health behavior. In S.L. Groenwald, M.H. Frogge, M. Goodman, & C.H. Yarboro (Eds.), *Cancer nursing,* 2nd edition (pp. 91–101). Boston: Jones & Bartlett.

Gary E. Bilski

CHAPTER 19

The Psychiatric Setting

When, against one's will, one is high-pressured into making a hurried decision, the best answer is always "No," because "No" is more easily changed to "Yes" than "Yes" is changed to "No."

—*Charles E. Nielsen (cited in Safire & Safir, 1990).*

INTRODUCTION

Defined simply, decisions are choices among alternatives. In reality, however, decisions involve much more than this. Some decisions are simple; others can be quite complex and complicated. Decisions represent the pathway by which we move from where we are now to where we will be at some future point. Clearly, different choices of actions produce different results. It is through our decision-making abilities that we can take charge and not be, as above, creatures of circumstance. Consequently, the significance of making decisions is evident.

Decision making has been described as a process (Anderson, 1988). First, a problem requiring a solution is identified. Next, alternative choices of action are identified, and the implications of implementing these choices are evaluated. The next step involves selecting the alternative that will produce the desired or optimal result. Following selection, the alternative is implemented, and the effectiveness of the choice is evaluated.

The importance of decision making has been emphasized, and the implications of decision making in a variety of clinical settings have been reviewed. The unique environment of each specialty, and the unique factors affecting the nature of the nurses' work in each clinical specialty setting influences the decision-making process.

Nursing is a science that concerns itself with the quality of life and its relationship to health (Wilson and Kneisl, 1992). In the psychiatric/mental health setting, nurses' concerns are focused on the individual's biopsychosocial health with increased emphasis on the client's feelings, his or her sense of identity, his or her sense of self-worth and personal integrity, his or her ability to express him- or herself, and his or her ability to achieve self-fulfillment. Psychiatric/mental health nursing is an interpersonal process. The primary aim of nursing in this setting is to promote and maintain behavior that encourages integrated functioning. Psychiatric/mental health nursing has been defined by the American Nurses Association (1976) as a specialized area of nursing practice based on scientific theories of human behavior and the art of purposeful use of self. Nursing in this specialty involves interventions that prevent and correct mental disorders and their sequelae and promote optimal mental health for individual members of society (American Nurses Association, 1976).

DECISION INFLUENCERS IN THE PSYCHIATRIC SETTING

In the psychiatric/mental health setting, many decisions are made that are relatively simple, and uninvolved. Other decisions are more complicated and involve more detailed analysis of choices and consequences. At times, the decisions nurses must make in the psychiatric setting allow time to closely examine choices; other decisions must be made more immediately. The opportunity to examine alternatives closely may not be available, and the nurse will be required to act quickly. The decisions made by the nurse in the psychiatric setting may be independent actions. The decision-making process, however, may require input from other nurses, other members of the healthcare team, and the recipients of nursing service.

Multiple Customers

In this setting the nurse has multiple customers. As in all other areas of nursing, the individual and family serve as the primary customers. The community may also be a consumer of nursing services in the psychiatric/mental health setting. In a psychiatric setting, nurses function as members of interdisciplinary treatment teams. Their work involves interrelations with other healthcare providers—physicians, psychologists, social workers, and allied health professionals. These individuals also represent customers of nursing service. Finally, nurses must recognize that their work increasingly involves relationships with representatives from those institutions and organizations that provide payment for clients' treatment. Their role as consumers of nursing service is becoming increasingly more evident and important.

Note for example the impact that managed care has had on healthcare practice. Case managers, representing managed care companies, are able to very strongly and actively influence the direction of patient care. More and more frequently, providers are coming to the realization that issues related to treatment modalities, level of care provided, as well as length of service or treatment, must involve input from those representatives. Clearly, this will impact on decision making by the nurse in the psychiatric setting.

Individuality

An individual's ability to make decisions is affected by many factors. One knows from experience that individuals can often be presented with the same information and use the same model for analysis of problems, and still reach independent and different decisions. The unique attributes of the individual affect the decision-making process. Smith, Carrol, Kefalas, and Watson (1980) have emphasized the unique attributes of the individual in decision making. "People make decisions by perceiving and evaluating; they perceive by sensation and intuition and they evaluate the perception by thinking and feeling." Individuals think and perceive differently, therefore they can, and do, arrive at different conclusions based upon individual differences that affect their perception and ability to evaluate information.

Value System

Marquis and Huston (1987) have identified four factors that impact on and influence nurses' decision making. Decision making is affected by, and can be limited by, the individual's value system. Our values influence how we see things. Our ability to gather and process information is affected by our belief system. Decision making involves making choices and judgments. Very often these can be value judgments. Personal values influence our perception and impact on our ability to make choices. Our beliefs very often tell us what is important and unimportant, what is significant and what is insignificant. In some situations, a range of choices may be restricted by the individual's belief system.

Scenario 19-1

Mary is a 33-year-old married female, mother of three small children. Mary has been married for twelve years. She presents to the assessment center with a history of depressed mood, and feelings of hopelessness and helplessness for the past several months. She describes sleep disturbances, and reports weight loss of approximately fifteen pounds during this time. Upon gathering information, the nurse learns that Mary has been feeling very unfulfilled with her marital relationship for the past several years. She describes feeling trapped, and states that getting married was "my biggest mistake." With further probing, the nurse questions if Mary has considered leaving the marriage. Emphatically, Mary states that she could never do this. She further describes an upbringing in a strict religious home that did not recognize divorce as an option. In this situation, it can be seen that the range of choices to solving problems has been restricted by the individual's belief system.

Experience

Life experiences have also been identified as influencing an individual's decision-making abilities (Marquis and Huston, 1987). Individuals carry forth their experiences from the past as they act on information in the present. Experiences broaden an individual's background, and open avenues for a variety of perceptions and choices in the decision-making process.

Individual preference and risk has also been identified as a key factor that affects the ability to make decisions (Marquis and Huston, 1987). Choices among alternatives may involve perceptions of risk by the individual. The degree to which an individual takes risks will limit the array of choices available.

In the above example, Mary's choices are limited by her belief system. Her choices in decision making are further limited by her willingness to take risks. Specifically, she "risks" questioning her own belief system, and "risks" the impact a decision may have on those who influenced her belief system.

Thinking Skills

Finally, thinking skills differ among individuals and impact on the decision-making process (Marquis and Huston, 1987). As all individuals are unique, thinking skills vary among individuals. Research has pointed out that individuals differ in their abilities to use systematic analysis and intuition in their decision-making patterns. The use of systematic analysis and/or intuition will influence perception of information and choices of alternatives as individuals move through the decision-making steps.

Successful decision making by nursing in the psychiatric mental health setting requires the ability to accurately identify problems, to carefully examine and select choices, and to implement those choices in a timely manner. Nurses must be fully aware of who their customers are as they make decisions. As most individuals are unique, most decisions in the psychiatric setting are unique. Consequently, no single decision-making model can be universally applied to decision making in this setting.

Interpersonal Skills

Decision making in the psychiatric setting will require the employment of well-developed interpersonal skills (Stuart and Sundeen, 1983). The decision-making process for nurses in the psychiatric setting requires the ability to effectively facilitate communication. The nurse must be able to deliver clear messages, and must be an effective listener. The nurse will be faced with aberrant or unusual behaviors, and must be able to demonstrate understanding and acceptance, and remain non-judgmental. Negotiation and conflict resolution skills will be required. In addition, the nurse will be required to influence others through positive role modeling in the decision-making process. Finally, a keen awareness of self is essential as decision making is employed in the psychiatric setting.

Personal Characteristics

In addition to interpersonal skills, Marquis and Huston (1987) have identified personal characteristics that enhance the decision-making process and aid in making successful decisions. Courage is required, as decision making will often involve taking risks. Since decisions require a focus on situations and the implications of those situations, sensitivity is an important characteristic. Decision making also requires the ability to implement solutions. Energy and desire to make things happen is required. Last, decision making is a problem-solving process. Because this often requires new ways of looking at the problem, as well as solutions, creativity is an essential characteristic.

Effective decision making requires a knowledge of the nature of the work and an understanding of the customers served. Nurses must be aware of the unique factors that influence their decision-making abilities. The nurse will rely on interpersonal skills and the development of essential personal characteristics to effectively make decisions. Psychiatric nursing has many unique factors that impact on decision making. It is essential to understand the implications of those factors as decision making is employed in the clinical setting.

CLINICAL DECISION MAKING

Before any decision can be reached, problems must be clearly identified. In the clinical setting, the psychiatric nurse must first focus attention on clearly defining the problem. It is important that this point be fully understood. The best solution for a poorly defined problem is no more effective than the wrong solution for a clearly defined problem. Drucker (1967) has identified that in any decision-making process, problems can be classified into general categories: unique problems—those that are one-time events, recurring problems—problems that occur routinely, and unique problems that become recurring. Nurses in the psychiatric clinical setting will be faced with similar categories of problems. The nature of the problem—unique or recurring—can influence further steps in the decision-making process, so it is important that nurses clearly identify problems.

Problem Identification

Kepner and Tregoe (1965) have identified a matrix that has useful applications for nurses in the problem identification step of the clinical decision-making process. The matrix involves analysis of the problem in three areas—problem symptoms, what the problem is, and what the problem isn't. In terms of problem symptoms, the problem should be examined by describing the nature of the problem, when symptoms occurred, where symptoms occurred, the extent of the symptoms, and any changes that have occurred. In addition to examining and attempting to identify what the problem is, an analysis should be made of what the problem is not. Questions that should be evaluated in the problem identification process should include: Have the symptoms occurred at any other time? Have the symptoms occurred anywhere else? Have symptoms not occurred when they should have? For the psychiatric nurse, using this procedure matrix can help focus the problem, based on when and how problem symptoms do and do not occur, as well as examine what changes may have led to the problem. During a comprehensive psychosocial assessment with a client, the nurse is in an ideal position to apply this process.

The problem identification step should also include an examination of the priority of the problems. Anderson (1988) describes a "to-do" list that should be utilized in the problem identification stage of the decision-making process. Problems should be identified and prioritized by examining the consequences of the problem (what are its effects?), the impact of the problem on the total organization (will it create a series of problems if not resolved?), time pressures and urgency (how much time is required to solve this problem and is that time available?), best utilization of the decisionmaker's time (does this represent the greatest return for effort), and lifespan of the problem (will this problem resolve itself without intervention?).

The usefulness of this analysis of problem identification and prioritization can be seen by examining some commonplace problems that occur on most inpatient psychiatric units. As identified earlier, nurses in the psychiatric setting provide care to individuals that present with disorders of mood, disorders of behavior, and disorders of thinking. At any given time on the inpatient setting, the nurse can be presented with a variety of "problem symptoms."

Scenario 19-2

David, a nurse providing care to patients on a psychiatric unit, is confronted simultaneously with several immediate client needs. Sean is a 32-year-old male who is withdrawn and isolating himself. Lisa is an 18-year-old female who is displaying unusual behavior and appears to be responding to internal stimuli. Mark is a 25-year-old male demonstrating aggressive behavior, and threatening to strike out at others. David recognizes that the withdrawn client, Sean, does not present an urgent need, and that the individual responding to internal stimuli needs only be observed, as the behavior has been brief and self-limiting. However, if David does not intervene with Mark, demonstrating the aggressive behavior, the problem itself may intensify and cause significant disruptions and additional problems, such as acting out in other individuals, within the milieu.

Clinical decision making in the psychiatric setting requires a thorough understanding of the client's unique state, taking into account individual psychological states as well as social factors. In the decision-making process, the first step involves identification of a problem requiring solution. Problem identification can present a stumbling block to the nurse in this clinical setting. Nursing actions and clinical decision making can be best implemented when there is mutual agreement between the caregiver and client. Often in the psychiatric setting, the nurse is confronted with situations in which there is not mutual agreement or identification of problems.

Scenario 19-3

John, a 29-year-old married male, had been brought to the hospital last evening by his wife. Over the course of the past week, John has shown increased energy levels and has had a progressively decreasing need for sleep. His increased energy level has resulted in John embarking on several home renovation projects simultaneously. Although he has very limited carpentry skills, John has expressed to his wife that he believes he can completely renovate their home by himself. His "projects" have been quite costly, and John has continued despite pleas by his wife to stop. Over the two days prior to admission, John has slept only brief periods. He has been up throughout the night and his hammering and loud antics have been disruptive to not only his family, but neighbors as well. In addition, he has become increasingly irritable. He denies that anything is wrong, and has expressed the belief that the neighbors are plotting against him, because he can "out-do" them in home improvement abilities. He also has stated that he knows that he really owns the neighborhood, and will evict the neighbors if their complaints continue. As John's wife pleaded with him to seek help, his irritability focused on her and he attempted to strike her. His admission to the hospital occurred following his wife's petition for an involuntary commitment.

In the psychiatric setting, the nurse is frequently faced with providing care to clients who have impaired judgment. Disorders of thinking and disorders of mood can seriously impair reality testing. Their ability to make rational choices can be faulty. Often, the disturbance of thought or mood results in the individuals' inability to recognize problems. It has been estimated that roughly 50 percent of individuals entering psychiatric hospitals are originally admitted on an involuntary basis (Stuart and Sundeen, 1983). This indicates an inability of the individual to recognize the need for treatment. Consequently, a common obstacle the psychiatric nurse encounters in decision making is working with clients who have divergent views of their problems.

Problem Identification and Sociocultural Factors

Problem identification is also influenced significantly by an individual's cultural background. Nurses must be aware not only of an individuals psychological state, but also of the sociological or sociocultural factors involved. This will impact on decision making. The following represents an example of how sociocultural factors affect problem identification in the decision-making process.

Wilson and Kneisl (1992) stress the importance of recognizing the clients' sociocultural heritage in providing clinical services. The importance is clearly seen in problem identification. In the psychiatric setting, the nurse must recognize that individuals behave according to unwritten customs and traditions. Failure to recognize these will impede the nurse in effective problem identification in the clinical decision-making process.

Scenario 19-4

Julia, an experienced oncology nurse, has requested consultation from the psychiatric clinical nurse specialist in her work with a patient and family under her care. The patient and family arrived from Puerto Rico about one year ago. The family does speak and understand English, but their ability to communicate is limited. Julia has become aware in rendering care to her patient that the patient's 22-year-old son has been very distraught with his mother's deteriorating condition. Julia has frequently observed the son weeping, and has often heard him talking to someone in the room when no other person was there. Julia's concerns about the son's mental health intensified after she observed the son one day alone in the room crying and talking aloud to someone. When Julia approached him and asked who he was speaking to, the son responded that he was talking with his father. Julia knew from the health history that the father had died several years ago. She requested the assistance of the psychiatric clinical nurse specialist, because she believed that the son might be hallucinating. After meeting with the patient's son, the clinical nurse specialist reassured Julia that the son's behavior was not abnormal. While he was clearly and appropriately depressed about his mother's condition, he was not experiencing hallucinations. The practice of speaking to the dead is an acceptable and commonplace activity in the Puerto Rican culture.

Identifying Alternatives

Once problems have been clearly identified, the next step in the decision-making process involves generating and examining alternatives. As stated earlier, decisions represent choices; the very definition of a decision implies that there must be at least two choices. Choices then are the pathway by which we move from where we are now to where want to be. It is essential for the decisionmaker to have a clear goal in mind when examining and choosing among alternatives. This point is illustrated in the following dialogue from Lewis Carroll's (1932) *Alice in Wonderland,*

Alice: Cheshire Cat, would you tell me, please, which way I ought to walk from here?

Cat: That depends a good deal on where you want to get to.

Alice: I don't care where.

Cat: Then it doesn't matter which way you walk.

To make an effective decision, it is essential to have an understanding of what outcome the clinician wishes to achieve. Outcomes represent the standard against which alternatives are evaluated and compared. For the nurse in the psychiatric setting, outcomes can be derived from the treatment planning process, from the theoretical knowledge base of the discipline, or from standards generated by professional organizations. In addition, outcomes may be influenced by clearly defined policies and procedures developed by the healthcare organization. In other cases, standards or outcomes can be influenced by external regulating organizations. Increasingly, third-party payers, especially managed care organizations, are influencing providers by defining expected outcomes.

Criteria for Selecting Alternatives

In some situations, the identification of alternative solutions may be dictated for the nurse in the psychiatric setting. Most times, however, problems are identified in which clearly defined alternatives are not that apparent. In choosing among alternatives to achieve a desired outcome, Kepner and Tregoe (1965) recommend that alternatives be evaluated using must and want criteria. *Must criteria* are those objectives that have to be satisfied before the alternative is accepted. *Want criteria* represent objectives that are desirable, but not necessary in achieving the desired outcome. In evaluating alternatives, if the must criteria do not exist, that alternative can be discarded immediately.

Kepner and Tregoe's want and must criteria can be useful to the psychiatric nurse in clinical decision making. This model forces the nurse to think through what a good solution to a problem might look like. It can also have an effect of limiting the array of alternatives to be evaluated. The usefulness of setting criteria for alternatives can be seen in the following clinical case study.

Scenario 19-5

Tim, a robust 25-year-old male, was admitted to the psychiatric hospital approximately three days ago for major depression. Several months ago, due to the failing economy, he lost his job as a construction worker, and has since then been unable to find work. Tim had always been a physically active individual. Tim identified that the physical demands of his job often helped him "work off" stress. He has had difficulty coping with inactivity since he lost his job. Additionally, his loss of employment has created financial hardship for his family. Tim's wife has recently assumed full-time employment. Tim subsequently has taken full responsibility for managing their home, and caring for the couple's 2-year-old child. Tim views himself as a failure, and has had considerable difficulty accepting the change in roles in the household. He has been increasingly restless and irritable, and has experienced difficulty sleeping. In his attempts to cope with uncomfortable feelings, Tim has been abusing alcohol. His irritability increased, and this in turn increased the tension within the marital relationship. Finally, after much persuasion by his wife, Tim sought professional help and accepted the recommendation of hospitalization.

During the first two days of hospitalization, Tim was withdrawn and isolated himself from others. He attended therapy sessions, and appeared to be actively listening to others, but disclosed little of himself. During his third hospitalization day, Tim appeared increasingly irritable and anxious. He could not tolerate group activities on this day, and stormed out of this session. Tim's behavior was frightening to some of the patients, and was alarming to staff as well. An immediate solution was required when Tim approached a nurse stating "You need to do something. I feel like I'm going to explode."

In this situation, the nurse recognized that alternatives must include the following objectives:

- Maintaining safety for both Tim and other patients
- Promoting a sense of increased control within Tim

Want criteria for this situation included:

- Promoting an opportunity for Tim to expend energy
- Assisting Tim in developing more effective coping skills

While solutions to use seclusion or to consult with the psychiatrist for increased medications were recommended by other staff, the nurse chose to have Tim spend individual time with the recreational therapist in the fitness room engaging in activities to "work off" his stress while the therapist helped him identify some ways to more effectively cope with his uncomfortable feelings of anxiety and irritability.

While alternative courses are being evaluated, it is essential to examine if the choices will achieve the desired outcome and meet established criteria. It is also essential that alternatives be examined in terms of what other consequences may occur. This is particularly important for nurses in the psychiatric setting since the significance of group and collective behavior impacts on the milieu. While most times, nurses in the psychiatric setting are aware of how the behavior of one patient can influence others, nurses are often less attentive to how their interventions with one patient can impact on the group collectively. For example, staff's limit setting on inappropriate behavior often is viewed by other patients as punitive and/or restrictive. This often promotes anger in other patients.

Implementation of Selected Alternatives

Once alternatives have been identified and criteria for successful solution applied to the problem, the next phase of the decision-making process involves implementation of the selected alternative. A common mistake made by many effective decisionmakers is to assume that implementation automatically follows selection of an alternative. Implementation involves seeing the chosen course of action through to its completion. The selected alternative may be a single action, or a series of actions that involves several sequential steps. The decision may be implemented by the person making the decision. In many cases, however, the decision may be delegated to others for implementation. The nurse, in the psychiatric setting, typically works as a part of a multidisciplinary team. Other healthcare providers, physicians, psychologists, social workers, and allied therapists, are integrally involved in patient care. For the nurse in the psychiatric setting, decision making is a collaborative process. It is essential that decisions be effectively communicated to all other healthcare providers involved in patient care. If the decision is not clearly communicated to others, the risk of the decision's failing increases.

Evaluation

The decision-making process does not end with implementation of the chosen course of action. Not all decisions are effective, and certainly the possibility exists that the chosen course of action will not work. For this reason, it is essential that the effectiveness of the decision be evaluated and monitored. Most times, this stage of the decision-making process simply involves observing if the actions have achieved the desired results.

For example, a nurse working with an individual experiencing panic states may choose to teach the client ways of managing anxiety through relaxation/stress reduction techniques. To monitor the effectiveness of this choice, the nurse should evaluate whether the individual is able to successfully use the technique during a future attack and successfully manage the symptoms.

In other situations, monitoring the effectiveness of the decision can be more involved. Monitoring of results can be a time-consuming process, and very often can be overlooked. Particularly for nurses, when faced with the need to continuously identify problems and make decisions in the clinical setting, monitoring the effectiveness of actions often is overlooked.

PITFALLS

Clinical decision making in psychiatric nursing has been presented as a series of steps that nurses, as decisionmakers, go through from beginning to end, involving problem identification, choosing among alternatives, and implementing the best possible solution. In reality, the process is not always that orderly and controlled. Anderson (1988) has identified the following limitations to application of the decision-making process. Many times the problem is not recognized. In the work setting where there is significant stimulation, as exists in most healthcare settings, an overload can occur that limits an individual's ability to see all problems clearly. Secondly, all information about the problem may be unavailable, or too difficult to obtain. Third, decisions often have to be reached immediately and the opportunity to fully explore all options doesn't exist. Often a quick decision is needed, not necessarily the best decision. Finally, individuals responsible for making decisions don't always have all the alternatives. Limitations in knowledge base and experience can and do restrict the nurses' ability to fully identify all alternatives.

Marquis and Huston (1987) have identified points of vulnerability in the decision-making process. Critical elements exist that can result in a poor quality decision. First, lack of a clear objective can lead to faulty decision making. Remember earlier Alice and the Cheshire Cat. Not knowing the destination makes it difficult to choose the correct route. Faulty data gathering impedes effective decision making. It is essential that the decisionmaker develop the ability to effectively obtain and process information. Lack of self-awareness also presents an obstacle to successful clinical decision making. One's decisions are influenced by individual values, therefore, to be effective in decision making, one must have a solid understanding of one's own value system. Failure to generate and examine all potential alternatives will also impede effective decision making. Finally, an inability to choose, or an inability to act on choices, will prohibit successful decision making. Earlier, it was identified that decision making involves risk taking. If an individual is unwilling to make choices, decision making cannot be effective.

SUMMARY

Decisions are the pathways by which we take charge of our circumstances. In the psychiatric setting, clinical decision making represents a vehicle by which the nurse can influence behavior to promote integrated functioning. Decision making in this setting is influenced by multiple customers. Additionally, individuality and value systems within the decisionmaker and experiences of the person making the decision will influence both the process and the outcome. Thinking skills and interpersonal skills will also have significant impact on decision making.

As nurses implement the decision-making process, they must be aware of pitfalls in the process. The process may at times not be orderly, and nurses must be able to use the decision-making process with limited information. Additionally, nurses should be aware of their own limitations and abilities. To effectively map out the right route, the nurse must know where to go and what is needed to get there.

REFERENCES

American Nurses Association, (1976) *Division on psychiatric and mental health nursing practice: Statement on psychiatric and mental health nursing practice.* Kansas City, MO: Author.

Anderson, C.R. (1988). *Building decision skills: Management skills, functions, and organization performance,* second edition, Boston: Allyn and Bacon.

Carroll, L. (1932). *Alice in wonderland,* adapted for the stage by Eva Le Gallienne and Florida Friebas, New York: Samuel French.

Drucker, P.F. (1967, Jan./Feb.). The effective decision. *Harvard Business Review* 92–98.

Kepner, C.H., & Tregoe, B.B. (1965). *The rational manager.* New York: McGraw-Hill.

Marquis, B.L., & Huston, C.J. (1987). *Management decision making for nurses.* Philadelphia: J.B. Lippincott Company.

Safire, W., & Safir, L. (1990). *Leadership.* New York: Simon & Schuster.

Smith, H.R., Carrol, A.B., Kefalas, A.G., & Watson, H.F. (1980). *Management: Making organizations perform.* New York, NY: Macmillian.

Stuart, G.W., & Sundeen, S.J. (1983). *Principles and practice of psychiatric nursing.* St. Louis, MO: C.V. Mosby Company.

Wilson, H.K., & Kneisl, C.R. (1992). *Psychiatric nursing,* Redwood City, CA: Addison-Wesley Nursing.

Julie Hensler-Cullen
Elaine Flynn
Julie Hyland

CHAPTER 20

The Rehabilitation Setting

Nurses put the able back into disabled when making decisions in the rehabilitation setting.

—*Anonymous*

INTRODUCTION

Medical rehabilitation in the United States surfaced as a specialty after World War II in response to the significant number of veterans who returned home maimed by the war's ravages. These men and women were often unable to return to the careers they had previously chosen, and thus, they needed to be trained in alternative professions. This significant national need gave birth to the era of rehabilitation, a segment of healthcare that has proliferated ever since.

Professional nurses, at the time of this new healthcare approach, were learning to adapt to a higher level of available technology and pharmaceuticals that revolutionized patient treatment and outcome. The ever-changing role of nursing in this healthcare environment was apparent. Sometimes patients only came to hospitals because they had the need for nursing expertise and intervention.

Paralleling the recognition that professional nurses were receiving in acute care settings, rehabilitation nurses were charting a new course on a team of rehabilitation professionals. Rehabilitation nurses were identifying patient goals, sharing those goals with other team members for valued input, and, most importantly, sharing those goals with the patient. This process of teamwork has been the hallmark of medical rehabilitation, and certainly has added to the unique aspects of rehabilitation nursing and clinical decision making.

The basic purposes of the interdisciplinary team are information-sharing and coordination of patient care; the more advanced purposes revolve around complex problem solving and accountability to patient outcomes. The team, through regular meetings, reviews patient progress and updates the treatment plan, one that will result in restoration of the disabled person to his or her maximum physical, emotional, social, spiritual, and vocational capacity (Willis-Sukosky, 1987).

A significant portion of any day in the life of a rehabilitation nurse is spent in making crucial decisions regarding client management or in justifying prior decisions to others, including interdisciplinary team members, family, and/or caregivers (Flannery and Thomas, 1990). Like the rehabilitation nurse's colleagues in other settings, expert clinical decision making is a valued and critical skill.

Decision making is an integral part of the rehabilitation nurse's role. For the purposes of this chapter, rehabilitation is defined as the process of providing opportunities for disabled individuals to develop skills necessary for optimum functioning (Hickey, 1981). The rehabilitation setting is collaborative in nature; a relationship of interdependence that recognizes the value of complementary roles of the interdisciplinary team members. This chapter will explore:

- The impact of three nursing theories on clinical decision making in the rehabilitation setting
- The team's function and process in decision making
- The effects of nurses' knowledge and experience on decision making

The use of nursing theory and clinical decision making in the rehabilitation setting is the initial focus of this chapter. Carnevali (1984) defines the diagnostic reasoning process for nursing as a complex, sometimes unconscious integration of critical thinking and the data collection process that clinicians use to identify and classify phenomena. The phenomena provide the foundation for subsequent treatment choices.

Theory is a powerful tool for explaining and predicting actions. It allows a systematic examination of events. Theoretical frameworks help describe the characteristics of a phenomenon or problem and specify the network of relationships between aspects of the phenomenon.

THEORIES IN CLINICAL DECISION MAKING

Theories guide or predict nursing action. By defining the problem within the context of a theory, the problem becomes more objective and obvious. Nursing theorists have attempted to provide nurses with tools that allow systematic analysis of an event and prescribe an appropriate scientific nursing treatment. Three nurse theorists and their works are most frequently cited as a basis for identifying nursing action in the rehabilitation setting. These are Orem's theory of self-care, Roy's theory of adaptation, and Neuman's theory of human systems. Readers are referred to any nursing theory text for a complete description of these theories.

The process of clinical decision making includes assessment, diagnosis, plans of care, interventions, and evaluation of care. The process of arriving at a nursing diagnosis can be applied to each theory.

The first theorist is Dorothy Orem (1980). Orem's *theory of self-care* describes self-care as a practice of learned behavior initiated or performed by the patient to maintain life, health, and well-being (Fields, 1987). The primary focuses are awareness of the universal self-care requisites of the patient and an evaluation of deviation of health and development or adaptation to disability. Self-care development is an ongoing process that is promoted by the nurse at appropriate times throughout the rehabilitation phase. Self-management is the goal, even when the patient's disability has rendered him or her completely dependent.

A rehabilitation patient's potential to manage his or her self-care is not related to a particular dysfunction, but rather to the patient's collective capability to participate in self-care as the self-care agent. The role of the nurse in rehabilitation is to evaluate and decide the individual's capability for self-care and his or her potential to achieve self-care agency. Specific nursing actions include making judgments about self-care activities, choosing methods of assistance, checking to see if selected interventions worked, and observing if other self-care deficits develop.

The second nursing theorist is Sister Callista Roy. Roy's (1976) *theory of adaptation* focuses on assessment and development of adaptive interventions to stabilize the client. The rehabilitation team's primary focus is on evaluation of the patient's adaptation to disability in four areas:

- Physiological
- Self-concept
- Role function
- Interdependence

The patient is viewed as a holistic system interacting with the environment. The team's decision making is centered on how to enhance or modify the adaptation of the patient. Roy's theory views reality as consisting of unified wholes that are greater than the sum of the parts. Roy concentrates on the use of adaptive modes to plan care. The team and the patient agree upon mutual goals.

The third nursing theorist presenting a framework for decision making by rehabilitation nurses is Neuman. Neuman's (1989) *human systems theory* addresses changes due to interactions between all the subsystems in the system. System in this paradigm is defined as a whole with interrelated parts, in which the parts have a function, and the system, as a totality, has a function (Putt, 1988). The disabled patient is seen as an open system constantly interacting with the environment and adapting to stressors. The goal of the rehabilitation team is to assist the person in attaining and maintaining an optimal level of wellness by enhancing adaptive mechanisms/processes and by reducing stress factors and modifying coping skills. The decision-making process includes the steps of diagnosis, goals, and outcomes. The rehabilitation team's evaluation would include assessment of the patient's and caregiver's stressors and actual and potential variances from wellness. Assessment data is collected to evaluate physiological, psychological, sociocultural, developmental, and spiritual variables and the interaction among the variables. The patient goals are derived from the team's evaluations and negotiation with the patient. Goals are developed to reduce the actual or potential stressors, helping the patient to move toward wellness and restoring equilibrium. Intervention strategies are identified to retain, attain, or maintain the system's stability.

The testing of these theories has not provided sufficient support for use of them alone to guide nurses in clinical decision making. Nurses must learn how to translate the "know that" of the paradigm into the "know how" of practice (Carper,

1978). Nursing theories give shape to the abstract components that define nursing and direct the goals of nursing care.

Scenario 20-1

LQ is a 36-year-old female who sustained a cervical fracture of the second, third, and fourth vertebrae, a basilar skull fracture, and quadriplegia as a result of a hit-and-run motor vehicle accident. The patient was initially treated in an acute care trauma center for 67 days and then transferred to a free-standing physical rehabilitation facility.

A review of the social history indicates that LQ is a recently divorced mother and primary custodian of four children ages 15, 13, 9, and 7. She is the youngest child of a family of ten. Her parents are living. She has been in a monogamous dating relationship for the last three months. Her boyfriend has been active in planning her discharge care.

During her acute care stay, LQ was declared legally incompetent, because she did not demonstrate the ability to understand and appreciate the nature and consequences of a particular healthcare decision. Her sister Eleanor was appointed legal guardian, with a durable power of attorney for healthcare. LQ was in the process of moving to a friend's home when she was injured by the automobile.

A review of the physical exam indicated that the patient was admitted with halo traction to stabilize the cervical fractures. She has no muscle strength in the neck. She was alert and oriented to person, place, and time. She had two Grade II decubiti on each iliac crest. She sustained a right temporal lobe skull fracture that remained open, approximately 3 by 5 centimeters in size. Her airway was maintained with a #6 Jackson tracheostomy. She was unable to speak because of her tracheostomy and poor muscle strength. Her bladder care was established using intermittent catheterization every four hours. The bowel program could not be established at the acute care hospital because of clostridium difficle diarrhea. The patient was experiencing six to eight liquid stools per day. The patient weighed 90 pounds and had lost 6 pounds since her initial injury. The patient had great difficulty swallowing and managing her secretions. The patient was receiving enteral tube feeding every six hours via gastrostomy tube.

The initial rehabilitation team meeting occurred within one day of the admission. At that time, LQ was experiencing intermittent febrile episodes. She also experienced orthostatic hypotension when her head was elevated 30 degrees or more. She needed to be maintained in a reclining position when out of bed to stabilize her blood pressure. She was unable to participate in any therapies due to the orthostatic hypotension. Her tracheostomy was plugged for 30 minutes every four hours. Her pulse oximeter reading was 93%. The patient was very tearful and depressed. Her ex-husband was attempting to obtain custody of their children, because he found out she had been declared legally incompetent. There was a disagreement among LQ's family about her children, discharge care, and general decision making. LQ was scared she would lose custody of her children and her independence.

The interdisciplinary team discussed the patient's ability to make and communicate healthcare decisions. The team consisted of a physical therapist, occupational therapist, physician, social worker, pharmacist, speech therapist, psychologist, and the registered nurse. The interdisciplinary team's flow of communication is both lateral or between disciplines, as well as vertical to the team leader. This is because the expected activity of the group is decision making and responsibility for developing the optimal plan of care. The problem focus and lateral flow of communication within the team is similar to the function of project teams and communication patterns of matrix organizations. The patient is considered part of this planning group and has a key role in the team's decision making.

The attending physician had evaluated LQ to determine her decision-making capacity. The physician used three key attributes:

- Understanding
- Judgment
- Communication

The physician asked three questions:

- Is LQ able to understand the information about her condition and the particular decisions to be made, including treatment options?
- Is LQ capable of judging how this information relates to her values and goals?
- Is LQ able to communicate her decisions in a consistent and meaningful manner?

Each member of the team had interviewed LQ to develop a treatment plan.

At the interdisciplinary team meeting, the team members discussed LQ's ability to communicate and understand informed decisions. LQ had a number of difficulties with sending and receiving communication because of her paralysis and tracheotomy. The professional staff from the Center for Communication Disorders had designed a sip-and-puff communication system. The system facilitated LQ's ability to answer yes/no questions and to enhance control of environmental equipment like the call light, bed control, and bedside lighting. LQ was able to communicate her understanding and implications of decisions through use of these assistive devices.

LQ expressed concern for self-control or autonomy and custody of her children. The attending physician, together with legal counsel, was able to regain competency status and maintain legal custody of LQ's children. The team recognized autonomy as a vital value for directing patient care services. Orem's theory of self-care was used to develop goals with LQ. The overall team goal was to manage and maintain LQ as her own independent self-care agency. LQ could not move anything but her mouth and head. She could not perform basic activities of daily living such as grooming, bathing, and dressing. The nurse, as a member of the rehabilitation team, must decide how he or she will coordinate LQ's care to facilitate the goal of self-care agency. The goal for LQ was to become wholly independent in directing her care. LQ's nurse, utilizing her expertise as a certified rehabilitation registered nurse (CRRN), developed a detailed plan of care that outlined a paradigm to increase LQ's autonomy in direct self-care activities. The plan detailed the individual nursing actions that each nurse would use to incorporate LQ into the decision-making process.

TEAM FUNCTION AND DECISION MAKING

In the rehabilitation hospital, each discipline evaluates the client's ability to adapt to his or her disability. At regularly scheduled team conferences, the individual team members present their evaluations as well as their plans of care. This process is ongoing from inpatient to outpatient stays; thus, there is an orderly progression of decision making that can be used to evaluate the outcome of patient care.

As a member of a rehabilitation team, the professional nurse relies on more than nursing models and theories to make judgments. The nurse indicates the area of practice that is nursing and distinct from that of the other health-related professions such as medicine, social work, or physical therapy (Fields, 1987). Nursing theories assist the rehabilitation nurse in defining nursing. However, in order to contribute as an expert member of the team, the rehabilitation nurse must have a sound scientific knowledge base in the behavioral and physical sciences related to the practice of nursing.

Fields (1987) notes that there is a need for practitioners to have common knowledge and shared skills, if each professional is to collaborate in the provision of healthcare. The rehabilitation nurse is the obvious fulcrum of shared knowledge, since the nurse must have or acquire skills possessed by the physician, physical therapist, social worker, psychologist, and others. In order to render treatment and evaluate the outcome of that treatment, the rehabilitation nurse must possess the skills and knowledge necessary to promote patient safety while simultaneously maximizing measurable results.

The treatment plan, designed by the team of rehabilitation providers, is a tool by which the patient's hospitalization is charted. Rehabilitation nurses provide the linkage between the patient, the treatment plan, and the treatment team. It is the rehabilitation nurse who, for instance, notes the patient's interaction with family in the evening hours or who witnesses the first success of an oft-attempted physical feat. These nurses provide the 24-hour-a-day feedback that the rehabilitation team requires in order to modify the patient's treatment plan.

The development of critical pathways in rehabilitation is an innovative approach to care that can be greatly influenced by the rehabilitation nurse. As the team of rehabilitation professionals design blueprints of the typical courses of treatment, the expert rehabilitation nurse can draw on a body of decision-making skills that will profoundly enhance the plans. In a shrinking healthcare reimbursement environment, such as the one we face approaching the twenty-first century, rehabilitation nurses must take the lead in defining measurable, functional outcomes for patients. When a course is designed, nurses must evaluate the course frequently via feedback from the other disciplines and make corrections accordingly. The goal is, and must be, to attain the highest achievable outcome(s) in a cost-responsible way. Every effort must be made by the team to avoid duplication of therapeutic interventions, thus improving team efficiency. Dealdlines and other timeframes are critical and all team members must share the awareness. Rehabilitation nurses, however, are the greatest predictors of how achievable those timeframes are, vis-à-vis their holistic view of the patient's accomplishments.

THE USE OF PRECEPTORS/MENTORS

Providing a nurse with the tools and knowledge to work in a system can and will occur as a result of a well-planned, comprehensive orientation program. However, the efficient application of this knowledge requires time and experience on the nurse's part. The effect of preceptor or mentor programs on mastering the process of decision making needs to be explored. Thomas O. Boyle (1990) reports that mentoring is beneficial for the mentor, the protégé, and, above all, the organization. Mentoring builds trust and loyalty and provides for better informed decision making among organizational members (Boyle, 1990).

Flannery and Thomas (1990) suggest that novice nurses have critical decisions validated through the mentor relationship by an expert nurse. Investigators have noted that the inexperienced problem solver neither generates as many alternatives for testing nor accomplishes alternative generation as early in the process as an experienced problem solver (Ekwo, 1977; Elstein, Shulman, and Sprafka, 1978). Flannery and Thomas (1990) concluded that these differences seem clearly related to the bank of knowledge and accumulated experiences of the problem solver.

Preceptor programs provide opportunities for orientation, induction, and socialization of the new nurse, as well as being a way to recognize outstanding staff nurses. Preceptors should be chosen for their superb nursing skills, their organizational and interpersonal skills, their interest in the orientation process, and, of course, expert decision-making skills. A highly motivated preceptor can assist the new nurse in gaining confidence and skill in the provision of nursing care, and can also provide a safe haven where the novice can feel free to acknowledge inexperience or lack of knowledge. Young, Theriault, and Collins (1989) posit that this one-to-one teaching relationship is the most effective mechanism for learning. Also, in one-to-one teaching, the process can be individualized to the specific needs of the learner and immediate feedback can be given to the learner (Young et al., 1989).

Preceptors are chosen and may even have to apply for this prestigious role. A formal orientation program for the preceptor should cover the purposes of the preceptor program, the role of the preceptor, principles of adult education, teaching-learning principles, the skills of empathy and feedback, and methods of evaluation of the preceptor.

The preceptor is instrumental in guiding the move to independence. Such a relationship allows the orientee to work and identify with a competent role model who is involved on a daily basis in decisions regarding patient care and unit management issues. In the early part of the program, the preceptor input is *continuous*. This input decreases as the new nurse takes on more responsibility.

One rehabilitation nurse who has served as a preceptor for new nurses on a spinal cord unit related the following anecdote that describes how she assisted a graduate nurse to develop competence in the care of spinal cord injured patients.

Scenario 20-2

Graduate nurse MF was caring for a 32-year-old spinal cord injured patient, DM. DM's care required keen attention to her bowel and bladder management. Bladder care involved DM having an indwelling, continuously draining urinary catheter. DM's bowel care was managed by administration of a rectal suppository given every other morning.

During two months of rehabilitation, DM experienced frequent episodes of autonomic dysreflexia. Autonomic dysreflexia is a dramatic complication of spinal cord injuries that starts when an afferent stimulus from some effector enters the cord and triggers off a reflex motor outflow that is widely disseminated. The afferent stimulus generally comes from the mucosa and muscle of distended bladder. The basic pathology in cord injuries in terms of the bladder is that the detrusor muscle does not develop sufficient emptying contractures, and sphincters do not relax. Thus bladder distention occurs. The autonomic nervous system reacts by constricting the blood vessels and causing the blood pressure to rise as high as 300/160!

MF's preceptor was very familiar with the nursing interventions required when a patient evidenced symptoms of dysreflexia. She started to plot DM's events to evaluate the pattern of the hypertensive episodes. The preceptor also noted that the patient experienced hypertension with vaginal or rectal stimulation.

MF learned well from the preceptor. During insertion of a rectal suppository, the experienced preceptor palpated a "mass" in the rectal area. This nurse notified the physician who examined the patient and diagnosed her with a peri-rectal abscess, an unusual occurrence, but one picked up by the astute experienced preceptor. The patient had the abscess drained and the hypertensive episodes subsided. This uncommon occurrence of the development of an abscess might not be one that a preceptor would routinely review with every orientee, and yet by just being with an experienced nurse, MF, the graduate nurse, was exposed to and developed her own competence in the care of the spinal cord injured patients.

SUMMARY

Decision making in rehabilitation nursing takes place in a multidisciplinary context. Members of the interdisciplinary team assess the patient and together with the patient decide on a plan of care that is most beneficial to the patient. The nurse contributes to the assessment and plan using her unique perspective and her knowledge of nursing theory and specific patient care needs and activities. The theories of Orem, Roy, and Neuman have all been integrated into rehabilitation nursing and provide a framework for decision making for the nurse. The use of mentors/preceptors for the novice nurse enhances the knowledge and decision-making ability needed to provide quality rehabilitiative nursing care.

REFERENCES

Carnevali, D.L. (1984). The diagnostic reasoning process. In D.L. Carnevali, P.H. Mitchell, N.F. Woods, and C.A. Tanner (Eds.), *Diagnostic reasoning in nursing.* Philadelphia: J.B. Lippincott Co.

Carper, B. (1978). Fundamental patterns of knowing. *Advances in Nursing Science, 1* (1), 13–23.

Ekwo, E. (1977). An analysis of the problem solving process of third year medical students. *Proceedings of the 16th annual conference on research in medical education.* Washington, DC: Association of American Medical Colleges.

Elstein, A., Shulman, L., & Sprafka, S., (1978). *Medical reasoning.* Cambridge, MA: Harvard University Press.

Fields, P.A. (1987). The impact of nursing theory on the clinical decision making process. *Journal of Advanced Nursing, 12,* 563–571.

Flannery, J., & Thomas, J. (1990). Focus on excellence: Decision making in rehabilitation nursing. *Rehabilitation Nursing, 15*(4), 187–190.

Hickey, J., (1981) *The clinical practical of neurological and neurosurgical nursing,* (pp. 301–324). Philadelphia: J.B. Lippincott.

Neuman, B. (1989). *The Neuman systems model* (2nd Ed.) Norwalk, CT: Appleton & Lange.

O'Boyle, T. (1990, June 12) Mentor-protege ties can be strained, *Wall Street Journal,* B1.

Orem, D. (1980). *Nursing: Concepts of practice* (2nd Ed.). New York: McGraw-Hill Book Company.

Putt, A.M. (1988). *General system theory applied to nursing.* Boston: Little, Brown.

Roy, C. (1976). *Introduction to nursing: An adaptation model.* Englewood Cliffs, NJ: Prentice-Hall.

Willis-Sukosky, N. (1987). *Rehabilitation nursing: Concepts and practice a core curriculum.* C. Mumma (Ed.) Evanston, IL: Rehabilitation Nursing Foundation.

Young, S., Theriault, J., & Collins, D. (1989) The nurse preceptor: Preparation and needs. *Journal of Nursing Staff Development, 5*(3), 127.

Renee P. McLeod

CHAPTER 21

The Primary Care Setting

To know you is to better understand you.
—*Anonymous*

INTRODUCTION

Clinical decisions that are made in a primary care setting are very different from clinical decisions that nurses make within a hospital setting. An environment of uncertainty is typical of all healthcare settings, but is magnified in the open, unstructured environment of primary care. Providers have less control over clinical situations and are dependent on patients to provide accurate information, follow instructions, and administer and monitor their own treatments. Factors that contribute to this environment were identified in one primary care setting by Brykczynski (1991) as including the following:

- Wide range in age of patients
- Diversity in objective signs and subjective symptoms
- Multicultural ethnicity of clientele
- Socioeconomic, educational, and language differences
- Varied treatments (lay and scientific)
- Lack of availability of medical records
- Staffing problems
- Communication gaps among providers and between providers and patients
- Long-term nature of care

These situations create an environment of ambiguity where clinical judgment skills become paramount. Making diagnostic clinical decisions in this environment is risky, but making a diagnosis and finding solutions to problematic patient situations also carries with it great rewards. The purpose of this chapter is to demonstrate ways nurse practitioners make decisions in the primary care setting, and discuss ways that clinical problem-solving skills can be improved.

Scenario 21-1

In clinical situations where everything is straight forward and routine, the practitioner may use established standard protocols to make decisions. For example, in the following patient scenario, Mr. Garrett comes to the office for care. He is Caucasian, speaks English and is well educated. He tells you that he was working in his garden yesterday and managed to "get into a pile of poison ivy." He now has a very itchy rash that covers both hands and arms up to his elbows; the rest of his body is unaffected and he does not have any other complaints. He is one of your regular primary care patients and you have a complete health history on file from previous visits. Your physical exam demonstrates a well-developed, healthy, 65-year-old man who has a linear, vesicular rash on both arms that is slightly excoriated. The decision-making process for the diagnosis and treatment of poison ivy exposure is straightforward and can easily be made using standard protocols.

However, it is not often the case that everything is simple and straightforward, and it is during these times that practitioners manage cases and make decisions by using their expertise and clinical experience.

DEFINITIONS

Primary care has been defined in a variety of ways. These definitions are derived from organizational, functional, professional, and academic perspectives. Primary care may be defined as a level of service that is community-based instead of hospital-based. Primary care has also been defined from a functional viewpoint: the primary care provider provides access, continuity, and integration of healthcare for the patient (Alpert and Charney, 1975). Primary care is also defined by the American Nurses Association (ANA) as the first point of contact with the health care system (ANA, 1985). (See Appendix A for "Assumptions" concerning the scope of practice of primary care nurses [ANA, 1985]).

Other definitions of primary healthcare include identification, management, and referral for healthcare problems, as well as health promotion and prevention of illness. Primary care is holistic, considering the needs, weaknesses, and strengths of the whole person and his or her support system. Because primary care is the first point of contact that a patient has with the healthcare system, it is also the point where a decision needs to be made to resolve the presenting healthcare problem.

Stoeckle (1987) uses a clinical definition to define primary care as "coordinated, comprehensive, and personal care, available on both a first-contact and continuous basis. It incorporates several tasks: medical diagnosis and treatment, psychological assessment and management, personal support, communication of information about illness, prevention, and health maintenance" (p. 1).

The nurse practitioner is a registered nurse prepared through a formal, organized educational program, usually a masters degree in nursing, to meet the guidelines for advanced practice established by the profession. The nurse practitioner is then licensed by the state to provide a full range of primary healthcare services. Nurse practitioners are patient-oriented rather than a disease-oriented, concentrating on preventive measures, such as immunizations and health assessments, as well as the diagnosis and management of commonly occurring acute and chronic conditions. Nurse practitioners engage in independent decision making about healthcare needs, and provide healthcare to individuals and groups across the lifespan. Therefore, nurse practitioners are ideally suited to provide primary care.

Collaboration

Hawkins and Thibodeau (1993) state that "inherent in the role of the advanced practitioner is accountability and responsibility for decisions made and actions rendered. This responsibility is retained even when a referral to another health care provider is indicated" (p. 9). "Since primary health care involves the delivery of health care from entry into the system and is also continuous and comprehensive, it necessitates collaboration among many health professions and with the patient" (ANA, 1985, p. 3).

Collaboration is a process in which two or more individuals work together, jointly influencing one another, for the attainment of a goal. Collaborative decision making is an act of selecting a choice among two or more possible alternatives for an action by a group of individuals mutually influencing the decision (Kim, 1983). In the primary care setting, collaboration occurs between the patient and the provider, as the provider works with the patient to attain the needed information to make a clinical decision and resolve the healthcare problem. Collaborative decision making occurs as the nurse practitioner involves other members of the healthcare team including the physician, social worker, or other medical specialist to provide comprehensive, holistic care for the patient on a long-term basis. Collaboration is an approach to professional-client relationships that requires moving beyond roles of professional dominance with the provider having all of the knowledge and client dependency on that knowledge as the only way to achieve health. Collaboration allows for the integration of personal information and experience and professional knowledge and experience in a way that optimizes the outcome of the decision.

COLLABORATION WITH THE PATIENT: THE HUNT FOR ALL THE FACTS

The chart on the door tells the practitioner that the next patient is Maria Sanchez, a 6-year-old girl who has presented herself with abdominal pain. She is here with her mother and a note states that she only speaks Spanish. She is a new patient to the practitioner, but she has been at the clinic before. Where does one begin?

To lay the foundation for the patient interview, the practitioner needs to start with the environment. The ideal setting would provide the patient with privacy, proper lighting, a comfortable quiet space that is the right temperature with no distracting equipment or decorations. The patient should be interviewed while still in her street clothes. The seating arrangements should allow the practitioner to make eye contact with the patient. The distance between the provider and the patient should be culturally appropriate. This can often be discovered by sitting on a rolling stool and moving closer or farther away from the patient until the patient's body language indicates that you are in the right spot. Be sure that enough time has been allowed for an interview to be free from interruptions. If the nurse remains standing and does not make eye contact with the patient during the interview, this may imply that the nurse is in a rush and does not have time or does not want to hear what the patient has to say.

At this point it is appropriate to talk about how to set up an interview when a translator is needed. If at all possible, a family member, especially a child should not be used as the translator. Family members may tend to misrepresent the patient's subjective views. Position the translator slightly behind the nurse and to one side so that the patient can make eye contact with the nurse and the translator without having to turn back and forth. Ideally, the translator will act as an interpreter who will guide the nurse so that questions are asked in a culturally appropriate manner without losing sight of the intent and content of the questions. The translator should translate the questions as close to verbatim as possible. The practitioner should be aware that age, gender, and socioeconomic differences between the patient and the translator can often be a problem. Just because a translator speaks another language does not mean that the translator knows anything about the culture of the patient.

Nurse practitioners need to develop a high level of interviewing skills that assist in obtaining an ideal history and avoid commonly made errors such as overuse of professional jargon, value-laden questions, inappropriate assurance, leading questions, and interrupting. Remember that body language, voice, expressions, and posture give the patient a particular message that can either help or hinder the interview process. Using a translator takes practice and a close working relationship with the translator to interview patients smoothly.

Do not underestimate the significance of continuing to develop and refine history-taking skills. Kraytman (1991) states that

> it has been estimated that the information gathered in the initial interview allows a correct diagnosis in over 50% of internal diseases. However, history taking is not just a process of collecting information on the onset and evolution of an illness. It must also give an insight into the patient's personality, the ability of the patient to cope with the medical problem, and the effects of the problem on the patient. It serves as the basis for the relationship between patient and interviewer (p. 1)."

With this information in mind, it is time to start the patient encounter. Barrows and Pickell (1991) recommend that at the start of the patient encounter, the practioner should pay systematic attention to all of the following methods of gathering data:

- Search for information from the patient's appearance, body language, age, sex, speech characteristics, and movement
- Observe for attitudes or other information that might be useful about friends or family members who have accompanied the patient
- Determine if the patient is implying something other than what he or she is expressing verbally
- Learn about the patient's attitude toward the practitioner and the encounter
- Look for evidence that may substantiate preliminary diagnoses

Scenario 21-2

You are now ready to go see Maria Sanchez, a 6-year-old Hispanic female. During the interview you discover that she went to the emergency room two weeks ago for facial paralysis and was diagnosed with "Bell's Palsy" secondary to an ear infection. She was placed on two weeks of antibiotics, and the facial paralysis and ear infection seem to have resolved without further difficulty. You investigate further and discover that she had a similar incident a year ago with a "staring spell," which the mother had mentioned to the provider at Maria's last well-child visit, but the provider had not seemed concerned. The mother also mentioned that she had similar spells as an infant, which she had mentioned during well-child visits. You find these documented in the chart, but no followup. The history reveals that in addition to complaining of a stomachache, Maria is waking up at night to go to the bathroom, has urgency, and some burning on urination. It is not unusual for your history to reveal a variety of problems that may or may not be related to the "chief complaint."

At this point it is time to make your first decision. Maria has been scheduled for a 15-minute sick visit, and the interview has already taken over the allotted time. You now must decide how you are going to proceed with this patient, and you haven't even started a physical exam.

How important is this new information? Why has it not been followed up on in the past? Is it because this patient is receiving her primary care with many different providers and therefore no one has looked at the total picture? What initial hypotheses have been generated by this information, and which hypothesis is the more important one? Could the two problems be related? Which problem takes precedence? Should you take the time to do a more comprehensive history and physical now, or schedule her to come back another day for a followup visit? Have you made any unwarranted assumptions? Have you assumed what the patient means by the words she is using? Translation errors are easy to make during the interview process. Have you been attentive to your own hidden biases?

Based on the information you have gathered so far, you should be able to generate an initial hypothesis or hypotheses. Your hypotheses will vary from those of other providers who might see this patient. The hypotheses generated are a product of your own unique experience and education. Hypotheses are labels that you use to guide your inquiry. These labels often do not fall into neat categories and may instead cover a wide variety of data in the provider's memory. This collection of facts includes a cluster of related data, based on the provider's education and experience with patients, that fit with a particular hypothesis. Examples of hypotheses are specific diagnoses (medical and nursing), social issues, syndromes, etiologic processes, and anatomic entities like fractured tibia. Barrows and Pickell (1991) call these hypotheses "individually authored titles," because they are only meaningful to the provider generating them from his or her long-term memory library. So be creative and generate all the hypotheses needed to help in the decision-making process.

The interview with Maria Sanchez has so far generated two main hypotheses that need further exploration. The first is a possible urinary tract infection. The second is a concern that there might be some sort of neurological disorder like epilepsy or a possible tumor occurring in this child. Before you can come to your final working hypothesis or diagnostic decision, additional information must be gathered. Based on the fact that the possible neurological symptoms have been occurring over a long period of time without significant harm, that the interview has taken longer than the time allotted, and the mother is currently more concerned about her daughter's abdominal pain, the decision is made to address this problem first.

USING CLINICAL SKILLS TO GATHER SUPPORTING DATA

The data gathered from the physical exam is usually the easiest part of the decision-making process. Physical assessment requires skill, tact, and should be geared to the age of the patient. Develop a systematic approach to the physical exam and perform it the same way every time. The practitioner needs to be sure that all of the equipment is in proper working condition and easily accessible. Proceed with the examination using all senses to be completely aware of the patient. Complete the exam as thoroughly as needed to fully explore all hypotheses. Be sure to look at the patient meticulously. This usually means that the physical should be conducted with the patient in a gown to facilitate the exam. If the exam is being conducted in a room that lacks privacy, a sectional approach may be used to undress and redress the patient so that a total body exam may be completed.

To complete the process of data gathering before the working diagnosis is formulated, consider what laboratory work would facilitate or add supporting data for the working hypotheses. Deciding what kind of lab work to order may require some negotiating with the patient. How is the patient going to pay for the visit? If the patient is the payer source, how much can he or she afford to pay? What lab work will allow the most information for the least cost? What lab work is the least intrusive and provides the least amount of risk and discomfort to the patient? What is the value of the information available from the test, will it change the treatment plan for the patient? "Tests ordered as a substitute for thinking, or tests ordered on the basis of unquestioned tradition, have served to escalate the cost of health care for all of us and expose countless patients to unnecessary costs and risks" (Barrows and Pickell, 1991, p. 143).

In the case of Maria, her mother does not have insurance and she is paying for the visit today. The nurse practitioner decides that a urine dipstick will provide enough information to support a working diagnosis. The urine shows leukocytes, nitrates, and a trace of blood.

Did the patient supply enough information to generate at least one working hypothesis or diagnosis? That decision must be made with limited information. Each patient is unique in response and reaction, and each disease will manifest itself differently in every person. To arrive at this decision, the practitioner must gather enough data to fit one of the hypotheses. The "fit" occurs when there is enough of the expected positive and negative findings to make the clinician feel that the hypothesis explains the problem. A perfect "fit" rarely happens in the real world, which is why one infrequently sees a textbook case!

> A diagnostic decision has to be made before you treat. In most instances, all the data you would like to have to make this decision are not available, despite a detailed and effective inquiry. You have to decide what in all likelihood is wrong with the patient so that you can care for the patient even if the diagnosis is not a sure thing. You have to play the odds in favor of the patient. There is risk and responsibility in this task (Barrows and Pickell, 1991, p. 149).

The information obtained from the history, physical exam, and laboratory testing of Maria has provided enough information, pending confirmation, to "fit" the working hypothesis or diagnosis of "urinary tract infection." This will allow the practitioner to treat this problem while waiting for confirmation from a culture and sensitivity of her urine. In this instance the nurse used the rule that "common things occur commonly."

Scenario 21-2, Continued

What if there was still some doubt about her diagnosis? This is certainly true as regards the second hypothesis of some sort of neurological disorder. Taking the decision-making process through a series of questions will provide one with an appropriate plan of action.

First, is there enough evidence in your problem synthesis to decide that one of the hypotheses can be accepted as tentative? The only evidence really available to document that Maria might have a neurological problem is concern on the part of her mother, which has been documented in the chart over time, and the unusual diagnosis of Bell's palsy in a 6-year-old. You decide there is not enough evidence to make a diagnosis based on the available information.

Second, is there enough evidence to suggest a likely diagnosis, pending confirmation by tests, response to treatment, or information from subsequent events? The answer to this question is no, but there does seem to be enough information to warrant further exploration.

Third, are there other hypotheses that need to be ruled out because they represent a potential threat of morbidity or mortality? Could Maria have a tumor?

Fourth, how necessary is it to reach a diagnosis at this time, or can the diagnosis be deferred for a period of time? "Tincture of time" often resolves many problems in medicine. In the case of Maria, the other providers had either chosen this solution, or failed to note the problem on either a problem summary sheet or the progress notes so another provider could continue the clinical reasoning process. By failing to note the problem, the flow of the clinical reasoning process was interrupted and problem synthesis did not continue, since new data was not entered for analysis. Therefore, the clinical decision making for this problem appears fractured. It has been difficult for anyone to make the connections necessary to fit the pieces of this puzzle together to complete the picture.

This demonstrates that a hypothesis may be carried and worked on by other providers or the primary care provider at later visits when the problem is not life threatening or critical. This is only possible if the information is documented in the chart in a manner that makes it easy to find. This is especially important when the patient presents, as Maria did, with several problems that need to be sorted out for action at subsequent visits. It also demonstrates the importance of communication and collaboration between providers when more than one person is seeing a patient in the primary care setting, or when the patient goes to other settings like the emergency room for treatment when the primary care provider is not available.

If no diagnosis is really possible, then the final working hypothesis for that patient encounter should be stated in very general terms followed by the possible, but as yet unsubstantiated more refined diagnoses (which may be ruled out by subsequent tests, consultations, reexaminations, etc.). Remember that if the therapies for the entertained hypotheses are the same, or if the prognoses are essentially the same, then further refinement of the diagnosis may not be necessary at this time. This is particularly important to remember when the practitioner needs to negotiate with the patient about the treatment plan, because the patient has limited money, limited education, or limited ability to understand and follow through with advice.

When the most obvious diagnosis is one that has a poor prognosis, like a tumor, or is not treatable, then it is important for the clinician to consider any and all treatable conditions, although unlikely, as the possible diagnosis. Treatable conditions should be treated first. The encounter with Maria has generated one treatable diagnosis (urinary tract infection) and one possible diagnosis (rule out a neurological problem like seizure disorder) that needs more data generated before a diagnostic decision can be made.

To complete the diagnostic decision-making process for the second hypothesis, it is essential to recognize that the clinician may not know what is wrong, and that there is a limit to the amount of knowledge and experience any clinician may have. When the inquiry strategy is exhausted, it is important to change one's thinking. This is a common problem encountered in primary care, and there are a number of strategies that can be used when this situation develops. There are many books and computer programs to help generate alternative hypotheses for consideration. The computer should be viewed as an important tool in the clinical decision-making process, and therefore an important addition to any practice.

Another option is to analyze the data gathered in a different way to see if it suggests two problems that might be separated. It is possible for a patient to have both chicken pox and asthma. The symptoms for one disease can confuse the diagnosis of another disease. Look for new cues from the data. This may mean returning to the patient to gather additional history information or to perform another physical examination. Find out what the patient thinks is going on. Finally, take all of the additional information and consult with a colleague. Collaboration with a physician or specialist provides the benefits of his or her knowledge and expertise. Often colleagues can direct inquiry strategies in a new way to provide the clinician with a different way of looking at the problem.

Collaboration with Other Professionals

In the primary care setting, it is often necessary for the generalist to refer the patient to a specialist for further work-up. Given the time limitations of this patient encounter, the possible risks and benefits to the patient, and the need to follow up on the information generated from the interview, the decision is made to refer Maria to a neurologist for a complete workup. The findings and treatments provided by the neurologist should be transmitted back to the primary care provider as part of the collaboration process. Additional diagnoses allow the primary care provider to take this information into consideration to guide further investigation, to select appropriate treatments, and to classify the patient's problems for record keeping and statistical purposes. This sort of collaborative decision making provides the most comprehensive, holistic care for the patient in a way that optimizes outcomes.

The last consideration when formulating a working diagnosis is to know the prevalence of disease in a patient population. Know the patients, their environment, and the diseases that are more likely in this population due to race, culture, jobs, and living conditions. If at all possible, the practitioner should live in the neighborhood where the practice is located.

The information gathered from the history and physical and the analysis of the data at hand has now provided the practitioner with two working hypotheses or diagnostic decisions for Maria that can now be incorporated into a treatment plan. This part of the patient encounter involves another decision making process called therapeutic decision making.

THERAPEUTIC DECISION MAKING: INVOLVING THE PATIENT IN THE TREATMENT PLAN

It is easy to assume that the most difficult part of the decision-making process has been accomplished once a diagnosis has been made. Actually, the clinician's most important decision is the management plan. If the patient is not committed to and actively involved in the management plan, there will not be a change in the patient's health. The first step in the therapeutic decision-making process is to determine if there are other problems, even nonmedical ones, that might affect the patient's response to treatment, recovery, sense of well-being, attitude, or ability to return to work or school. In the case of Maria, explore other issues with the mother, because the family will be responsible for Maria's treatment. If there are problems occurring with the family, they will affect the outcome, and Maria's response to treatment.

Exploring these issues and making sure that there are no unexplained complaints, findings on examinations, or laboratory results (present or past) that need further analysis before ending the patient encounter are particularly important in today's managed care environment. These few extra minutes reviewing the patient's chart and talking to the patient may prevent the patient from receiving extra office visits, or expensive laboratory tests that are unnecessary. Taking extra time will also prevent the kind of fractured care evident in Maria's case, because she is seeing different primary care providers and no one is looking at the whole picture or adding data necessary to continue the clinical reasoning process over time.

Next, consider objectives for treatment. Is it to correct some underlying pathology, relieve symptoms, prevent complications, or cure the patient? Other reasons for treatment include assuring the patient or patient's family that something is being done, and assuring that the most appropriate treatment is given. If treatment objectives are not known, then one will never be able to evaluate treatment effectiveness. Other considerations include the cost and risks to the patient. Are there side effects to the treatment that might prevent the patient from following through with the treatment? Is the treatment convenient? When dealing with children, care should be taken in selecting medications that taste good and are easily dosed to maximize compliance. If the mother cannot remember to give the medication four times a day for ten days then will it matter if the medication is given only two times a day for five or six days? What if the child spits out the medication or refuses to take it after four days of treatment, or a sibling breaks the bottle of medicine?

When developing a treatment plan, it is imperative to actively involve the patient. If the patient is not committed to the plan, he or she will not be motivated to follow through with the recommendations provided. What are the patient's reasons for seeking treatment? Management of the patient's problem must be directed to the patient as a person, as a member of a family, and as a member of society. For example, in Maria's case, does her mother understand the diagnosis of a urinary tract infection? Is there information that has not been gathered that might affect the treatment outcome? For example, the inability of Maria's mother to pay for the recommended antibiotic. Does the mother understand the need to refrigerate the antibiotic, and how to properly administer the medication? Does the child have difficulty taking medication, and what was Maria's prior response to antibiotic treatment? If written educational material is going to be provided, one must gather additional data concerning educational level, reading level, and language of the patient and family members.

The ability to manage Maria's possible neurological problem will depend on the practitioner's ability to educate Maria's mother to the importance of going to the neurologist even though transportation and ability to pay may prevent her from following through with recommendations. The practitioner must collaborate with the patient and family to find solutions that motivate the patient, minimize barriers, and increase patient autonomy.

Be certain that the chosen treatment plan offers a better outcome than no treatment. To do this one must understand the natural course of the disease being treated, including the likelihood of progress, complications, and new symptoms. Without this information, the practitioner will be unable to educate the patient on the appropriate time to return for care or call for advice. Remember that in primary care, the practitioner will not be the person who must make the decision to take the medication or return for treatment. This is the patient or patient's family's responsibility. It is the practitioner's responsibility to give the patient the information needed to enable the patient to take appropriate, logical, and reasoned actions in dealing with her problems, and to enhance healthy behaviors. One must have the active, willing, and informed participation of the patient to achieve a successful outcome for the treatment plan.

> Compliance is not as much affected by the patient's knowledge about his illness or health as it is by the patient's motivation, previous experiences, biases, cultural background, social and environmental factors, and sometimes by the personality effects of the disease process itself (Barrows and Pickell, 1991, p. 192).

Developing a therapeutic treatment plan and managing the medical problem are accomplished through collaboration with the patient. To attain treatment goals, a partnership must be developed between the practitioner and the patient. To work effectively with the patient on a continuous basis and provide coordinated, comprehensive, and personal care, the practitioner must help the patient understand the problem and its treatment.

DECIDING WHEN TO CLOSE THE PATIENT ENCOUNTER

The time needed for any patient encounter varies. Most primary care providers have time constraints imposed on them. The decision-making process discussed allows for flexibility in the time needed in any one patient encounter. In the primary care setting where the nurse practitioner plans to follow the patient over time, many treatment decisions or educational needs of the patient may be deferred to another visit when the patient may be more receptive.

Barrows and Pickell (1991) have developed the following criteria to assist the practitioner with the decision to come to closure with the patient:

- Accurate, effective, and efficient diagnostic and treatment decisions have been made at this particular stage of the provider-client encounter
- No more information is available in this setting at this time on which to base decision making
- The patient's situation is urgent, and requires immediate treatment
- Followup has been arranged, and appropriate evaluation and management for other problems has been planned and arranged.

After closing the encounter, it is important to document in the patient's record everything that went on during the time spent with the patient. The documentation should tell others and remind the practitioner of the decisions that were made and why they were made. This should include the treatment goals and any unresolved matters that need followup at future visits. This information should be written in a format that is legible and includes all of the pertinent data without rambling on in a way that prevents others from finding the important information in the notes. A problem summary sheet at the beginning of the chart is an excellent place to keep pertinent data accessible without plowing through the chart, as long as it is updated each time the patient comes in for care. Proper documentation of the reasoning process and diagnostic decisions will assist the practitioner and any other provider who might see the patient to continue the clinical reasoning process during future encounters. Followup visits with the patient duplicate the decision-making process discussed in this chapter: The practitioner starts with the patient and any additional records, then continues with the patient interview to add additional data to evaluate the patient's response to treatment and to generate any additional hypotheses to be acted on. This ensures continuity of care, allows the practitioner to evaluate the effectiveness of treatment decisions, and ultimately improves the health of the patient.

IMPROVING CLINICAL DECISION-MAKING SKILLS

Developing a system to provide for self-improvement and lifelong learning is important to become and stay an expert clinician. The records of patient encounters can provide the practitioner with a tool for self-improvement. After each patient encounter, take the time to carefully review the clinical decision-making process. Barrows and Pickell (1991) suggest considering the following and writing down any significant answers:

1. Did you recognize the problem well enough to pull together an initial concept?
2. Did you understand the symptoms and signs that were presented?
3. Were you able to come up with reasonable initial hypotheses?
4. Did you have sufficient information about those hypotheses to inquire against them?
5. Did you know good laboratory or diagnostic tests to separate the hypotheses?
6. Did you order redundant or unnecessary tests?
7. Could you decide whether the patient's problems matched your hypotheses?
8. Did you know which tests and treatment to employ?
9. Did you know what results to expect if your hypothesis was correct?
10. Of those tests you did consider, were you comfortable with your knowledge of their benefit/cost aspects? Could you decide on closure?
11. If the problem was urgent, was your inquiry focused, efficient, and effective?
12. Was your treatment based on a knowledge of the probable course of the suspected illness in this patient and did it consider all the benefit/cost aspects? (p. 203–204).

This review should occur right after a patient encounter, while all of the facts are fresh in the practitioner's mind. As this process is continued after every patient encounter, experience in assessment is gained and the practitioner will become more aware of shortcomings and educational needs (Barrows and Pickell, 1991).

SUMMARY

This chapter has provided the nurse practitioner with a step-by-step approach to the clinical decision-making process in primary care. Appendix B summarizes these steps as "Pearls for Developing Clinical Reasoning Skills in the Primary Care Setting." Key to this process is collaboration with the patient, family, and other health care professionals if needed. Through experience and self-reflection, the practitioner continually develops increased knowledge and skills that improve decision-making ability.

REFERENCES

Alpert, J., & Charney, E. (1975). *The education of physicians for primary care.* DHEW publication No. 74-31B. Washington, DC: U.S. Government Printing Office.

American Nurses Association. (1985). *The scope of practice of the primary health care nurse practitioner.* Kansas City, MO: Author.

Barrows, H.S., & Pickell, G.C. (1991). *Developing clinical problem-solving skills: A guide to more effective treatment.* New York: Norton.

Brykczynski, K. (1991). Judgment strategies for coping with ambiguous clinical situations encountered in primary family care. *Journal of the American Academy of Nurse Practitioners, 3,* 79–84.

Hawkins, J., & Thibodeau, J. (1993). *The advanced practitioner: Current practice issues.* New York: Tiresias Press.

Kim, H.S. (1983). Collaborative decision making in nursing practice: A theoretical framework. In P.L Chinn (Ed.), *Advances in nursing theory development.* Rockville, MD: Aspen.

Kraytman, M. (1991). *The complete patient history* (2nd Edition). New York: McGraw-Hill.

Stoeckle, J. (1987). Tasks of primary care. In A.H. Goroll, L.A. May, & A.G. Mulley (Eds.), *Primary care medicine: Office evaluation and management of the adult patient.* Philadelphia: Lippincott.

APPENDIX A

Assumptions

1. Primary healthcare is an integral part of the healthcare delivery system that is taking an even more important role with healthcare reform.
2. The nurse practitioner is a client advocate in the primary healthcare setting who functions independently and interdependently.
3. Nurse practitioners practice nursing by managing all health problems encountered by the client (the management may include referral), and are accountable for health and cost outcomes.

Adapted from: American Nurses Association. (1985). *The Scope of Practice of the Primary Health Care Nurse Practitioner. Kansas City, MO: Author.*

APPENDIX B

Pearls for Developing Clinical Reasoning Skills in the Primary Care Setting

1. To develop an accurate initial concept, look carefully for important initial information as the patient encounter begins.
2. Generate a complete set of hypotheses in every patient encounter, carefully watching their degree of specificity and their complimentarity. Be sure to watch out for hidden biases.
3. Use your creativity, and your inductive skills, to develop these hypotheses.
4. Use your critical deductive skills to inquire in a manner that will establish the more likely hypothesis.
5. Generate new hypotheses whenever your inquiry becomes unproductive or new data makes your present hypotheses less likely.
6. Carefully assemble a problem synthesis from the significant data obtained from your hypothesis-guided inquiry.
7. Employ consistent and accurate clinical skills.
8. In both your hypotheses-generation and inquiry strategies, be guided by an awareness of the basic pathophysiologic mechanisms that may be operative in your patient's problem.
9. Think of past patient experiences similar to the one you are facing now, and what was productive or unproductive about them.
10. Force yourself to make diagnostic and therapeutic decisions even in situations where there is ambiguity or lack of important information.
11. In your choice of subsequent tests and a management plan, be aware of benefit/cost factors.
12. Consider carefully the educational needs of your patient and employ the appropriate educational strategy.
13. As you work with your patient, constantly ask yourself if you have all the facts or skills you need to evaluate and care for your patient and to keep yourself contemporary with medical knowledge.
14. Note the areas you need to study, and go to appropriate resources to gain the information and skills you need.
15. Apply newly acquired knowledge and skills to the problem, and note how you would have handled the problem differently after review.

INDEX

Abel, R.L., 92
Accountability, of team, 196
Actual cost per patient day, 149
Acute care, 243–257
  allocation of beds, 248–249
  competent versus incompetent, 245–248
  decreasing length of stay, 252–253
  delegation, 253–255
  formulating opportunities, 255–256
  intuitive decision making, 256–257
  nursing care hours versus bed allocation, 250–251
  patient advocacy, 244–245
  room changing, 249–250
Adaptive approach, 44
Advanced Directives, 247–248
Algorithms, 61–62
Allocation of beds, 248–249
American Association of Critical Care Nurses, 225
American Nurses Association (ANA), 261
  Code for Nurses, 271
Anderson, C., 48
Anderson, C.R., 287, 293
Angehern, A.A., 208
ANSOS Budget Module, 214
ANSOS Staffing and Scheduling System, 214
Applications in clinical practice
  acute care, 243–257
  critical care, 225–241
  maternal and child care, 259–275
  oncological nursing, 277–282
  primary care, 305–317
  psychiatric setting, 283–294
  rehabilitation, 295–303
Artificial intelligence, 120
Assisting patients with decision making, 18–21, 18(Table 1-4), 20(Fig. 1-2)
Austin, S., 92
Autocratic leadership style, 181, 182
Autonomy, 102, 102(Table 7-1)
  and empowerment, 193–195
Baldridge, J.V., 26
Barrows, H.S., 308, 310, 315, 316
Baylor Plan, 190
Becker, C.B., 91
Becker, P.H., 102, 103, 105, 106
Bedside decision making, 117–118
Beneficence, 102, 102(Table 7-1)
Benner, P., 10, 11, 12, 61, 120, 231, 232
Bennis, W., 179
Berger, K., 270
"Best member," 72
Blanchard, K.H., 183, 199
Block, P., 193, 194, 195
Bona fide occupational qualification, 165
Boss, leadership style of, 186
Bottger, P.C., 72
Boyle, Thomas O., 301
Brainstorming, 54–55
Brainwriting, 55
Brennan, P.F., 119, 121
Broad span of control, 249
Brykczynski, K., 305
Bryson, J.M., 133, 134, 137
Budget development, 146–162
  capital, 154, 158, 158(Table 10-4), 159
  cash, 146, 147(Table 10-1)
  operating, 146–154, 150–153(Table 10-2), 155–157(Table 10-3)
  program, 159–162
Budgets, 144–146
  capital, 145
  cash, 145
  operating, 145
  program, 145–146
Bureaucratic model, 33–36, 34(Table 2-4)
  change features, 34–35
  other components, 35
  pros and cons, 35–36
  underlying features and process, 33–34
Burke, S., 103

Capital budget, 145
development of, 154, 158, 158(Table 10-4), 159
Carnevali, D.L., 12, 14, 15, 16, 117, 231, 296
Carroll, A.B., 285
Cash budget, 145
development of, 146, 147(Table 10-1)
Cassel, R.N., 61
Central tendency or leniency effect, 165
Chaffee, E.E., 25, 26
Chandler, G.E., 193
Childs, B.W., 121
Choice, as decision making stage, 62
Clinical decision making, material health and pediatric nursing, 262–267
communication, 263–265
competency, 262–263
death, 265–266
focus on the family, 267
standards of practice, 262
time constraints, 266–267
Clinical decision making, psychiatric setting, 287–293
client's sociocultural heritage, 289–290
criteria for selecting alternatives, 290–292
evaluation, 292–293
identifying alternatives, 290
implementation of selected alternatives, 292
problem identification, 287–289
Clinical practice council (CPC), 203–204
Cloning effect, 165
Cohen, M.D., 36
Collaboration, 307
with other professionals, 313
with patient, 307–310, 315
Collaborative model, 16–18, 16(Table 1-3)
assessment of problem, 16–17
care plan formulation, 17
care plan implementation, 17–18
diagnostic workup, 17
differential diagnosis, 17
final diagnosis, 18
treatment, 18
Collectivism, 89–91
Collegial model, 31–33, 31(Table 2-3)
change features, 32
other components, 33
pros and cons, 33
underlying features and process, 32
Collins, D., 301
Collins, R.R., 63
Coming to conclusions, 44
Committee as a group, 85
Communication skills, in critical care nursing, 239
Communication style, effect of culturalism on, 89–91, 90(Table 6-1)
Competency, 228–229
Competent versus incompetent patient, 245–248
Complacency, 71
CompuServe, 217
Computer applications for nursing care, 115
Computer-assisted decision support, 113–127
applications for nursing care, 115–116
beside decision making, 117–118
coordination of care, 116
deciding to automate, 121–125
decision-making systems, 118–120
extending nursing's commitment to computerization, 125–126
problems with expertise, 120–121
Computerized patient record (CPR), 117
Computers, and decision making, 118–120
decision to automate, 121–125
Computer-supported decision making, 207–221
additional software applications, 216
data manipulation, 212–215
decision data, 209–212
information sharing systems, 216–217
need definition, 208–209
using technology to support decisions, 217–221
Conflict and decisions, 68
Conflict resolution model. *See* political model
Consequentialist theory, 100

Considered decisions, 43
Content-focused approach, 85
Content validity of data, 209
Context frequency, 62
Contextual/situational sphere, 108
Continuum of leadership behaviors, 182–183, 183(Table 12-2)
Coordination of care, using computers, 116–117
Corcoran, S., 18
Cost attributes, 160
Cost-benefit analysis, 50
Cost center, 148
Costello-Nickitas, D.M., 193
Council on Computer Applications in Nursing, 126
Councilor model, 202–203
Counseling and discipline, 171–175
  cautions, 173–174
  disciplinary process, 172–173
  discipline and substance abuse, 174–175
  grievance process, 173
Covey, S.R., 195, 196, 198
Cox, K.R., 115
Creative process of decision making, 5(Table 1-1), 7–8
  felt need, 7
  preparation, 7
  incubation, 7
  illumination, 7
  verification, 7
Creativity in decision making, encouraged by leader, 190
Critical care, 225–241
  communication skills and decision making, 239
  ethical issues, 234–236
  factors affecting clinical decision making, 228–232
  leadership factors, 236–237
  legal issues, 232–234
  regulatory bodies governing decision making, 225–228
  staffing issues, 238–239
Critical incident technique, 169
Critical path method (CPM), 50
Cue clusters, 15
Cultural factors, effects of, 87–96
  culturalism and communication, 89–91, 90(Table 6-1)
  culturalism and nursing administration, 92–93
  culture of nursing, 92
  gender as a culture, 88–89
  hospital culture, 94–95
Culturalism and nursing administration, 92–93
Culture of nursing, 92
Curtain, L.L., 272
Curtis, D.V., 26
Cybernetic model, 38–41, 39(Table 2-6)
  needs assessment, 38, 39–40
  program implementation, 38, 40
  results assessment, 38, 40–41

Dallery, A.B., 106
Databases, 214
Data frame, 120
Data manipulation, 212–215
  data trail, 212–213
  methods of data refinement, 213–215
Data requirements, defining, 208–209, 209(Table 14-1)
Davis, D.L., 64
dBase IV, 214
Death, coping with, 265–266
Decisional balance sheet, 53
Decision analysis, 65, 66(Table 4-1)
Decision data, 209–212
  characteristics, 209–210
  formats, 211
  sources, 210–211
  timeliness, 211–212
Decision influencers in the psychiatric setting, 284–287
  experience, 285–286
  individuality, 285
  interpersonal skills, 286
  multiple customers, 284
  personal characteristics, 286
  thinking skills, 286
  value system, 285
Decisionmaker individual, 62–63
Decision making
  assisting patients with, 18–21
  collaborative model, 16–18

Decision making (*cont.*)
computer-assisted decision support, 113–127
creative process, 7–8
cultural factors, effects of, 87–96
diagnostic, 12–16
emergency process, 8–9
ethical, 97–111
group, 77–86
individual, 59–75
intuitive process, 10–12
multiattribute utility process, 9–10
organizational level, 25–42
routine process, 4–7
scope of practice model, 21–22, 23
significance of, 4
strategies, 43–58
Decision-making models, 139–141
Decision packages, 50–51
Decision rule, 62
Decision stages, 61–62
choice of best alternative, 62
information processing, 61–62
perception and information gathering stage, 61
Decision support system (DSS), 208
software, 216
Decision tree, 44–45, 46(Fig. 3-1)
Decker, P.J., 8, 190
Decreasing length of stay, 252–253
Defensive avoidances, 71
Delbecq, Andre, 55
Del Bueno, D.J., 165
Delegation of patient care, 253–255
Delphi method, 54
Democratic leadership style, 181, 182
Deontological approach, 100
Dewey, John, 109
Diagnostic decision making, 12–16, 13(Fig. 1-1)
assigning a diagnosis, 15–16
collection of the database, 14
cue clusters, 15
diagnostic explanations or concepts, 15
entry into the data field, 14
no fit situation, 16
pre-encounter data, 14
Diagnostic related groups (DRGs), 33, 144
Disciplinary process, 172–173
Dispute process, 92–93, 93(Table 6-2)
Draper, E., 231
Dreyfus, H. and S., 11, 232
Drucker, P.F., 287

Ecker, G.P., 26
Education council, 204
Elimination by aspects, 52
Elstein, A.S., 11, 12, 16
Emergency decision–making process, 8–9
Empowerment, 193–206
and autonomy, 193–195
creating a mission and a vision of leadership, 198–199
participative management, 199–201
professional practice models, 201
shared governance, 201–205
team building, 195–197
traditional leadership, 199
Entrepreneurial strategy, 44
Equal Employment Opportunity Commission (EEOC), 174
Erikson, Erik, 79–80
Essay technique, 169
Ethical decision making, 97–111, 98(Table 7-1)
contextual/situational sphere, 108
ethical principles, 102–103, 102(Table 7-1)
ethical theory, 99–102
guide for, 108–110
moral developmental theory, 103–104
nursing theory, 104–106
patient's role, 107
social/interactional sphere and nursing, 106–107
Ethical decision-making process, 108–110, 108(Table 7-3)
moral decision making, 108, 109–110
moral perspective, 108, 109
moral reflection, 108, 109
moral sensitivity, 108, 109
plurality of perspective, 108, 109
Ethical issues
critical care nursing, 234–236
maternal child and pediatric nursing, 270–272

Ethical theory, 99–102
  deontological approach, 100
  situational perspective, 101–102
  utilitarian approach, 100–101
Ethics, 99
Etzioni, A., 53
Evaluating the results, 44
Executive information system (EIS), 208
Executive or coordinating council (CC), 204
Expectations, 164
Expert system, 119–121
  inference engine, 119
  knowledge base, 119
  problems with, 120–121
External environment, assessing, 134–135

Face validity of data, 209
Factors affecting clinical decision making, 228–232
  competency, 228–229
  intuition, 231–232
  nurse/physician relationships, 231
  stress, 229–231
  validation, 232
Felstiner, W.L.F., 92
Financial decision making, 143–162
  budget development, 146–162
  budgets, 144–146
Financial viability score, 154
Fink, Steven, 68, 70
Finkler, S., 149
Finnegan, S., 201
Fitzpatrick, Joyce, 92
Flannery, J., 301
Followers, effectiveness of, 184–185
Forced choice rating, 169
Framing, 43
Frankena, W.K., 101
Frequency of recurrence, 62
Full time equivalencies (FTEs), 145, 148, 210

Gadow, S., 18
Gantt chart, 45–46, 47(Fig. 3-2)
Garbage can model, 36–38, 36(Table 2-5)
  change features, 37
  other components, 37–38
  pros and cons, 38
  underlying features and process, 36–37
Gathering intelligence, 43–44
Gender as culture, 88
Gillies, D.A., 82, 182
Gilligan, C., 104
Graphic rating scale, 169
Grievance process, 173
Group behavior, and leadership effectiveness, 187
Group decision making, 54, 77–86, 78(Table 5-1)
  committee as group, 85
  group process, 79–80
  individual as group member, 77–79
  Oermann's model, 80–82
  Tuchman and Jensen's model, 82–85
Group process, 79–80
Groupthink, 72

Halo or horn effect, 165, 170–171
Harbison, J., 65
Hardware, 114–115
Harris, B.L., 90
Hauser, M., 168
Hawkins, J., 307
Heimlich maneuver, 8
Hersey, P., 183
Heuristics, 62
Hierarchical relationships, 120
High-context communication, 91
Hiring, 163–168
  interview process, 164, 165–168
  obstacles and pitfalls, 164–165
  reference check, 168
Hospital culture, 94–95
Huber, G.P., 9, 54
Huckaby, L.M.D., 68
Humanistic contextual perspective, 105, 106
Humanistic ethic of human care, 104–106
Human resource management, 163–178
  counseling and discipline, 171–175
  hiring, 163–168
  performance appraisals/evaluation, 168–171
  recruitment and retention, 175–177
Human systems theory, Neuman's, 297

Huston, C.J., 285, 286, 293
Hypervigilance, 71
Hypotheses, 309–310

Incrementalism, 53
Individual as group member, 77–79
Individual decision making, 59–75
  conflict and decisions, 68
  dangers in, 72
  decisionmaker, 62–63
  defined, 60
  modified rational approach, 66
  monitoring decisions, 73–74
  Myers-Briggs Type Indicator, 63–65
  other issues, 72–73
  rational decision making, 65–66
  risk and decision making, 67–68
  role of nurse, 60–61
  role of stress, 68–72
  strengths in, 72–73
  wrong decisions, 73
Individual dominance, 72
Individualism, 89–90
Information conditions, 62
Information processing, 61–62
Information sharing systems (ISS), 216–217
Input devices, 114
Interactive software programs, 216
Interface, 117
Internal environment, assessing, 135, 137
Interview process, 164, 165–168
Intuition, 62, 231–232
Intuitive decision making, 256–257
Intuitive decision-making process, 10–12, 11(Table 1-2)
  aspects of intuitive judgment, 11–12
  common sense understanding, 12
  deliberate rationality, 12
  pattern recognition, 11, 12
  sense of salience, 12
  similarity recognition, 11, 12
  skilled knowhow, 12
Ives, J.R., 134

Janis, I., 52, 53
Jein, R.F., 90
Job description, 168
Job knowledge questions, 166
Job sample/simulation questions, 166
Johnson, S., 199
Joint Commission on Accreditation of Healthcare Organizations (JCAHO), 225, 227, 228, 260, 263
Jones, D., 168
Jung, C., 63
Justice, 102, 102(Table 7-1)

Kaluzny, A.D., 38, 41
Kaus, W., 231
Kaye, H., 74
Kefalas, A.G., 285
Kelley, R.E., 184, 185
Kepner, C.H., 287, 291
Kitzman, H., 116
Kohlberg, L., 103, 104
Kohls, L.R., 91
Korpman, R., 122
Kouzes, J.M., 139
Kraytman, M., 308

Laissez-faire leadership, 183
Lancaster, J. and W., 180
Leadership, 179–191, 198–199, 236–237, 272–275
  boss's style of, 186
  in critical care nursing, 236–237
  decision-making obstacles, 188–190
  group behavior, 187
  in maternal child and pediatric nursing, 272–275
  situational considerations, 187–188
  strengths of subordinates, 186–187
  theory, 180–186
  traditional, 199
  versus management, 198–199
Leadership theory, 180–186
  attributes of followers, 184–185, 185(Table 12-3)
  behavior, 181–186, 183(Table 12-2)
  maturity of group members, 183–184
  traits and skills, 180, 181(Table 12-1)
Learning systems, 120
Legal guardian, 269
Legal issues
  critical care nursing, 232–234
  maternal child and pediatric nursing, 268–270
Leske, J.S., 116

Leung, K., 90
Lind, E.A., 90
Living Will laws, 248
Local area network (LAN), 217
Lohman, R., 50
Loomis, M., 86
LOTUS 1-2-3, 214
Low-context communication, 91
Lower, M.S., 115
Luthi, H.J., 208
Lyons, N., 104

Magnuson, B.A., 193
Malley, J.C., 64
Management, distinguished from leadership, 198–199
Management by objectives, 169
Management council, 203
Mann, L., 52, 53, 89
Manthey, M., 57
Maraldo, P., 176
March, J.G., 36
Marquis, B.L., 285, 286, 293
Marr, P.B., 116
Marriner-Tomey, A., 7, 8, 44, 46, 54, 55, 183
Mason, D.J., 193, 194
Maternal and child health, 259–275
  clinical decision making, 262–267
  ethical issues, 270–272
  leadership, 272–275
  legal issues, 268–270
  oversight by regulatory boards, 260–262
Medical Intensive Care Unit (MICU), 26–28
Medicare, 143, 144
MEDLINE, 214
Mentors, use of, 300–302
Microsoft Project, 214
Microsoft Word, 213
Microstat, 215
Miller, D., 57
Mintzberg, H., 44
Mission statement, 198
Mixed scanning, 53
Modeling system, 119
Modified rational approach, 66
Monitoring decisions, 73–74
Moral decision making, 108, 109–110
Moral developmental theory, 103–104
  care perspective, 104
  justice perspective, 103–104
Moral perspective, 108, 109
Moral reflection, 108, 109
Moral sensitivity, 108, 109
Moral standards, 99
Motivation, lack of, 189
Multiattribute utility model (MAU), 9–10
  attribute, 9
  formula, 10
  utility, 9–10
  weight, 10
Multiattribute utility theory (MAUT), 144, 159–162, 161(Tables 10-5 and 10-6), 177
Myers-Briggs Type Indicator, 63–65
  sensing-intuiting index, 63–64
  thinking-feeling index, 64–65

Narrow span of control, 249
National League of Nursing, 260
Nauert, L.B., 115
Neuman, B., 297
Noddings, N., 104
No fit situation, 16
Nominal group technique, 55
Non-maleficence, 102, 102(Table 7-1)
Nonprogrammed decisions, 63
Nurse
  and control of information systems, 126
  decisionmaker, 60–61
  and ethical care, 104–106
  member of rehabilitation team, 300
  patient advocate, 18–21, 18(Table 1-4), 107
  relationship with physician, 231, 255–256
Nurse extenders, 238
Nurse Practice Act, 261, 263
Nursing
  and social/interactional sphere, 106–107, 107(Table 7-2)
  culture of, 92
  extending commitment to computerization, 125–126
  role in strategic planning process, 141–142

Nursing administration and culturalism, 92–93
Nursing care hours (NCH), 250–251
Nursing Informatics, 126
Nursing Minimum Data Set (NMDS), 116

Oermann's Model, 80–82
  orientation stage, 80
  termination stage, 82
  working stage, 81
Oncology nursing, 277–282
  crucial factors, 278
  decision making during treatment process, 280–281
  disease process, 278
  patient's preferences, 279–280
  physician's philosophy, 278–279
Open architecture systems, 117
Open-ended questions, 166–167
Open systems view, 207
Operating budget, 145
  development of, 146–154, 150–153(Table 10-2), 155–157(Table 10-3)
Operational decisions, 43
Operational planning, 131–132
Optimizing, 52
Orem, Dorothy, 296–297
Organizational/cultural conditions and effect on leadership, 188–189
Organizational models, 25–42
  bureaucratic, 33–36
  collegial, 31–33
  cybernetic, 38–41
  garbage can, 36–38
  political, 28–31
  rational, 26–28
Organization for Obstetric, Gynecologic, and Neonatal Nurses, 261
Output devices, 114
Ozbolt, J.G., 115

Padrick, K.P., 16
Paired comparison ranking, 169
Parentalism, 107
Participative leadership, 182–183
Participative management, 199–201
Paternalism, 107
Patient
  preference in cancer treatment, 279–280
  role in decision making, 107
Patient advocacy, 244–245
  nurse and, 107
Patient interview, 308
Patient Self-Determination Act of 1990, 233
Pediatric healthcare, 259
Peplav, H., 126
Perception and information gathering stage, 61
Performance appraisals/evaluation, 168–171
  evaluation, 169–170
  instrument types, 168–169
  process of evaluation, 170–171
Personal biases, 164
PERT chart, 46–49, 49(Fig. 3-3)
Physician, relationship with nurse, 231
Pickell, G.C., 308, 310, 315, 316
Planning approach, 44
Plurality of perspective, 108, 109
Political model, 28–31, 29(Table 2-2)
  change features, 30
  other components, 30–31
  pros and cons, 31
  underlying features and process, 29–30
Porter-O'Grady, T., 195, 201, 202
Posner, B.Z., 139
Practical model of decision making, 66
Preceptors, use of, 300–302
Primary care setting, 305–317
  closing the patient encounter, 315–316
  collaboration with other professionals, 313
  collaboration with patient, 307–310
  definitions, 306–307
  improving clinical decision-making skills, 316, 319
  therapeutic decision making, 313–315
  using clinical skills to gather supporting data, 310–313
Process-focused approach, 85
PRODIGY, 217

Professional practice at unit level, 205
Professional practice models, 201
Program budget, 145–146
  development of , 159–169,
    161(Tables 10-5 and 10-6)
Programmed decision, 62
Project management, 214
Prospective payment system (PPS), 144
Psychiatric/mental health setting,
    283–294
  clinical decision making, 287–293
  decision influences, 284–287
  pitfalls, 293
Psychological strategies, 51–57
  group, 54–55
  individual, 51–54
  individual or group, 56–57
Putzier, D., 16

Quality Assessment and Improvement
    (QA&I) committee, 34–35
Quality improvement council (QIC),
    204
Quality of service score, 154
Quantitative strategies, 44–51
  cost-benefit analysis, 50
  critical path method (CPM), 50
  decision packages, 50–51
  decision tree, 44–45
  Gantt chart, 45–46, 47
  PERT chart, 46–49
Quattro-Pro, 214

Radford, M., 89
RAM (read and write memory), 114
Rank order method, 169
Rational decision making, 65–66
  decision analysis, 65, 66(Table 4-1)
Rational model, 26–28, 27(Table 2-1)
  change features, 27–28
  other components, 28
  pros and cons, 28
  underlying features and process,
    26–27
Recruitment and retention, 175–177
  plan for, 176
  retention incentives, 176
Reductionism, 44
Reductionist perspective, 105
Reference check, 168
Regulatory agencies, 260–262
Rehabilitation setting, 295–303
  team function and decision making,
    300
  theories in clinical decision making,
    296-299
  use of preceptors/mentors, 300–302
Request for Proposal (RFP), 122, 123
Research council, 204
Restraining patients, 246–247
Retention. *See* Recruitment and
    retention
Reu, L., 231
Revenue attributes, 160
Riley, G.L., 26
Risk, and effect on decision making,
    67–68, 187–188
ROM (read only memory), 114
Room changing, 249–250
Routine process of decision making,
    4–6, 5(Table 1-1)
  identification of problem, 4–5
  seeking alternatives, 5
  selection of an alternative, 5
  implementing the decision, 5
  evaluation, 6
Rowland, B. and H., 43
Roy, Sister Callista, 297
Russo, J.E., 43
Rutkowski, B., 174
Ryan, S.A., 116

SAS, 215
Satisficing, 51–52
Scanlan, J.M., 193
Scarcity of key resources, 189
Scenario development, 56–57
Schmidt, W.H., 182
Schoemaker, P., 43
Schon, D.A., 105
Schwartz, P., 56, 57
Scope of practice model, 21–22,
    23(Fig. 1-3)
Semantic net, 120
Sensing-intuiting index, 63–64
Shared governance, 201–205
  clinical practice council (CPC),
    203–204

Shared governance (*cont.*)
 councilor model, 202–203
 education council, 204
 executive or coordinating council (CC), 204
 management council, 203
 professional practice at unit level, 205
 quality improvement council (QIC), 204
 research council, 204
Sheridan, D., 168
Shulman, L.S., 11
Simon, H., 51–52
Simpson, A.L., 208
Sinclair, V.G., 121
Situational questions, 166
Situation analysis, 4
Skill, lack of, 189
Smart Forecast II, 214
Smith, H.R., 285
Social/interactional sphere and nursing, 106–107, 107(Table 7-2)
 patient advocacy, 107
Software, 115
Sprafka, S., 11
Spreadsheets, 213–214
SPSS-PC, 215
Staffing issues
 in critical care nursing, 238
 energy of staff, 238–239
 nurse extenders, 238
Stages of human psychosocial development, 79
Stakeholders, 134
State Board of Nursing, 225, 226, 227
Statistical packages, 214–215
Steiner, G.A., 135
Stevens, B., 44, 45
Stoeckle, J., 307
Stogdill, R.M., 180
Stoner, J.A.F., 63
Strasen, L., 45, 48, 50, 135
Strategic issues
 identifying, 137–138
 managing, 138–139
Strategic planning process, 131–142
 assessing external environment, 134–135
 assessing internal environment, 135–137
 clarifying organizational mission and values, 133, 134
 establishing vision for the future, 139
 formulating strategies to manage issues, 138–139
 identifying organizational mandates, 133
 identifying strategic issues, 137–138
 initiating and agreeing on process, 133
 versus operational planning, 131–132
Strategies, 43–58
 psychological, 44, 51–57
 quantitative, 44–51
Stress, 229–231
Stress, role of, 68–72, 69(Fig. 4-1)
 complacency, 71
 defensive avoidance, 71
 hypervigilance, 71
 vigilant decision making, 70
Structured questions, 165
Subordinates, and response to leadership, 186–187
Substance abuse, and discipline, 174–175
Sullivan, E.J., 8, 190
Supporting decisions using technology, 217–221
 building credibility, 220
 concerns and counterarguments, 217–220
 issue definition, 217
 operation and evaluation plan, 220
Swallow-hard decisions, 43
SWOT analysis (Strengths, Weaknesses, Opportunities and Threats), 134–137, 136(Fig. 9-1)
Synectics, 190
Systems theory, 180
System unit, 114

Tannenbaum, R., 182
Tanner, C.A., 10, 11, 12, 16, 231
Team building, 195–197, 197(Table 13-1)
 group-building roles, 196–197
 group maintenance roles, 197
Team function and decision making, 300
Ten-second decisions, 43

Theory of adaptation, Roy's, 297
Theory of self-care, Orem's, 296–297
Theriault, J., 301
Thibodeau, J., 307
Thinking-feeling index, 64–65
Thomas, J., 301
Thomas, M.D., 12, 14, 15, 16, 117, 231, 232
Thompson, C.B., 116
Total Quality Management (TQM), 184
Total relationship score, 154
Transactional leadership style, 184
Transformational leadership style, 184
Tregoe, B.B., 287, 291
Tuchman and Jensen's model, 82–85
  adjoining, 84–85
  forming, 82
  norming, 83
  performing, 84
  storming, 83
Turnover attributes, 160
Tversky, A., 52

Uncertainty, and effect on decision making, 188
Utilitarian approach, 100–101

Validation, 232
Value analysis, 144
Value analysis matrix, 154, 158, 158(Table 10-4)
Van de Ven, Andrew, 55
van Dissel, B.J., 73
Variance report, 149, 154, 155–157(Table 10-3)
Veney, J.E., 38, 41
Vigilant decision making, 70
Vision, 195
  for the future, 139
  statement, 198

Wagner, D., 231
Watson, H.F., 285
Werley, H.H., 116
Westfall, U.E., 16
Williams-Brinkman, M., 270
"Win-lose" strategy, 89
"Win-win" strategy, 89
Woolery, L., 120
Word Perfect, 213
Word processing, 213
Work requirement questions, 166
Wrong decisions, 73

Yetton, P.W., 63, 72
Young, S., 301
Yukl, G.A., 180, 184

Zimmerman, J., 231